Cross-sectional Anatomy of Acupoints

For Churchill Livingstone

Commissioning Editor: Inta Ozols
Project Manager: Neil A. Dickson
Project Controller: Nicola S. Haig
Indexer: Nina Boyd
Design Direction: Judith Wright
Sales Promotion Executive: Hilary Brown

Cross-sectional Anatomy of Acupoints

Eachou Chen MD MPH

Subject Editor
Andrew Flower BA MRTCM MRCHM

CHURCHILL LIVINGSTONE
EDINBURGH HONG KONG LONDON MADRID MELBOURNE NEW YORK AND TOKYO 1995

CHURCHILL LIVINGSTONE
Medical Division of Longman Group Limited

Distributed in the United States of America by Redwing Book
Company, 44 Linden Street, Brookline, Massachusetts
01246.

First published 1995

ISBN 0 443 04974 2

British Library Cataloguing in Publication Data
A catalogue record for this book is available from the British
Library.

Library of Congress Cataloging in Publication Data
Chen, Eachou.
    Cross-sectional anatomy of acupoints/Eachou Chen;
subject editor, Andrew Flower.
        p.   cm.
    Includes index.
    ISBN 0-443-04974-2
    1. Acupuncture points.   2. Anatomy, Surgical and
topographical.   I. Title.
    [DNLM: 1. Acupuncture Points.   2. Anatomy.   WB
369 C51554c 1994]
RM184.5.C414   1994
615.8'92—dc20
DNLM/DLC
for Library of Congress   94-27579

The
publisher's
policy is to use
**paper manufactured
from sustainable forests**

Produced by Longman Singapore Publishers (Pte) Ltd.
Printed in Singapore

Contents

Preface

Cross-sectional Anatomy of Acupoints combines modern anatomy and acupuncture, integrating traditional Chinese medicine and Western medicine, as well as providing useful clinical information. A total of 378 acupoints are discussed in this book: 71 acupoints with cross-sectional anatomy of the upper extremities, 84 acupoints of the lower extremities, 63 acupoints of the head, eight acupoints of the neck, 137 acupoints of the trunk and 15 high risk acupoints. The most commonly used acupoints are depicted with illustrations and text; the remaining acupoints are explained by text only. Each illustration describes in detail its specific structure, including the nerve supplied, the muscles, the vessels and the adjacent important organs, as well as the safe depth, the direction and the angle of needle insertion required to prevent inappropriate needle technique which may induce adverse acupuncture reactions.

With special thanks to the Shanghai College of Traditional Medicine, Inc. and Dr Zhen-Guo Yan, without whose permission to use illustrations from *Illustration of Common Acupoints of Basic Anatomy*, as well as *Cross Sectional Anatomy of Acupoints* and *Layers Anatomy of Acupoints* as major references, this book would never have been completed.

1994   E.C.

Editor's note
Safety

For guidelines on the safe clinical practice of acupuncture, please refer to *Clean Needle Technique for Acupuncturists: a manual* (third edition), published by the National Commission for the Certification of Acupuncturists, Washington DC, USA.

Introduction
A short history of acupuncture

Acupuncture is one of the most important therapies of traditional Chinese medicine. In using needles and moxibustion to treat disease it is essential to select and locate points precisely but also to use appropriate manipulation of the needle in accordance with the nature of the disease and the chosen point. The treatment of disease through superficial acupoints is made possible by activating the meridian network and thereby moving and recuperating the Qi and Blood. The exact location of each acupoint and its method of use are most important in obtaining the maximum benefit in treatment.

The classic Chinese medicine textbook *Huang Di Nei Jing* (The Yellow Emperor's Internal Classic), probably compiled around 100 BC, which explains the meridian system connecting the Zang and Fu (visceral organs) internally and all acupoints externally, included 160 acupoints with 25 single acupoints and 135 bilateral acupoints. Until 282 AD, *Zhen Jiu Jia Yi Jing* (A B C Classic of Acupuncture and Moxibustion) by Huang-Fu Mi was the only complete acupuncture textbook and included 349 acupoints with 49 single acupoints and 300 bilateral acupoints. *Tong Ren Shu Xue Zhen Jiu Tu Jing* (Illustrated Manual of Acupoints of the Bronze Figure) by Wei-Yi Wang (1026), who designed a bronze human statue engraved with the standardized meridians and collaterals as well as acupoints as a teaching model, included 354 acupoints with 51 single acupoints and 303 bilateral acupoints. In 1601, *Zhen Jiu Da Cheng* (Great Compendium of Acupuncture and Moxibustion), a comprehensive summing up of experiences and achievements of acupuncture and moxibustion by Ji-Zhon Yang, included 359 acupoints with 51 single acupoints and 308 bilateral acupoints. *Yi Zong Jin Jian* (The Golden Mirror of Medicine) by Qian Wu (1742) consists of 361 acu-points with 52 single acupoints and 309 bilateral acupoints.

CHARACTERISTICS OF CROSS-SECTIONAL ANATOMY

In the last 30 years, many articles and books have been published about the anatomical structures of acupoints. However, most of them use layer dissection, in which the structure of acupoints may be moved during observation, which cannot reflect precisely the nature of the anatomical layers and structures affected during needle manipulation, and cannot adequately demonstrate the needle route from the skin to the tip of the needle.

The acupoints in this book are described according to bone length measurements and the most common superficial locational method. Each acupoint is located on the superficial surface of a corpse which is then frozen to −30 to −50°C. Multi-cross sections of each acupoint are then taken to demonstrate the anatomical structure of the different layers affected by the angle, depth and range during needle insertion and manipulation.

FUTURE TRENDS IN ACUPOINT ANATOMY

Most traditional Chinese medical schools or acupuncture schools should develop a new systemic and local anatomical curriculum to improve traditional Chinese medical anatomy. The recent trends of anatomical development include:
a. Integration of research into acupoint structure and function. This not only applies to layer anatomy of acupoints, cross-sectional anatomy of acupoints, CAT scan, descriptive anatomy of acupoints, tissue structure receptor observation of acupoints, but also to the use of histological differentiation, electron microscopy, autoradiography, micro-element measurement, electrophysiology, immunology and biochemistry. Integrating all of them from gross, light and electron microscopy to molecular and quantum biology, from corpse to living-body, from appearance to function, and from basic science to clinical medicine can result in highly rewarding research.

b. Research of the spatial configuration and appearance of the acupoint. Research and analysis of the spatial distribution of each layer of blood vessels, nerves, and muscles.

c. Research of clinical Chinese medicine in applying anatomical knowledge, integrating Tui Na (Chinese massage), acupuncture, Chinese traumatology and Chinese surgery, using the previously described research methods in section A to analyze common diseases according to anatomical knowledge gained in Chinese medical departments to produce a specific Chinese medical anatomy.

d. Sorting out references of Chinese medical anatomy and body length measurement.

MEASUREMENT OF ACUPOINTS

In clinic, there are four methods used to measure the acupoint: finger inch measurement, superficial measurement, convenient measurement and bone length measurement.

1. Finger inch measurement

a. *Middle finger inch measurement.* Ask the patient to join the tip of the middle finger to the tip of the thumb to make a ring. At the lateral side of the middle phalange of the middle finger, the distance between the proximal crease and the distal crease of the middle phalange is 1 inch. Usually this method is applied to the lower back and the four limbs.

b. *Thumb inch measurement.* The patient's thumb joint diameter is 1 inch. Usually this method is applied to the four limbs.

c. *Finger breadth measurement.* Ask the patient to close the four fingers together; the breadth at the proximal middle phalanges is 3 inches. Usually this method is

applied to the upper and lower limbs, the abdomen and the back (Fig. I.1).

The finger inch measurement is one of the most commonly used measurements and should be adjusted according to the individual patient.

2. Superficial measurement

a. *Skin crease measurement.* Skin creases are found most commonly at the joint areas and are useful in acupoint measurement. For example: flexing the elbow, Quchi [LI 11, Chuchih] is located in the fossa of the radial side of the skin crease of the elbow. Weizhong [BL 40, Weichung] is located in the middle of the skin crease of the popliteal fossa and between the tendons of the biceps femoris and semitendinosus muscles. Chengfu [BL 36, Chengfu] is located inferior to the skin crease of the inferior buttock.

b. *Bony measurement.* This method is used with bony protuberances and fossae which can be observed or palpated. For example: Dazhui [GV 14, Tachui] is located inferior to the spinous process of the seventh cervical vertebra. Jugu [LI 16, Chuku] is located in the fossa between the acromion of the scapula and the spine of the scapula. With the palm facing downwards, Yanglao [SI 6, Yanglao] is located at the highest point of the styloid process of the ulna; or flexing the elbow and holding the palm facing the chest, Yanglao [SI 6, Yanglao] is located on the radial side of the styloid process of the ulna.

c. *Muscular measurement.* This method is used with the superficial musculature, aided by observation and palpation. For example: Chengshan [BL 57, Chengshan] is located in the midpoint at the inferior border of the gastrocnemius muscle in the fossa of a reverse V shape while fully extending the leg. Neiguan [PC 6, Neikuan] is located 2 inches above

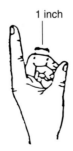

1 inch

1 inch

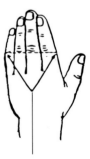

3 inches

Fig. I.1 Finger breadth method.

the palmar wrist crease between the tendons of the flexor carpi radialis and palmaris longus muscles. Renying [ST 9, Jenying] is located at the same height as the larynx, on the anterior margin of the sternocleidomastoid muscle, and 1.5 inches lateral to the laryngeal protuberance.

d. *Miscellaneous measurement*. Apart from skin creases, bony and muscular measurements, there are many other landmarks which can be used in acupoint location, such as hairlines, finger and toenails, the umbilicus, the nipple and the five sense organs. For example: Touwei [ST 8, Touwei] is located 0.5 inch posterior to the anterior hairline, and 4.5 inches lateral to the midline of the head. Dadun [Liv 1, Tatun] is located on the lateral side of the big toe, and about 0.1 inch lateral and proximal to the nail root. Zhongwan [CV 12, Chungwan] is located on the midline of the abdomen, and 4 inches above the umbilicus. Shanzhong [CV 17, Shanchung] is located on the midline of the chest, level with the fourth intercostal space. Yingxiang [LI 20, Yinghsiang] is located at the intersection of the midpoint of the lateral ala nasi and the nasolabial groove, 0.5 inch lateral to the nostril.

3. Convenient measurement

Convenient measurement is a very simple and easily applied method used very often in clinic. For example, for Xuehai [SP 10, Xuehai], ask the patient to sit down and flex the knee. Put the palm on the patient's knee, the middle finger on the lateral thigh and the thumb on the medial thigh at a 45° angle. Xuehai [SP 10, Xuehai] is then located at the tip of the thumb. Lieque [LU 7, Liehchueh] is located by asking the patient to cross both thumbs and index fingers with one hand's index finger pressing superiorly on the styloid process of the radius of the other hand. Lieque [LU 7, Liehchueh] is then located in the fossa at the index finger tip.

4. Bone length measurement

One of the commonest measurements in clinic. A certain portion of the body, often defined by bone length, is divided into a particular length, then local points are located by using these as proportional units to measure the patient. Thus a traditional 'inch' varies in length according to which part of the body is being considered. For example: Jianshi [PC 5, Chienshih] is located 3 inches above the skin crease of the wrist, between the tendons of the flexor carpi radialis and palmaris longus muscles. From the skin crease of the wrist to the skin crease of the elbow is 12 inches,

which is divided into 12 units (inches). Jianshi [PC 5, Chienshih] is located in the third unit (inch) above the skin crease of the wrist.

The great advantage of the bone length measurement is its accuracy and specificity to each patient. No matter if the patient is male or female, old or young, tall or short, fat or skinny, this measurement can be used with all. The most common bone length measurements are shown in Figure I.2 and Table I.1.

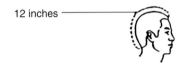

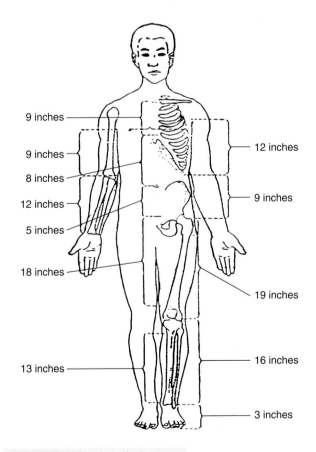

Fig. I.2 Bone length method.

Table I.1 Bone length measurement

Location	Origin and insertion	Bone length unit	Measurement method
Head	From the front hairline to the posterior hairline	12 inches	Straight inch
	Between the two corners of the hairline	9 inches	Horizontal inch
	From the midpoint of the two eyebrows to the front hairline	3 inches	Straight inch
	Between the two mastoid process posteriorly to the ear	9 inches	Horizontal inch
	From the front hairline to the inferior margin of the mandibular mental	10 inches	Straight inch
	Between the two highest points of the zygomatic bone	7 inches	Horizontal inch
Neck	From the posterior hairline to the spinous process of the seventh cervical vertebral (Dazhui [GV 14])	3 inches	Straight inch
Chest	From the superior margin of the sternum (jugular notch) to the junction of the body and the xiphoid process of the sternum	9 inches	Straight inch
	Between the two nipples	8 inches	Horizontal inch
Abdomen	From the umbilicus to the junction of the body and the xiphoid process of the sternum	8 inches	Straight inch
	From the umbilicus to the superior margin of the pubic symphysis	5 inches	Straight inch
Lateral side of trunk	From the middle of the axilla to the eleventh rib.	12 inches	Straight inch
	From the eleventh rib to the greater trochanter of the femur.	9 inches	Straight inch
Lumbar region	From the posterior midline to the vertebral margin of the scapula	3 inches	Horizontal inch
	From the spinous process of the first thoracic vertebra to the inferior margin of the median sacral crest	9 inches	Straight inch
Upper extremities	From the skin crease of the anterior axilla to the skin crease of the elbow	9 inches	Straight inch
	From the skin crease of the elbow to the skin crease of the wrist	12 inches	Straight inch
Lower extremities	From the superior margin of the pubic symphysis to the superior margin of the medial supracondyle of the femur (superior margin of the patella)	18 inches	Straight inch
	From the greater trochanter of the femur to the middle of the knee (level with the knee joint)	19 inches	Straight inch
	From the inferior gluteal line to the middle skin crease of the popliteal fossa	14 inches	Straight inch
	From the inferior margin of the medial condyle of the tibia to the highest point of the medial malleolus of the tibia	13 inches	Straight inch
	From the middle of the knee to the highest point of the lateral malleolus of the fibula	16 inches	Straight inch
	From the highest point of the lateral malleolus of the fibula to the sole of the foot	3 inches	Straight inch

1

Cross-sectional anatomy of the upper extremities

The upper extremities consist of the shoulder, the arm, the elbow, the forearm, the wrist, and the hand. The upper extremities are attached to the pectoral girdle, the neck and the thorax and are defined by the anterior margin of the deltoid muscle, the posterior margin of the deltoid muscle, the line between the anterior and posterior axillary folds of the lateral thoracic wall which forms an inferior borderline.

For the purposes of measurement during acupuncture treatment, the distance from the anterior axillary fold to the skin crease of the elbow is taken as 9 inches and the distance from the skin crease of the elbow to the distal skin crease of the wrist is taken as 12 inches.

1.

(CHUKU) JUGU, LI 16, HAND YANG MING LARGE INTESTINE MERIDIAN

Location
In a seated position, the point is located on the medial side of the acromioclavicular joint, in the fossa between the acromion process of the scapula and the acromial extremity of the clavicle.

Needle and moxibustion method
Slightly lateral perpendicular insertion 0.8–1.0 inch.
— *Needle sensation:* soreness and distension in the scapular joint.
— *Moxibustion dosage:* 3–7 cones; stick 5–20 minutes.

Cross-sectional anatomy of the needle passage
(Fig. 1.1)
a. *Skin:* the branches of the lateral supraclavicular nerve containing fibers from the fourth cervical nerves (C4) innervate the skin.
b. *Subcutaneous tissue:* includes the previously described skin nerve branches.
c. *Acromioclavicular ligament:* the ligament is superior to the bursa of the acromioclavicular joint. It is attached to the acromion process of the scapula and spine of the scapula. If the needle is slightly laterally inserted, it will directly enter the bursa of the acromioclavicle.
d. *Supraspinatus muscle:* the branches from the suprascapular nerves containing fibers from the fifth and sixth cervical nerves (C5, C6) innervate the supraspinatus muscle.

Functions
Expels Wind and clears away Cold, relaxes the muscles and tendons and eases movement of the joint.

Clinical indications
Diseases of the scapular joint and surrounding soft tissue, hematemesis, tuberculosis of the cervical lymph nodes, childhood convulsions, toothache.

2.
(NAOSHU) NAOSHU, SI 10, HAND TAI YANG SMALL INTESTINE MERIDIAN

Location
In a seated position with the arm adducted, the point is located on the posterior side of the scapula. Draw a line from Jianzhen [SI 9] or the lateral posterior axillary crease, to the fossa just below the inferior margin of the acromion process of the scapula where the point is located.

Needle and moxibustion method
Perpendicular insertion, slightly anterior inferior direction, 1.0–2.0 inches.
— *Needle sensation:* local soreness and distension, sometimes radiating to the shoulder.
— *Moxibustion dosage:* 3–7 cones; stick 5–20 minutes.

Cross-sectional anatomy of the needle passage
(Fig. 1.2)
a. *Skin:* the branches from the lateral supraclavicular nerve containing fibers from the fourth cervical nerve (C4) innervate the skin.
b. *Subcutaneous tissue:* includes the previously described skin nerve branches.
c. *Posterior deltoid muscle:* the branches from the axillary nerve containing fibers from the fourth and sixth cervical nerves (C4, C6) innervate the deltoid muscle.
d. *Infraspinatus muscle:* the branches from the suprascapular nerve containing fibers from the fifth and sixth cervical nerves (C5, C6) innervate the infraspinatus muscle. The needle is inserted to the posterior wall of the shoulder joint bursa, through the joint bursa and into the joint cavity, where it will directly contact the head of the humerus bone.

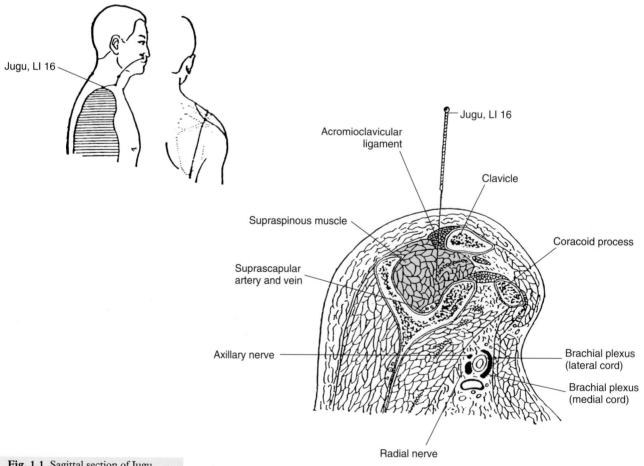

Jugu, LI 16

Acromioclavicular ligament

Jugu, LI 16

Clavicle

Supraspinous muscle

Coracoid process

Suprascapular artery and vein

Axillary nerve

Brachial plexus (lateral cord)

Brachial plexus (medial cord)

Radial nerve

Fig. 1.1 Sagittal section of Jugu.

Functions

Removes phlegm-heat, and alleviates pain and numbness.

Clinical indications

Cardiovascular disease, hemiplegia, hypertension, shoulder joint pain, soft tissue inflammation of shoulder joint, shoulder soreness and weakness, sweating.

3.

(CHIENCHIEN) JIANQIAN, EX-UE 48, EXTRA POINT OF THE UPPER EXTREMITIES (also known as Jianneiling)

Location

In a seated position with the arm adducted, the point is located on the anterior part of the deltoid muscle at the midpoint between the lateral part of the inferior margin of the anterior axilla and Jianyu [LI 15].

Needle and moxibustion method

Medial inferior oblique insertion 1.0–1.5 inches, at an angle of 50°.

— *Needle sensation:* local soreness and distension, or an electrical sensation radiating from the upper extremities to the fingertips.
— *Moxibustion dosage:* 3–7 cones; stick 5–20 minutes.

Cross-sectional anatomy of the needle passage

(Fig. 1.3)
a. *Skin:* the branches from the supraclavicular nerve containing fibers from the fourth cervical nerve (C4) innervate the skin.
b. *Subcutaneous tissue:* includes the previously described skin nerve branches.
c. *Anterior deltoid muscle:* the branches from the axillary nerve containing fibers from the fifth and sixth cervical nerves (C5, C6) innervate the deltoid muscle.
d. *Tendon of long head of biceps brachii muscle:* the tendon originates from the scapular joint bursa, crosses the anterior superior head of the humerus, runs inferior along the intertubercular groove of the humerus, and ends in the middle arm together with the short head of biceps brachii muscle. The tendon of the long head of the biceps brachii muscle is covered with a

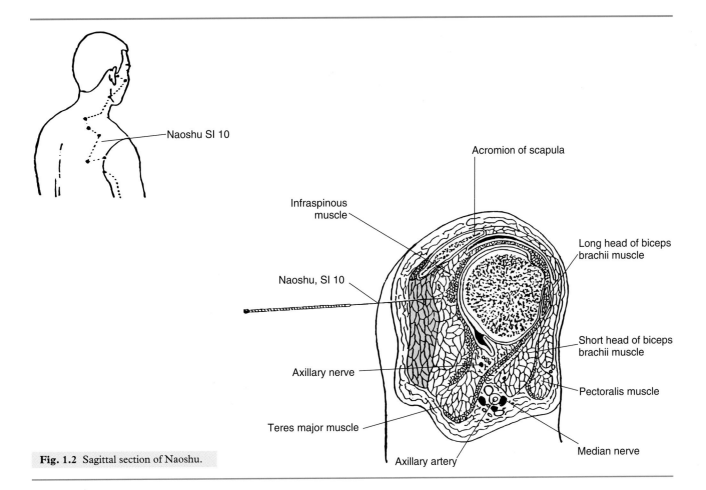

Fig. 1.2 Sagittal section of Naoshu.

synovial sheath, while crossing the intertubercular groove of the humerus. The branches from the musculocutaneous nerve containing fibers from the fifth and sixth cervical nerves (C5, C6) innervate the biceps brachii muscle.

The anterior humeral circumflex artery and vein pass under the tendon of the long head of the biceps brachii muscle and are attached close to the surface of the humerus.

Clinical indications
Hemiplegia, hypertension, shoulder joint pain, soft tissue inflammation of the shoulder joint.

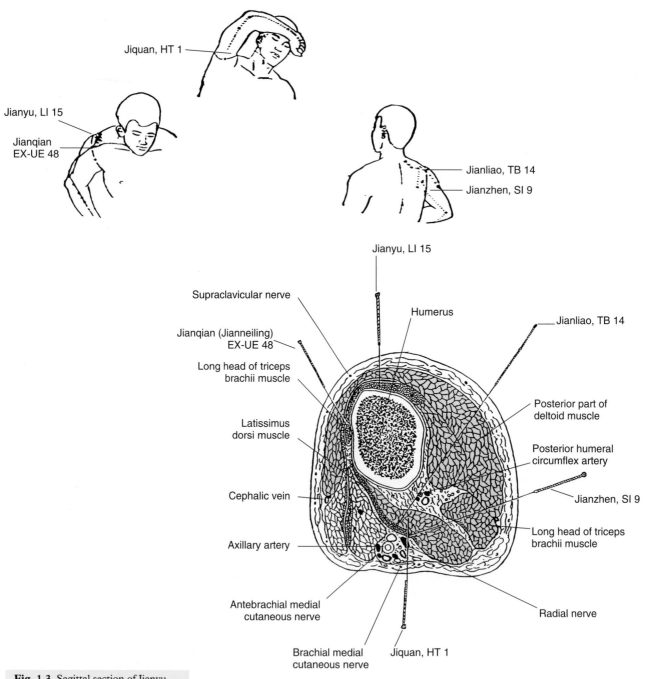

Fig. 1.3 Sagittal section of Jianyu, Jiquan, Jianzhen, Jianliao and Jianqian.

4.

(CHICHUAN) JIQUAN, HT 1, HAND SHAO YIN HEART MERIDIAN

Location
In a seated position, with the arm abducted and exposing the armpit, the point is located in the middle of the axilla, and posterior to the axillary artery. WARNING: Avoid the axillary artery.

Needle and moxibustion method
Perpendicular insertion 1.0–1.5 inches.
— *Needle sensation:* local soreness and distension, or a strong electrical sensation radiating to the forearm.
— *Moxibustion dosage:* 3–5 cones; stick 10 minutes. However, generally no moxibustion is used for this point.

Cross-sectional anatomy of the needle passage
(Fig. 1.3)
a. *Skin:* the lateral cutaneous branches of the second intercostal nerve innervate the skin.
b. *Subcutaneous tissue:* includes the previously described skin nerve branches.
c. The needle is punctured through deep fascia into the axilla. If the needle is inserted into the brachial plexus or its branches, an electrical sensation radiates to the forearm.
d. *Latissimus dorsi muscle:* the branches from the thoracodorsal nerve from the brachial plexus containing fibers from the sixth, seventh, and eighth cervical nerves (C6, C7, C8) innervate the latissimus dorsi muscle.
e. *Teres major muscle:* the branches from the subscapular nerve containing fibers from the fifth and sixth cervical nerves (C5, C6) innervate the teres major muscle.

Warning
a. Avoid the axillary artery by using one finger tip as a guide to find the axillary artery and then insert the needle just medial and posterior to it.
b. Avoid vigorous and repeated lifting of the needle. The axillary region consists of soft connective tissue and the axillary vein adhered to deep fascia. Accidentally puncturing the axillary vein will cause hematoma.

Functions
Regulates the flow of Qi to promote Blood circulation, removes Blood Stasis and resolves masses.

Clinical indications
Angina pectoris, shoulder joint inflammation, soft tissue inflammation of the shoulder joint, pleurisy, jaundice, depression, nausea.

5.

(CHIENYU) JIANYU, LI 15, HAND YANG MING LARGE INTESTINE MERIDIAN

Location
In a seated position with the arm adducted, the point is located on the margin of the shoulder at the midpoint of the superior margin of the deltoid muscle, in the fossa between the highest point of the acromion process of the scapula and the greater tuberosity of the humerus; or in a seated position and abducting the arm to shoulder height, two fossae will appear on the shoulder – and the anterior one is Jianyu [LI 15].

Needle and moxibustion method
Perpendicular insertion: keep the needle at 90° perpendicular insertion 0.5–0.8 inch (treating supraspinatus muscle inflammation).
— *Needle sensation:* local distension and soreness, sometimes radiating to the wrist.
   Medial oblique insertion: keep the needle at 50°, 1.5-2.0 inches.
— *Needle sensation:* local distension and soreness, or radiating to the shoulder joint.
   Inferior oblique insertion: keep the needle at 50° inferior oblique insertion 1.5–2.0 inches; or anterior medial inferior and posterior medial inferior insertions (treating periarthritis of shoulder).
— *Needle sensation:* soreness and distension at the wrist.
— *Moxibustion dosage:* 3–5 cones; stick 5–15 minutes.

Cross-sectional anatomy of the needle passage
(Fig. 1.3)
Perpendicular insertion:
a. *Skin:* the branches from the lateral supraclavicular nerve containing fibers from the fourth cervical nerve (C4) innervate the skin.
b. *Subcutaneous tissue:* includes the previously described skin nerve branches.
c. *Deltoid muscle:* the needle is inserted into the middle superior part of the deltoid muscle. The branches from the axillary nerve containing fibers from the fifth and sixth cervical nerves (C5, C6) innervate the deltoid muscle.
d. *Subdeltoid bursa of deltoid muscle:* the synovial bursa between the deep deltoid muscle and the greater tuberosity of the humerus, which frequently communicates with the subacromial bursa.
e. *Tendon of supraspinatus muscle:* the tendon is attached to the superior part of the greater tuberosity of the humerus. The branches from the suprascapular nerve containing fibers from the fifth cervical nerve (C5) innervate the supraspinatus muscle.

Medial oblique insertion:

a–c same as perpendicular insertion.

d. *Subacromial bursa:* the synovial bursa between the acromion process of the scapula and the supraspinatus muscle, which frequently communicates with the subdeltoid bursa.

e. *Supraspinatus muscle:* the branches from the suprascapular nerve containing fibers from the fifth cervical nerve (C5) innervate the supraspinatus muscle. The function of this muscle is to abduct the shoulder joint.

Inferior oblique insertion:

a–d same as medial oblique insertion.

e. The needle is inserted through the subdeltoid bursa, then into the deltoid muscle.

Functions

Clears and activates the channels and collaterals, eases joint movement and alleviates pain.

Clinical indications

Hemiplegia, hypertension, shoulder joint pain, supraspinatus muscle inflammation, periarthritis of shoulder, urticaria, sweating.

6.

(CHIENCHEN) JIANZHEN, SI 9, HAND TAI YANG SMALL INTESTINE MERIDIAN

Location

In a seated position with the arm adducted, the point is located at the posterior, inferior shoulder one inch above the posterior end of the axillary fold.

Needle and moxibustion method

Keeping the needle in an anterior direction, at 70° to the skin, use an anterior inferior oblique insertion 2.0–2.5 inches.

— *Needle sensation:* local soreness and distension, or sometimes an electrical sensation radiating to the shoulder and the fingertips.

— *Moxibustion dosage:* 3–7 cones; stick 5–20 minutes.

Cross-sectional anatomy of the needle passage
(Fig. 1.3)

a. *Skin:* the lateral cutaneous branches of the intercostal nerve containing fibers from the second thoracic nerve (T2) innervate the skin.

b. *Subcutaneous tissue:* includes the previously described skin nerve branches.

c. *Posterior part of deltoid muscle:* the branches from the axillary nerve containing fibers from the fifth and sixth cervical nerves (C5, C6) innervate the posterior deltoid muscle.

d. *Long head of triceps brachii muscle:* the branches from the radial nerve containing fibers from the seventh and eighth cervical nerves (C7, C8) innervate the long head of the triceps brachii muscle.

e. *Teres major muscle:* the branches from the subscapular nerve containing fibers from the fifth and sixth cervical nerves (C5, C6) innervate the teres major muscle.

f. *Latissimus dorsi muscle:* the branches from the thoracodorsal nerve containing fibers from the sixth, seventh, and eighth cervical nerves (C6, C7, C8) innervate the latissimus dorsi muscle.

g. *Axilla:* the needle is inserted posterior to the axillary artery into the radial nerve, a branch of the brachial plexus. An electrical sensation radiating to the dorsal part of the upper extremities and fingertips is felt.

Warning

a. To avoid pneumothorax, the needle can only be inserted in a perpendicular direction; a medial direction is absolutely contraindicated.

b. After the needle is inserted into the axilla, to avoid hematoma, do not vigorously and repeatedly lift and thrust the needle.

Functions

Wakes up the patient from unconsciousness by clearing Heat, and promotes Blood circulation to remove Blood Stasis.

Clinical indications

Shoulder and surrounding soft tissue inflammation, hemiplegia, deafness, dizziness, headache, toothache, numbness of the hand.

7.

(CHIENLIAO) JIANLIAO, TB 14, HAND SHAO YIN TRIPLE BURNER MERIDIAN

Location

In a seated position, the point is located on the posterior inferior part of the acromion of the scapula about 1 inch posterior to Jianyu [LI 15]. If the patient abducts the arm, two fossae will appear at the shoulder, the posterior one of which is Jianliao [TB 15].

Needle and moxibustion method

Perpendicular insertion: abducting the arm, perpendicular insertion to Jiquan [HT 1] 1.5–2.5 inches, (treating arthritis of the shoulder).

Oblique insertion: with inferior oblique insertion for 2 inches, the needle point can be directed either side (treating periarthritis of the shoulder).

— *Needle sensation:* local soreness and distension,

radiating to the whole shoulder, and an electrical sensation radiating to the distal part of the upper extremities.
— *Moxibustion dosage:* 3–7 cones; stick 5–15 minutes.

Cross-sectional anatomy of the needle passage
(Fig. 1.3)
Perpendicular insertion:
a. *Skin:* the branches from the lateral supraclavicular nerve containing fibers from the fourth cervical nerve (C4) innervate the skin.
b. *Subcutaneous tissue:* includes the previously described skin nerve branches.
c. *Posterior deltoid muscle:* the branches from the axillary nerve containing fibers from the fifth and sixth cervical nerves (C5, C6) innervate the deltoid muscle.
d. *Teres minor muscle:* the branches from the axillary nerve containing fibers from the fifth cervical nerve (C5) innervate the teres minor muscle.
e. *Axillary nerve and posterior humeral circumflex artery and vein:* the needle is inserted into the surrounding structures of the axillary nerve and posterior humeral circumflex artery and vein. If the needle is inserted into the axillary nerve, a branch of the posterior cord of the brachial plexus, an electrical sensation radiates to the shoulder and posterior arm. The posterior humeral circumflex artery and vein are continuations of the axillary artery and vein respectively, and run together with the axillary nerve.
f. *Teres major muscle:* the branches from the subscapular nerve of the brachial plexus containing fibers from the fifth and sixth cervical nerves (C5, C6) innervate the teres major muscle.
g. *Latissimus dorsi muscle:* the branches from the thoracodorsal nerve containing fibers from the sixth, seventh, and eighth cervical nerves (C6, C7, C8) innervate the latissimus dorsi muscle. The needle is inserted into the axillary cavity and an electric sensation radiates to the distal part of the upper extremities, if the needle is inserted into the brachial plexus or its branches in the axillary cavity.
Oblique insertion:
a-d same as perpendicular insertion.
e. *Long head of triceps brachii muscle:* the branches from the radial nerve of the sixth, seventh, and eighth cervical nerves (C6, C7, C8) innervate the triceps brachii muscle.

Functions
Expels Wind and clears away Cold, and promotes Blood circulation to relieve pain.

Clinical indications
Periarthritis of shoulder, arthritis of shoulder, cerebrovascular accident, hemiplegia, hypertension, pleurisy.

8.

(NAOHUI) NAOHUI, TB 13, HAND SHAO YANG TRIPLE BURNER MERIDIAN

Location
In a seated position with the arm adducted, the point is located on the dorsal side of the arm 3 inches below the acromion process of the scapula. Draw a line between Jianliao [TB 14] and the olecranon process of the ulna, and the point is located 3 inches below Jianliao [TB 14], in the fossa between the tuberosity of the lateral head of the triceps brachii muscle and the tuberosity of the deltoid muscle.

Needle and moxibustion method
Perpendicular insertion 0.5–0.8 inch.
— *Needle sensation:* local distension and numbness radiating to the distal part of the arm.
— *Moxibustion dosage:* 3–7 cones; stick 10 minutes.

Cross-sectional anatomy of the needle passage
a. *Skin:* the branches of the posterior brachial cutaneous nerve containing fibers from the eighth cervical nerve (C8) innervate the skin.
b. *Subcutaneous tissue:* includes the previously described skin nerve branches.
c. *Triceps brachii muscle, long head and lateral head:* the needle is passed between the long head and lateral head of the triceps brachii muscles. The branches of the radial nerve containing fibers from the sixth, seventh and eighth cervical nerves (C6, C7, C8) innervate the muscle.
d. *Deep brachial artery and vein:* the deep brachial artery, together with the deep brachial vein, is a branch of the brachial artery. The needle is passed to the radial side of the deep brachial artery and vein.
e. *Radial nerve:* the branches from the brachial plexus containing fibers from the fifth to eighth cervical nerves (C5, C6, C7, C8) supply the radial nerve. If the needle punctures the radial nerve, a strong electrical sensation starts from the lateral side of the forearm and the lateral dorsal side of the hand and radiates to the fingers.
f. *Triceps brachii muscle, medial head:* the branches of the radial nerve containing fibers from the the sixth, seventh, and eighth cervical nerves (C6, C7, C8) innervate the muscle.

Functions
Dredges the channels to promote Blood circulation, subdues inflammation and dissipates Blood Stasis.

Clinical indications
Shoulder pain, pleurisy, frozen shoulder, common cold.

9.

(TIENCHUAN) TIANQUAN, PC 2, HAND JUE YIN PERICARDIUM MERIDIAN

Location

In a supine position and slightly abducting the arm, the point is located 2 inches below the anterior skin crease of the axilla. Draw a line between the anterior skin crease of the axilla and Chize [LU 5] and the point is located 7 inches above Chize [LU 5], and between the fossa of the short head and long head of the biceps muscle.

Needle and moxibustion method

Perpendicular insertion 1.0–1.5 inches or use a triangular needle to induce bleeding.
— *Needle sensation:* local soreness and distension.
— *Moxibustion dosage:* 3–5 cones; stick 10 minutes.

Cross-sectional anatomy of the needle passage

a. *Skin:* the branches from the medial brachial cutaneous nerve containing fibers from the first thoracic nerve (T1) innervate the skin.
b. *Subcutaneous tissue:* includes the previously described skin nerve branches.
c. *Biceps brachii muscle, long head and short head:* the branches from the musculocutaneous nerve containing fibers from the fifth and sixth cervical nerves (C5, C6) innervate the muscle. The needle is passed between the long head and short head of the biceps brachii muscle.
d. *Musculocutaneous nerve:* the needle is passed on the lateral side of the musculocutaneous nerve. The branches from the brachial plexus containing fibers from the fifth, sixth, and seventh cervical nerves (C5, C6, C7) supply the nerve.
e. *Brachialis muscle:* the branches from the musculocutaneous nerve containing fibers from the fifth and sixth cervical nerves (C5, C6) innervate the muscle. The needle is passed into the muscle.
f. *Tendon of coracobrachialis muscle:* the branches from the musculocutaneous nerve containing fibers from the fifth, sixth, and seventh cervical nerves (C5, C6, C7) innervate the muscle.

Functions

Regulates the flow of Qi to promote Blood circulation, promotes lactation and removes Blood Stasis. \

Clinical indications

Heart pain, tachycardia, pleurisy, cough, nausea, shoulder pain, bronchitis.

10.

(PINAO) BINAO, LI 14, HAND YANG MING LARGE INTESTINE MERIDIAN

Location

In a seated position, with the arm adducted and the elbow flexed, the point is located at the inferior margin of the deltoid muscle. First locate Quchi [LI 11] and Jianyu [LI 15], then draw a line between these two points. The point is located 7 inches above Quchi [LI 11].

Needle and moxibustion method

Perpendicular insertion 0.5–1.0 inch; or insert the needle horizontally along the anterior posterior margin of the humerus bone 1.0–1.5 inches.

Oblique insertion: Insert the needle superiorly and obliquely 1–2 inches towards the deltoid muscle (treating eye disease).
— *Needle sensation:* local soreness and distension.
— *Moxibustion dosage:* 3–7 cones; stick 5–15 minutes.

Cross-sectional anatomy of the needle passage

(Fig. 1.4)
Perpendicular insertion:
a. *Skin:* the lateral brachial cutaneous nerve containing fibers from the fifth cervical nerve (C5) innervates the skin.
b. *Subcutaneous tissue:* includes the previously described skin nerve branches.
c. *Deltoid muscle:* the branches from the axillary nerve containing fibers from the fifth and sixth cervical nerves (C5, C6) innervate the deltoid muscle. If the needle is inserted along the anterior margin of the humerus it passes into the long head of the biceps brachii muscle. If the needle is inserted along the posterior margin of the humerus it passes into the lateral head of the triceps brachii muscle.
Superior oblique insertion:
a–b same as perpendicular insertion.
c. *Deltoid muscle:* the needle inserts into the deltoid muscle if angled slightly higher than for perpendicular insertion.

Functions

Removes obstruction in the channels, improves visual acuity, and promotes the circulation of Qi to dissipate Blood Stasis.

Clinical indications

Shoulder pain, paralysis of the upper extremities, eye diseases, tuberculosis of the lymph nodes.

11.

(TIENFU) TIANFU, LU 3, HAND TAI YIN LUNG MERIDIAN

Location

In a supine or seated position, the point is located on the medial side of the arm 3 inches below the skin crease of the axilla, and at the lateral side of the biceps brachii muscle, at the same height as the nipples.

Needle and moxibustion method

Perpendicular insertion 0.5–1.0 inch.
— *Needle sensation:* local soreness and numbness or radiating to the distal part of the arm.
— *Moxibustion dosage:* 3–7 cones; stick 5 minutes.

Cross-sectional anatomy of the needle passage

a. *Skin:* the branches from the lateral brachial cutaneous nerve containing fibers from the sixth cervical nerve (C6) innervate the skin.
b. *Subcutaneous tissue:* includes the previously described skin nerve branches.
c. *Cephalic vein and muscular branch of brachial artery:* the muscular branch of the brachial artery stems from the radial collateral branch of the profundus artery.
d. *Biceps brachii muscle, long head:* the branches from the musculocutaneous nerve containing fibers from the fifth and sixth cervical nerves (C5, C6) innervate the muscle. The needle passes lateral to the long head of the biceps brachii muscle.
e. *Brachialis muscle:* the branches from the median nerve containing fibers from the fifth and sixth cervical nerves (C5, C6) innervate the muscle.

Functions

Regulates the function of the Lung Qi, removes Heat and expels Wind.

Clinical indications

Asthma, cerebrovascular disease, epistaxis, vomiting, malaria, vertigo.

12.

(HSIAPAI) XIABAI, LU 4, HAND TAI YIN LUNG MERIDIAN

Location

In a supine or seated position with the elbow flexed, the point is located on the radial side of the biceps brachii muscle, and 5 inches above the skin crease of the elbow (Chize LU 5).

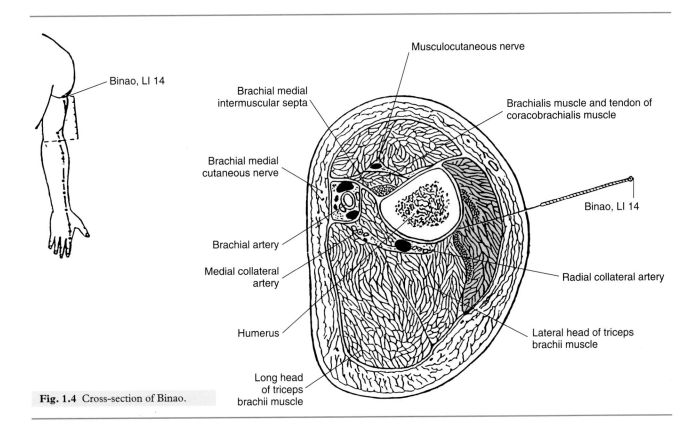

Fig. 1.4 Cross-section of Binao.

Needle and moxibustion method

Perpendicular insertion 0.5–1.0 inch.

— *Needle sensation:* local distension and soreness radiating to the distal part of the arm.

— *Moxibustion dosage:* 3–7 cones; stick 10–20 minutes.

Cross-sectional anatomy of the needle passage

a. *Skin:* the branches from the lateral brachial cutaneous nerve containing fibers from the fifth cervical nerve (C5) innervate the skin.

b. *Subcutaneous tissue:* includes the previously described skin nerve branches.

c. *Cephalic vein and muscular branch of brachial artery:* the muscular branch of the brachial artery stems from the radial collateral branch of the profunda artery.

d. *Biceps brachii muscle, long head:* the branches from the musculocutaneous nerve containing fibers from the fifth and sixth cervical nerves (C5, C6) innervate the muscle. The needle passes lateral to the long head of the biceps brachii muscle.

e. *Brachialis muscle:* the branches from the median nerve containing fibers from the fifth and sixth cervical nerves (C5, C6) innervate the muscle. The needle is passed into the lateral side of the brachial muscle.

Functions

Clears and activates the channels and collaterals, and regulates the function of Lung Qi.

Clinical indications

Cough, chest tightness, nausea, pleurisy, tachycardia.

13.

(HSIAOLO) XIAOLUO, TB 12, HAND SHAO YANG TRIPLE BURNER MERIDIAN

Location

In a seated position with the elbow flexed, the point is located on the dorsal side of the arm, 4.5 inches above the olecranon process of the ulna. Draw a line between the olecranon process of the ulna and Jianliao [TB 14]. The point is located at the midpoint between Qinglengyuan [TB 11] and Naohui [TB 13].

Needle and moxibustion method

Perpendicular insertion 0.3–0.5 inch.

— *Needle sensation:* local soreness and distension.

— *Moxibustion dosage:* 3–5 cones; stick 10 minutes.

Cross-sectional anatomy of the needle passage

a. *Skin:* the branches from the posterior brachial cutaneous nerve containing fibers from the fifth

cervical nerve (C5) innervate the skin.

b. *Subcutaneous tissue:* includes the previously described skin nerve branches.

c. *Triceps brachii muscle, long head:* the branches from the radial nerve containing fibers from the sixth, seventh and eighth cervical nerves (C6, C7, C8) innervate the muscle.

d. *Muscular branch of radial nerve, middle collateral artery and vein:* the middle collateral artery, together with the middle collateral vein, is a branch of the deep brachial artery.

e. *Triceps brachii muscle, medial head:* the branches from the radial nerve containing fibers from the sixth, seventh, and eighth cervical nerves (C6, C7, C8) innervate the muscle.

Functions

Regulates and promotes Blood circulation, and dispels Wind.

Clinical indications

Headache, neck pain, frozen shoulder, toothache.

14.

(CHINGLING) QINGLING, HT 2, HAND SHAO YIN HEART MERIDIAN

Location

In a seated position, with the elbow flexed, the point is located on the ulnar side of the arm 3 inches above Shaohai [HT 3].

Needle and moxibustion method

Perpendicular insertion 0.3–0.5 inch.

— *Needle sensation:* local soreness and numbness.

— *Moxibustion dosage:* 3–7 cones; stick 10 minutes.

Cross-sectional anatomy of the needle passage

a. *Skin:* the branches from the medial brachial cutaneous nerve containing fibers from the second thoracic nerve (T2) innervate the skin.

b. *Subcutaneous tissue:* includes the previously described skin nerve branches and ascending cephalic vein. The branches from the medial cord of the brachial plexus from fibers containing the eighth cervical and first thoracic nerves (C8, T1) supply the medial brachial cutaneous nerve. The cephalic vein joins the brachial vein.

c. The needle is inserted on the dorsal side of the superior ulnar collateral artery, ulnar nerve and triceps brachii muscle. The needle is inserted on the ventral side of the brachial artery and vein, and the median nerve. The branches from the radial nerve containing fibers from the sixth to eighth cervical nerves (C6, C7, C8) innervate the triceps brachii muscle. The superior ulnar collateral artery is a branch of the brachial artery. The branches from the brachial plexus containing the fibers from the seventh and eighth cervical and first thoracic nerves (C7, C8, T1) supply the ulnar nerve. The branches from the brachial plexus containing fibers from the fifth cervical to first thoracic nerves (C5, C6, C7, C8, T1) supply the median nerve.

d. *Brachialis muscle:* the branches from the musculo-cutaneous nerve containing fibers from the fifth and sixth cervical nerves (C5, C6) innervate the muscle. The needle is passed on the medial side of the muscle.

e. *Medial brachial intermuscular septum:* the needle is inserted at the anterior part of the septum.

Functions
Reduces fever, removes Dampness, relaxes rigidity of local muscles and tendons and relieves rigidity of the joints.

Clinical indications
Jaundice, chills, shoulder pain, precordial pain.

15.
(SHOUWULI) SHOUWULI, LI 13, HAND YANG MING LARGE INTESTINE MERIDIAN

Location
With the elbow flexed, the point is located above the lateral condyle of the lateral humerus on the line between Quchi [LI 11] and Jianyu [LI 15], and 3 inches above Quchi [LI 11].

Needle and moxibustion method
Perpendicular insertion 1.0–1.5 inches.
— *Needle sensation:* soreness and distension radiating to the forearm.
— *Moxibustion dosage:* 7–15 cones; stick 15 minutes.

Cross-sectional anatomy of the needle passage
a. *Skin:* the branches from the posterior antebrachial cutaneous nerve containing fibers from the sixth cervical nerve (C6) innervate the skin.
b. *Subcutaneous tissue*: includes the previously described skin nerve branches.
c. *Brachialis muscle:* the branches from the radial nerve containing fibers from the fifth and sixth cervical nerves (C5, C6) innervate the muscle.

Functions
Reduces fever, resolves Phlegm, and promotes the flow of Qi to remove Blood Stasis.

Clinical indications
Cough, pneumonia, rheumatoid arthritis, elbow pain, shoulder pain.

16.
(CHIENLENGYUAN) QINGLENGYUAN, TB 11, HAND SHAO YANG TRIPLE BURNER MERIDIAN

Location
With the elbow flexed, the point is located 1 inch above the fossa of the olecranon process of the ulna.

Needle and moxibustion method
Perpendicular insertion 0.3–0.5 inch.
— *Needle sensation:* local soreness and distension.
— *Moxibustion dosage:* 3–5 cones; stick 10 minutes.

Cross-sectional anatomy of the needle passage
a. *Skin:* the branches from the posterior antebrachial cutaneous nerve containing fibers from the sixth cervical nerve (C6) innervate the skin.
b. *Subcutaneous tissue:* includes the previously described skin nerve branches.
c. *Tendon of triceps brachii muscle:* the branches from the radial nerve containing fibers from the seventh and eighth cervical nerves (C7, C8) innervate the muscle. The needle passes through the middle of the inferior part of the muscle.
d. *Superior ulnar collateral artery and vein:* the needle passes superior to the ulnar collateral artery and vein. The superior collateral artery, together with the superior collateral vein, is a branch of the brachial artery.

Functions
Reduces fever and relieves jaundice, and clears the collaterals to alleviate pain.

Clinical indications
Headache, chills, frozen shoulder, migraine, axillary pain, common cold, cholecystitis, hepatitis.

17.
(CHOULIAO) ZHOULIAO, LI 12, HAND YANG MING LARGE INTESTINE MERIDIAN

Location
With the elbow flexed, the point is located about 1 inch slightly superior and lateral to Quchi [LI 11], or 1 inch above the lateral epicondyle of the humerus.

Needle and moxibustion method

Perpendicular insertion 1.0–1.5 inch.
— *Needle sensation:* local numbness and distension.
— *Moxibustion dosage:* 3–5 cones; stick 15 minutes.

Cross-sectional anatomy of the needle passage

(Fig. 1.5)
a. *Skin:* the branches from the posterior antebrachial cutaneous nerve containing fibers from the fifth cervical nerve (C5) innervate the skin.
b. *Subcutaneous tissue:* includes the previously described skin nerve branches.
c. *Triceps brachii muscle:* the branches from the radial nerve containing fibers from the sixth, seventh, and eighth cervical nerves (C6, C7, C8) innervate the triceps brachii muscle. After the needle is inserted through the subcutaneous tissue, if the needle is slightly directed to the anterior margin of the humerus bone, it will not pass into the triceps brachii muscle but into the brachioradialis muscle.

Functions

Clears and activates the channels and collaterals, relaxes local muscles and tendons and eases movement of the elbow joint.

Clinical indications

Arm and elbow pain, inflammation of the lateral epicondyle of the humerus, cough, malaria, numbness of the elbow, tennis elbow.

18.

(TIENCHING) TIANJING, TB 10, HAND SHAO YANG TRIPLE BURNER MERIDIAN, CONVERGING POINT

Location

With the elbow flexed at 90°, the point is located in the fossa 1 inch above the olecranon process of the ulna.

Needle and moxibustion method

Perpendicular insertion 0.5–1.0 inch.
— *Needle sensation:* local soreness and distension.
— *Moxibustion dosage:* 3–5 cones; stick 5–15 minutes.

Cross-sectional anatomy of the needle passage

(Fig. 1.5)
a. *Skin:* the branches from the posterior brachial cutaneous nerve containing fibers from the fifth cervical nerve (C5) innervate the skin.
b. *Subcutaneous tissue:* includes the previously described skin nerve branches.
c. *Tendon of triceps brachii muscle:* the branches from the radial nerve containing fibers from the sixth, seventh, eighth cervical nerves (C6, C7, C8) innervate the triceps brachii muscle. The medial collateral branch of the deep brachial artery and vein cross laterally to the point.

Functions

Clears away Wind Heat, and removes and eliminates masses.

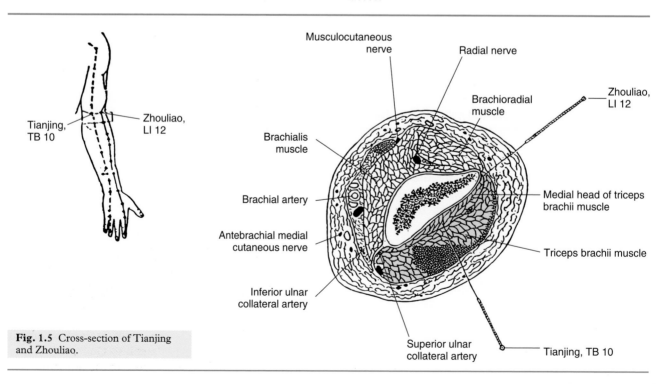

Fig. 1.5 Cross-section of Tianjing and Zhouliao.

Clinical indications

Migraine, tonsillitis, elbow joint and surrounding soft tissue disease, urticaria, cervical lymph node tuberculosis, cough, bronchitis, depression.

19.

(CHUCHIH) QUCHI, LI 11, HAND YANG MING LARGE INTESTINE MERIDIAN, CONVERGING POINT

Location

With the elbow flexed at 90°, the point is located at the anterior lateral elbow joint, in the midpoint between the radial side of the skin crease of the elbow and the lateral epicondyle of the humerus.

Needle and moxibustion method

With the elbow flexed, perpendicular insertion 1.0–1.5 inches (treating paralysis of the upper extremities).
— *Needle sensation:* local soreness and distension, or sometimes an electrical sensation radiating to the finger tips or the shoulder.

Perpendicular insertion penetrating to Shaohai [HT 3] 2.0–2.5 inches.

— *Needle sensation:* local soreness and distension, and sometimes an electrical sensation radiating to the shoulder or the fingers.

Perpendicular insertion: slightly oblique downwards insertion 1.5–2.5 inches.
— *Needle sensation:* after Qi arrives, twist the needle heavily several times and the sensation radiates to the antebrachium or sometimes to the shoulder.
— *Moxibustion dosage:* 3–7 cones (WARNING: Don't perform directly on the joint); stick 5–20 minutes.

Cross-sectional anatomy of the needle passage
(Fig. 1.6)
a. *Skin:* the branches from the posterior antebrachial cutaneous nerve containing fibers from the sixth cervical nerve (C6) innervate the skin.
b. *Subcutaneous tissue:* includes the previously described skin nerve branches.
c. *Extensor carpi radialis longus and brevis muscles:* the branches from the radial nerve containing fibers from the sixth and seventh cervical nerves (C6, C7) innervate the extensor carpi radialis longus and brevis muscles. These two muscles are firmly attached to the anterior wall of the elbow joint bursa.
d. *Brachioradialis muscle:* the branches from the radial

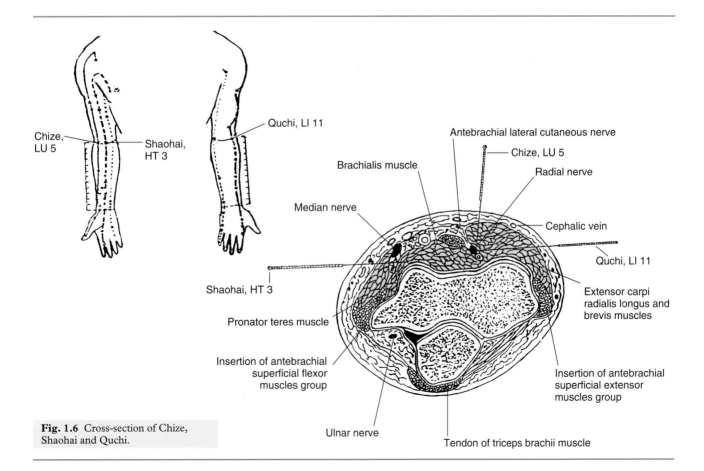

Fig. 1.6 Cross-section of Chize, Shaohai and Quchi.

Chize, LU 5

Shaohai, HT 3

Quchi, LI 11

Antebrachial lateral cutaneous nerve

Brachialis muscle

Chize, LU 5

Radial nerve

Median nerve

Cephalic vein

Quchi, LI 11

Shaohai, HT 3

Extensor carpi radialis longus and brevis muscles

Pronator teres muscle

Insertion of antebrachial superficial flexor muscles group

Insertion of antebrachial superficial extensor muscles group

Ulnar nerve

Tendon of triceps brachii muscle

nerve containing fibers from the fifth and sixth cervical nerves (C5, C6) innervate brachioradialis muscle.

e. *Radial nerve and anterior branch of radial collateral artery and vein:* the radial nerve descends between the brachioradialis muscle, triceps brachii muscle tendon and brachialis muscle. If the needle is inserted into the radial nerve, a strong electrical sensation will start from the lateral side of the forearm and lateral dorsal side of the hand and radiate to the fingertips. If this happens, stop inserting the needle immediately. The radial collateral artery, together with the radial collateral vein, is a branch of the deep brachial artery, which bifurcates in the elbow joint to form anterior and posterior branches.

f. *Brachialis muscle:* the branches from the musculocutaneous nerve containing fibers from the fifth and sixth cervical nerves (C5, C6) innervate the brachialis muscle.

Functions
Expels Wind to relieve Exterior Syndromes, clears Heat and regulates the flow of Qi to promote Blood flow.

Clinical indications
High fever, hypertension, measles, anemia, hyperthyroidism, upper extremities pain, hemiplegia, allergy, skin disease, tonsillitis, pleurisy, tooth pain.

20.

(CHIHTSE) CHIZE, LU 5, HAND TAI YIN LUNG MERIDIAN, CONVERGING POINT

Location
With an open hand and slightly flexing the elbow, the point is located on the skin crease of the elbow, in the fossa at the radial side of the tendon of the biceps brachialis muscle.

Needle and moxibustion method
Perpendicular insertion 0.5–1.0 inch.
— *Needle sensation:* local soreness and distension, or sometimes an electrical sensation radiating to the forearm.
— *Moxibustion dosage:* 5–7 cones; stick 5–10 minutes.

Cross-sectional anatomy of the needle passage
(Fig 1.6)
a. *Skin:* the branches from the lateral antebrachial cutaneous nerve from the musculocutaneous nerve containing fibers from the sixth cervical nerve (C6) innervate the skin.
b. *Subcutaneous tissue:* includes the previously described

skin nerve branches and the cephalic vein. The cephalic vein joins the axillary vein.

c. *Brachioradialis muscle:* the branches from the radial nerve containing fibers from the fifth and sixth cervical nerves (C5, C6) innervate the brachioradialis muscle.

d. *Tendon of biceps brachii muscle:* the needle is passed radial to the tendon of the biceps brachii muscle. The branches from the musculocutaneous nerve containing fibers from the fifth and sixth cervical nerves (C5, C6) innervate the muscle.

e. *Radial nerve and anterior branch of radial collateral artery and vein:* the radial nerve descends between the brachioradialis muscle, triceps brachii muscle tendon, and brachialis muscle. The branches from the brachial plexus containing fibers from the fifth to eighth cervical nerves (C5, C6, C7, C8) supply the radial nerve. If the needle is inserted into the radial nerve, a strong electrical sensation will start from the lateral side of the forearm and the lateral dorsal side of the hand and radiate to the fingertips. If this happens, stop inserting the needle immediately. The radial collateral artery, together with the radial collateral vein, is a branch of the deep brachial artery, which bifurcates in the elbow joint to form anterior and posterior branches.

f. *Brachialis muscle:* the branches from the musculocutaneous nerve containing fibers from fifth and sixth cervical nerves (C5, C6) innervate the muscle.

Functions
Clears Lung Heat, relieves sore throat and alleviates pain.

Clinical indications
Cough, asthma, pneumonia, bronchitis, pleurisy, hematemesis, sore throat, elbow pain, erysipelas, childhood coma, mastitis.

21.

(SHAOHAI) SHAOHAI, HT 3, HAND SHAO YIN HEART MERIDIAN, CONVERGING POINT

Location
With the elbow flexed at 90°, the point is located on the ulnar side of the skin crease of the elbow, and at the midpoint between the medial epicondyle of the humerus and the ulnar side of the tendon of the biceps brachialis muscle.

Needle and moxibustion method
Perpendicular insertion 0.5–1.5 inches.
— *Needle sensation:* local soreness and distension, or an

electrical sensation radiating to the wrist.

— *Moxibustion dosage:* 3–5 cones (WARNING: No direct moxibustion on the joint); stick 5–10 minutes.

Cross-sectional anatomy of the needle passage
(Fig. 1.6)

a. *Skin:* the anterior branches from the medial antebrachial cutaneous nerve containing fibers from the first thoracic nerve (T1) innervate the skin.

b. *Subcutaneous tissue:* includes the previously described skin nerve branches. The ascending cephalic vein lies adjacent to the point.

c. *Pronator teres muscle:* the branches from the median nerve containing fibers from the sixth and seventh cervical nerves (C6, C7) innervate the pronator teres muscle.

d. *Median nerve and ulnar recurrent artery and vein:* the median nerve passes posterior to the pronator teres muscle. The needle is passed posterior to the median nerve. If the needle is slightly directed to the anterior, it will be inserted into the median nerve. The needle response of the median nerve is a strong electric sensation radiating to the finger tips. The needle is passed anterior to the ulnar recurrent vein.

e. *Brachialis muscle:* the branches from the musculocutaneous nerve containing fibers from the fifth and sixth cervical nerves (C5, C6) innervate the brachialis muscle.

Functions

Promotes Blood circulation, regulates the flow of Qi, and relieves mental stress.

Clinical indications

Headache, epilepsy, angina pectoris, pleurisy, caries, toothache, dizziness, tuberculosis.

22.

(CHUTSE) QUZE, PC 3, HAND JUE YIN PERICARDIUM MERIDIAN, CONVERGING POINT

Location

With the elbow flexed, the point is located in the middle of the skin crease of the elbow and on the medial side of the tendon of the biceps brachii muscle, or at the midpoint between Chize [LU 5] and Shaohai [HT 3].

Needle and moxibustion method

Perpendicular insertion 0.5–0.7 inch or use a triangular needle to induce bleeding (treating acute gastroenteritis).

— *Needle sensation:* local distension and soreness,

sometimes radiating to the middle finger. WARNING: Avoid artery.

— *Moxibustion dosage:* 3–7 cones; stick 15 minutes.

Cross-sectional anatomy of the needle passage
(Fig. 1.6)

a. *Skin:* the branches from the medial antebrachial cutaneous nerve containing fibers from the first thoracic nerve (T1) innervate the skin.

b. *Subcutaneous tissue:* includes the previously described skin nerve branches and basilic vein.

c. *Tendon of the biceps brachii muscle:* the branches from the musculocutaneous nerve containing fibers from the fifth and sixth cervical nerves (C5, C6) innervate the muscle. The needle passes medial to the tendon of the biceps brachii muscle.

d. *Brachial artery and vein, and median nerve:* the needle passes on the radial side of the brachial artery and vein, and median nerve. The brachial artery, together with the brachial vein, is a branch of the axillary artery. The branches from the brachial plexus containing fibers from the fifth to eighth cervical and first thoracic nerves supply the median nerve. WARNING: Avoid puncturing the artery.

e. *Brachialis muscle:* the branches from the musculocutaneous nerve containing fibers from the fifth and sixth cervical nerves (C5, C6) innervate the muscle.

Functions

Removes Heat from the Lung and regulates the function of the Stomach, and promotes the circulation of Qi to alleviate pain.

Clinical indications

Myocarditis, bronchitis, elbow pain, tuberculosis, urticaria, precordial pain, tachycardia, stomach pain, vomiting.

23.

(HSIAOHAI) XIAOHAI, SI 8, HAND TAI YANG SMALL INTESTINE MERIDIAN, CONVERGING POINT

Location

With the elbow flexed, the point is located in the fossa between the olecranon of the ulna and the medial epicondyle of the humerus, and at the sulcus for the ulnar nerve of the humerus.

Needle and moxibustion method

Inferior oblique insertion 0.5–1.0 inch.

— *Needle sensation:* soreness and numbness radiating to the little finger.

— *Moxibustion dosage:* 5–7 cones; stick 15 minutes.

Cross-sectional anatomy of the needle passage

a. *Skin:* the branches from the medial antebrachial cutaneous and the medial brachial cutaneous nerves containing fibers from the first thoracic nerve (T1) innervate the skin.

b. *Subcutaneous tissue:* includes the previously described skin nerve branches.

c. *Superior ulnar collateral artery and vein:* the superior ulnar collateral artery, together with the vein, is a branch of the brachial artery.

d. *Ulnar nerve:* the ulnar nerve passes along the sulcus of the ulnar nerve of the humerus. The branches from the brachial plexus containing fibers from the seventh and eighth cervical and first thoracic nerves (C7, C8, T1) supply the ulnar nerve. If the needle is inserted into the nerve, an electrical sensation radiates to forearm and fingers.

Functions

Reduces fever and promotes resuscitation, and improves Blood circulation to remove Blood Stasis. Calms the mind.

Clinical indications

Headache, neck stiffness, elbow pain, shoulder pain, toothache, deafness, dizziness, convulsion, gingivitis.

24.

(SHOUSANLI) SHOUSANLI, LI 10, HAND YANG MING LARGE INTESTINE MERIDIAN

Location

With the elbow flexed, the point is located on the radial side of the elbow on the line between Quchi [LI 11] and Yangxi [LI 5], and 2 inches below Quchi [LI 11]; or clenching the hand firmly and flexing the elbow, the point is located in the fossa of the brachioradialis muscle.

Needle and moxibustion method

Perpendicular insertion: 0.8–1.2 inches.
— *Needle sensation:* local distension and numbness which can radiate to the forearm, hand and wrist.
— *Moxibustion dosage:* 3–7 cones; stick 5–20 minutes.

Cross-sectional anatomy of the needle passage

a. *Skin:* the branches from the lateral antebrachial cutaneous nerve containing fibers from the sixth cervical nerve (C6) innervate the skin.

b. *Subcutaneous tissue:* includes the previously described skin nerve branches.

c. *Extensor carpi radialis longus muscle:* the branches from the radial nerve containing fibers from the sixth and seventh cervical nerves (C6, C7) innervate the muscle.

d. *Extensor carpi radialis brevis muscle:* the branches from the radial nerve containing fibers from the sixth and seventh cervical nerves (C6, C7) innervate the muscle.

e. *Extensor digitorum muscle:* the needle passes on the dorsal side of the muscle. The deep branches from the radial nerve containing fibers from the sixth, seventh and eighth cervical nerves (C6, C7, C8) innervate the muscle.

f. *Supinator muscle and deep branch of radial nerve:* the branches from the radial nerve containing fibers from the fifth and sixth cervical nerves (C5, C6) innervate the muscle. The deep branch of the radial nerve contains fibers from the fifth to eighth cervical nerves (C5, C6, C7, C8).

Functions

Expels Wind to clear the collaterals, and regulates the function of the Stomach and Intestines.

Clinical indications

Abdominal pain, diarrhea, toothache, elbow stiffness, hemiplegia, shoulder stiffness, facial palsy, mumps.

25.

(SHANGLIEN) SHANGLIAN, LI 9, HAND YANG MING LARGE INTESTINE MERIDIAN

Location

With the elbow flexed, draw a line between Quchi [LI 11] and Yangxi [LI 5]. The point is located 3 inches below Quchi [LI 11], and 9 inches above Yangxi [LI 5].

Needle and moxibustion method

Perpendicular insertion 0.5–1.0 inch. Oblique insertion 0.5–1.0 inch.
— *Needle sensation:* local soreness and numbness radiating to the forearm and hand.
— *Moxibustion dosage:* 3–7 cones; stick 15 minutes.

Cross-sectional anatomy of the needle passage

a. *Skin:* the branches from the posterior brachial cutaneous nerve containing fibers from the sixth cervical nerve (C6) innervate the skin.

b. *Subcutaneous tissue:* includes the previously described skin nerve branches.

c. *Brachioradialis and tendon of extensor carpi radialis longus muscle:* the needle is inserted between the palmar side of the brachioradialis muscle and the tendon of the extensor carpi radialis longus muscle. The branches from the radial nerve containing fibers from the fifth and sixth cervical nerves (C5, C6) innervate the brachioradialis muscle. The branches from the radial nerve containing fibers from the sixth and seventh cervical nerves (C6, C7) innervate the extensor radialis longus muscle.

d. *Extensor carpi radialis brevis muscle:* the branches from the radial nerve containing fibers from the sixth and seventh cervical nerves (C6, C7) innervate the muscle.

e. *Supinator muscle:* the branches from the radial nerve containing fibers from the sixth and seventh cervical nerves (C6, C7) innervate the muscle.

f. *Extensor digitorum muscle:* the needle is inserted on the dorsal part of the extensor digitorum muscle. The posterior interosseous branches from the radial nerve containing fibers from the sixth, seventh and eighth cervical nerves (C6, C7, C8) innervate the muscle.

g. *Abductor pollicis longus muscle:* the branches from the radial nerve containing fibers from the sixth and seventh cervical nerves (C6, C7) innervate the muscle.

Functions
Clears and activates the channels and collaterals, reduces fever and removes Dampness.

Clinical indications
Gonorrhea, headache, shoulder pain, hand numbness, cystitis, enteritis, abdominal pain.

26.
(HSIALIEN) XIALIAN, LI 8, HAND YANG MING LARGE INTESTINE MERIDIAN

Location
With the elbow flexed, draw a line between Quchi [LI 11] and Yangxi [LI 5]. The point is located 4 inches below Quchi [LI 11], and 8 inches above Yangxi [LI 5].

Needle and moxibustion method
Perpendicular insertion 0.5–1.0 inch. Oblique insertion 0.5–1.0 inch.
— *Needle sensation:* local soreness and numbness which can radiate to the forearm and hand.
— *Moxibustion dosage:* 3–7 cones; stick 15 minutes.

Cross-sectional anatomy of the needle passage
a. *Skin:* the branches from the posterior brachial cutaneous nerve containing fibers from the sixth cervical nerve (C6) innervate the skin.

b. *Subcutaneous tissue:* includes the previously described skin nerve branches.

c. *Brachioradialis muscle:* the branches from the radial nerve containing fibers from the fifth and sixth cervical nerves (C5, C6) innervate the muscle.

d. *Tendon of extensor carpi radialis longus muscle:* the

needle is inserted on the palmar side of the tendon of the extensor carpi radialis longus muscle. The branches from the radial nerve containing fibers from the sixth and seventh cervical nerves (C6, C7) innervate the muscle.

e. *Extensor carpi radialis brevis muscle:* the branches from the radial nerve containing fibers from the sixth and seventh cervical nerves (C6, C7) innervate the muscle.

f. *Supinator muscle:* the branches from the radial nerve containing fibers from the fifth and sixth cervical nerves (C5, C6) innervate the muscle.

Functions
Reduces fever, expels Wind, and promotes the circulation of Qi to alleviate pain.

Clinical indications
Abdominal pain, headache, dizziness, bronchial asthma, bronchitis, tuberculosis, mastitis, enteritis, cystitis, elbow pain, periumbilical pain.

27.
(SZUTU) SIDU, TB 9, HAND SHAO YANG TRIPLE BURNER MERIDIAN

Location
With the elbow flexed, the point is located on the dorsal side of the forearm, 5 inches below the olecranon process of the ulna, at the midpoint between the radius and the ulna.

Needle and moxibustion method
Perpendicular insertion or oblique insertion 0.5–1.0 inch.
— *Needle sensation:* soreness and distension radiating to the elbow and dorsum of the hand.
— *Moxibustion dosage:* 3–5 cones; stick 10 minutes.

Cross-sectional anatomy of the needle passage
a. *Skin:* the branches from the posterior and medial antebrachial cutaneous nerves from the branch of the seventh cervical nerve (C7) innervate the skin.

b. *Subcutaneous tissue:* includes the previously described skin nerve branches.

c. *Extensor carpi ulnaris muscle and extensor digitorum communis muscle:* the needle is inserted between the extensor carpi ulnaris and extensor digitorum communis muscles. The branches from the radial nerve containing fibers from the seventh and eighth cervical nerves (C7, C8) innervate these muscles.

d. The needle is inserted on the radial side of the posterior interosseous nerve, artery and vein. The posterior interosseous nerve branches from the radial nerve. The posterior interosseous artery is a division from the common interosseous artery of the radial artery. The posterior interosseous vein joins the radial vein.

e. *Flexor and extensor pollicis longus muscles:* the posterior interosseous branches from the radial nerve containing fibers from the sixth and seventh cervical nerves (C6, C7) and from the seventh and eighth cervical nerves (C7, C8) innervate the flexor and flexor pollicis longus muscles, respectively.

f. *Dorsal antebrachial interosseous membrane:* the branches from the posterior interosseous nerve innervate the dorsal antebrachial interosseous membrane.

Functions

Improves hearing, and reduces fever to relieve sore throat.

Clinical indications

Deafness, migraine, tinnitus, toothache, forearm pain, sore throat, tonsillitis, nephritis, numbness of the upper extremities, arthritis of the elbow.

28.

(KUNGTSUI) KONGZUI, LU 6, HAND TAI YIN LUNG MERIDIAN, CLEFT POINT

Location

In a seated or supine position, draw a line between Chize [LU 5] and Taiyuan [LU 9]. The point is located 7 inches above Taiyuan [LU 9] on the medial side of the forearm.

Needle and moxibustion method

Perpendicular insertion 1.0–1.5 inches.
— *Needle sensation:* local distension and numbness radiating to the distal part of the arm.
— *Moxibustion dosage:* 3–5 cones; stick 15 minutes.

Cross-sectional anatomy of the needle passage

a. *Skin:* the branches from the lateral antebrachial cutaneous nerve containing fibers from the fifth and sixth cervical nerves (C5, C6) innervate the skin.

b. *Subcutaneous tissue:* includes the previously described skin nerve branches and cephalic vein. The cephalic vein joins the basilic vein.

c. *Brachioradialis muscle:* the branches from the radial nerve containing fibers from the sixth and seventh cervical nerves (C6, C7) innervate the muscle.

d. *Flexor carpi radialis muscle:* the branches from the radial nerve containing fibers from the sixth and seventh cervical nerves (C6, C7) innervate the muscle. The needle is inserted on the radial side of the radial artery and vein, and the superficial branch

of the radial nerve. The radial artery is a division of the brachial artery. The radial veins together with the radial artery join the brachial vein. The superficial branch of the radial nerve contains fibers from the sixth, seventh and eighth cervical nerves (C6, C7, C8).

e. *Pronator teres muscle:* the branches from the median nerve containing fibers from the sixth and seventh cervical nerves (C6, C7) innervate the muscle. The needle is inserted on the lateral side of the pronator teres muscle.

f. *Extensor carpi radialis longus and brevis muscles:* the branches from the radial nerve containing fibers from the sixth and seventh cervical nerves (C6, C7) innervate the extensor carpi radialis longus and brevis muscles. The needle passes on the medial side of these muscles.

Functions

Reduces fever, descends rebellious Qi of the lungs and regulates lung Qi to arrest bleeding and relieves acute cough and breathlessness.

Clinical indications

Headache, hoarseness of the voice, cough, sore throat, elbow pain, fever, tuberculosis, acute asthma attack and nosebleed.

29.

(CHIHCHENG) ZHIZHENG, SI 7, HAND TAI YANG SMALL INTESTINE MERIDIAN, CONNECTING POINT

Location

With the elbow flexed, draw a line between Yanggu [SI 5] and Xiaohai [SI 8]. The point is located 5 inches above Yanggu [SI 5] and 7 inches below Xiaohai [SI 8], on the dorsal side of the forearm on the medial side of the border of the ulna.

Needle and moxibustion method

Perpendicular insertion 0.5–0.8 inch.
— *Needle sensation:* local soreness and distension and radiating to the hand.
— *Moxibustion dosage:* 3–5 cones; stick 10 minutes.

Cross-sectional anatomy of the needle passage

(Fig. 1.7)

a. *Skin:* the branches from the medial antebrachial cutaneous nerve containing fibers from the first thoracic nerve (T1) innervate the skin.

b. *Subcutaneous tissue:* includes the previously described skin nerve branches.

c. *Flexor carpi ulnaris muscle:* the branches from the

ulnar nerve containing fibers from the sixth and seventh cervical nerves (C6, C7) innervate the muscle. The needle passes on the medial side of the flexor carpi ulnaris muscle.

d. *Flexor digitorum profundus muscle:* the branches from the ulnar nerve containing fibers from the sixth cervical and first thoracic nerves (C6, T1) and from the median nerve containing fibers from the eighth cervical and first thoracic nerves (C8, T1) innervate the muscle.

e. *Anterior interosseous membrane:* the needle punctures the anterior wall of the interosseous membrane.

Functions
Reduces fever and removes Heat from the Blood, and clears and activates the channels and collaterals.

Clinical indications
Headache, common cold, hysteria, schizophrenia, acne, mumps, diabetes mellitus, elbow joint pain, finger pain, fever, neck stiffness.

30.
(HSIMEN) XIMEN, PC 4, HAND JUE YIN PERICARDIUM MERIDIAN, CLEFT POINT

Location
In a seated or supine position, with the hand open and outstretched. The point is located in the middle of the medial side of the forearm. Find Daling [PC 7] first, and draw a line between Daling [PC 7] and the ulnar side of the tendon of the biceps brachii muscle on the cubital crease. The point is located 5 inches above Daling [PC 7] along this line.

Needle and moxibustion method
Perpendicular insertion 1.0–1.5 inches.
— *Needle sensation:* local numbness and distension, or electric sensation radiating to the fingertips.
— *Moxibustion dosage:* 5–7 cones; stick 5–15 minutes.

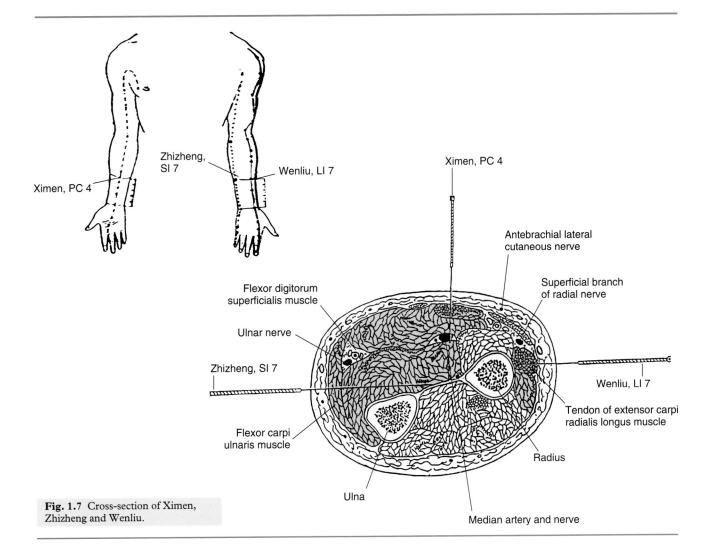

Fig. 1.7 Cross-section of Ximen, Zhizheng and Wenliu.

Cross-sectional anatomy of the needle passage
(Fig. 1.7)

a. *Skin:* the branches from the lateral antebrachial cutaneous nerve (C6) innervate the skin.

b. *Subcutaneous tissue:* includes the previously described skin nerve branches and median antebrachial vein.

c. *Flexor carpi radialis muscle:* the branches from the median nerve containing fibers from the sixth and seventh cervical nerves (C6, C7) innervate the flexor carpi radialis muscle.

d. *Flexor digitorum superficialis muscle:* the median nerve branches of the seventh cervical to first thoracic nerves (C7, C8, T1) innervate the flexor digitorum superficialis muscle.

e. *Median nerve and median artery:* the median nerve passes between the flexor digitorum superficialis muscle and flexor digitorum profundus muscle. If the needle is inserted into the median nerve, a strong electrical sensation radiates to the fingertips. Don't insert the needle any further. The median artery, a branch of the anterior interosseous artery descending together with the median nerve, supplies nutrient to the median nerve.

f. *Flexor digitorum profundus muscle:* the branches from the interosseous nerve, a branch of the median nerve, containing fibers from the seventh cervical to first thoracic nerves (C7, C8, T1), innervate the radial side of the flexor digitorum profundus muscle. The branches from the ulnar nerve containing fibers from the eighth cervical and first thoracic nerves (C8, T1) innervate the ulnar side of the flexor digitorum profundus muscle.

g. *Palmar side of anterior interosseous membrane:* the branches from the anterior interosseous nerve, a branch of the median nerve, innervate the anterior interosseous membrane. This artery and vein together with the anterior interosseous nerve pass into the superficial interosseous membrane. The needle is inserted into the radial margin of these structures.

Functions
Regulates the flow of Qi, clears heat at the Ying level, and relieves mental stress.

Clinical indications
Rheumatic heart disease, myocarditis, angina pectoris, tachycardia, mastitis, pleurisy, hysteria, diaphragm muscle spasm.

(WENLIU) WENLIU, LI 7, HAND YANG MING LARGE INTESTINE MERIDIAN, CLEFT POINT

Location
With the elbow flexed, the point is located on the posterior, lateral side of the forearm on the line between Yangxi [LI 5] and Quchi [LI 11], about 5 inches above Yangxi [LI 5].

Needle and moxibustion method
Perpendicular insertion 0.3–0.5 inch. Superior oblique insertion 0.5–1.0 inch.
— *Needle sensation:* local distension and numbness which can radiate to the hand.
— *Moxibustion dosage:* 3–5 cones; stick 5–15 minutes.

Cross-sectional anatomy of the needle passage
(Fig. 1.7)

a. *Skin:* the branches from the lateral antebrachial cutaneous nerve containing fibers from the sixth cervical nerve (C6) innervate the skin.

b. *Subcutaneous tissue:* includes the previously described skin nerve branches. The needle is passed anterior to the cephalic vein, a branch of the axillary vein.

c. *Tendon of extensor carpi radialis longus muscle:* the branches from the radial nerve containing fibers from the sixth and seventh cervical nerves (C6, C7) innervate the extensor carpi radialis longus muscle.

d. *Extensor carpi radialis brevis muscle:* the branches from the radial nerve containing fibers from the sixth and seventh cervical nerves (C6, C7) innervate the extensor carpi radialis brevis muscle.

Functions
Reduces fever and expels Wind, and clears the channels to promote Blood circulation.

Clinical indications
Headache, pharyngitis, epistaxis, mouth and tongue pain, abdominal pain, flatulence, psychosis, shoulder pain, back pain, facial edema, stomatitis.

(SANYANGLO) SANYANGLUO, TB 8, HAND SHAO YANG TRIPLE BURNER MERIDIAN

Location
With the elbow flexed, the point is located on the dorsal side of the forearm 4 inches above the skin crease of the dorsal wrist, at the midpoint between radius and ulna, or 1 inch above Zhigou [TB 6].

Needle and moxibustion method

Perpendicular insertion 0.5–1.0 inch.

— *Needle sensation:* local distension and numbness radiating to the hand.

Oblique insertion: penetrating through to Ximen [PC 4] 2.0–3.0 inches.

— *Needle sensation:* antebrachial numbness radiating to the fingertips, or sometimes radiating to the shoulder.

— *Moxibustion dosage:* 5–7 cones; stick 10 minutes.

Cross-sectional anatomy of the needle passage

a. *Skin:* the branches from the medial and posterior antebrachial cutaneous nerves containing fibers from the seventh cervical nerve (C7) innervate the skin.

b. *Subcutaneous tissue:* includes the previously described skin nerve branches.

c. *Extensor digitalis muscle:* the posterior interosseous branches from the radial nerve containing fibers from the sixth, seventh and eighth cervical nerves (C6, C7, C8) innervate the muscle.

d. *Abductor and extensor pollicis longus muscles:* the needle is passed between the abductor and extensor pollicis longus muscles. The posterior interosseous branches from the radial nerve containing fibers from the sixth and seventh cervical nerves (C6, C7) innervate both muscles.

e. The needle is passed on the radial side of the posterior interosseous nerve, artery and vein. The posterior interosseous nerve is a branch of the radial nerve.

f. *Dorsal antebrachial interosseous membrane:* the branches from the posterior interosseous nerve innervate the dorsal antebrachial interosseous membrane.

Functions

Reduces fever, dispels Wind, and activates the collaterals to alleviate pain.

Clinical indications

Caries, deafness, fever and chills, common cold, lower back pain, arm pain.

33.

(CHIENSHIH) JIANSHI, PC 5, HAND JUE YIN PERICARDIUM MERIDIAN, RIVER POINT

Location

With the hand open, the point is located on the palmar side of the forearm 3 inches above the skin crease of the wrist, between the tendons of the flexor carpi radialis and palmaris longus muscles. Alternative method: find Daling [PC 7] first and the point is located 3 inches above Daling [PC 7].

Needle and moxibustion method

Perpendicular insertion 0.5–1.5 inches.

— *Needle sensation:* local numbness and distension which can radiate to the fingertips.

Oblique insertion: slightly proximally to the radial side 1.5–2.0 inches (treating trunk disease).

— *Needle sensation:* after Qi is obtained, twisting the needle heavily several times causes distension and soreness to radiate to the elbow or the axilla.

— *Moxibustion dosage:* 3–5 cones; stick 5–15 minutes.

Cross-sectional anatomy of the needle passage

(Fig. 1.8)

a. *Skin:* the branches from the medial antebrachial cutaneous nerve containing fibers from the eighth cervical nerve (C8) innervate the skin.

b. *Subcutaneous tissue:* includes the previously described skin nerve branches.

c. *Tendon of flexor carpi radialis and palmaris longus muscles:* the branches from the median nerve containing fibers from the sixth and seventh cervical nerves (C6, C7) innervate the flexor carpi radialis and palmaris longus muscles.

d. *Flexor digitorum superficialis muscle:* the branches from the median nerve containing fibers from the seventh cervical to first thoracic nerves (C7, C8, T1) innervate the flexor digitorum superficialis muscle.

e. *Flexor digitorum profundus muscle:* the branches from the anterior interosseous nerve, a branch of the median nerve containing fibers from the seventh cervical to first thoracic nerves (C7, C8, T1), innervate the radial side of the flexor digitorum profundus muscle. The needle is inserted on the radial side of the flexor digitorum profundus muscle. The branches from the ulnar nerve containing fibers from the eighth cervical and first thoracic nerves (C8, T1) innervate the ulnar side of the flexor digitorum profundus muscle.

f. *Pronator quadratus muscle:* the anterior interosseous nerve, a branch of the median nerve containing fibers from the seventh cervical to first thoracic nerves (C7, C8, T1), innervates the pronator quadratus muscle.

g. *Palmar anterior interosseous membrane:* the branches from the anterior interosseous nerve from the median nerve innervate the lateral anterior interosseous membrane. If the needle is very deeply inserted, it will penetrate through the interosseous membrane to Zhigou [TB 6].

Functions

Regulates the flow of Qi to promote Blood circulation, and clears away Heart Fire to tranquilize the mind.

Clinical indications

Rheumatic heart disease, myocarditis, angina pectoris, hepatitis, stomach disease, malaria, epilepsy, psychosis, hysteria, schizophrenia, infantile convulsion, tachycardia, uterine bleeding, dysmenorrhea, irregular menstruation, endometritis.

34.

(CHIHKOU) ZHIGOU, TB 6, HAND SHAO YANG TRIPLE BURNER MERIDIAN, RIVER POINT

Location

With the elbow flexed, the point is located on the dorsal side of the forearm, 3 inches above the skin crease of the dorsal wrist, at the midpoint between the radius and the ulna. Alternative method: locate Yangchi [TB 4] first; the point is then located 3 inches above Yangchi [TB 4].

Needle and moxibustion method

Perpendicular insertion 1.0–1.5 inches.
— *Needle sensation:* local soreness and distension, radiating to the elbow, or sometimes an electric sensation radiating to the fingertips.
— *Moxibustion dosage:* 3–7 cones; stick 10 minutes.

Cross-sectional anatomy of the needle passage (Fig. 1.8)

a. *Skin:* the branches from the posterior antebrachial cutaneous nerve from the branches of the seventh cervical nerve (C7) innervate the skin.

b. *Subcutaneous tissue:* includes the previously described skin nerve branches.

c. *Extensor digiti minimi muscle:* the branches from the posterior interosseous nerve, a branch of the radial nerve containing fibers from the sixth, seventh and eighth cervical nerves (C6, C7, C8), innervate the extensor digiti minimi muscle.

d. *Extensor pollicis longus muscle:* the branches from the

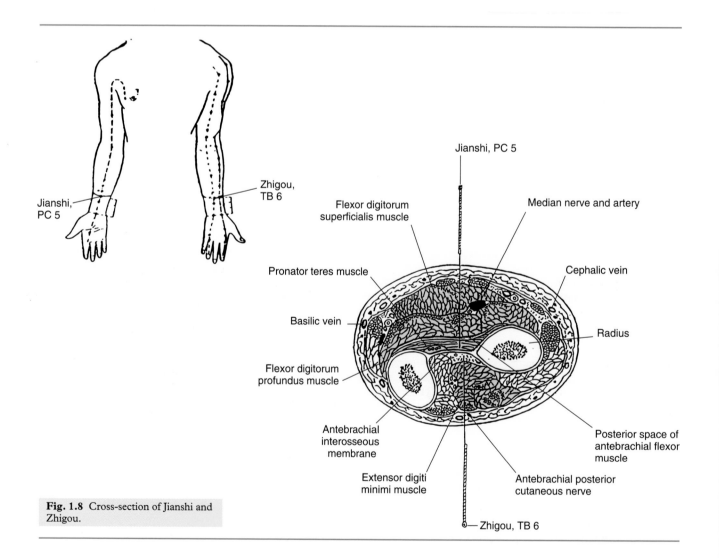

Fig. 1.8 Cross-section of Jianshi and Zhigou.

posterior interosseous nerve, a branch of the radial nerve containing fibers from the sixth, seventh and eighth cervical nerves (C6, C7, C8), innervate the extensor pollicis longus muscle.

e. The needle passes on the radial side of the posterior interosseous nerve, artery and vein: the posterior interosseous nerve is a branch of the radial nerve. If the needle is slightly directed to the ulnar side, it will pass into the interosseous nerve. The posterior interosseous nerve runs together with the posterior interosseous artery and vein.

f. *Dorsal antebrachial interosseous membrane:* the branches from the posterior interosseous nerve innervate the dorsal antebrachial interosseous membrane. If the needle is inserted deeply, it will penetrate through the anterior interosseous membrane to Jianshi [PC 5].

Functions

Reduces fever, and regulates and promotes the function of the intestines and Stomach.

Clinical indications

Angina pectoris, common cold, conjunctivitis, tinnitus, deafness, neurogenic vomiting, tonsillitis, pleurisy, intercostal nerve pain, habitual constipation, neck stiffness, shoulder and arm soreness, insufficiency of breast milk.

35.

(HUITSUNG) HUIZONG, TB 7, HAND SHAO YANG TRIPLE BURNER MERIDIAN, CLEFT POINT

Location

In a seated and supine position with the forearm pronated, the point is located on the dorsal side of the forearm, 3 inches above the skin crease of the dorsal wrist, and 1 inch lateral to Zhigou [TB 6].

Needle and moxibustion method

Perpendicular insertion 0.8–1.2 inches.
— *Needle sensation:* local soreness and distension radiating to the hand.
— *Moxibustion dosage:* 3–7 cones; stick 10 minutes.

Cross-sectional anatomy of the needle passage

a. *Skin:* the branches from the lateral and medial antebrachial cutaneous nerves containing fibers from the eighth cervical nerve (C8) innervate the skin.
b. *Subcutaneous tissue:* includes the previously described skin nerve branches.
c. *Extensor carpi ulnaris muscle:* the posterior interosseous branches from the radial nerve containing

fibers from the sixth, seventh and eighth cervical nerves (C6, C7, C8) innervate the muscle.

d. *Extensor indicis proprius muscle:* the posterior interosseous branches from the radial nerve containing fibers from the sixth, seventh and eighth cervical nerves (C6, C7, C8) innervate the muscle.

e. The needle passes on the radial side of the posterior interosseous nerve, artery and vein. The posterior interosseous nerve is a branch of the radial nerve. The posterior interosseous artery arises from the common interosseous artery and runs together with the posterior interosseous artery and vein.

f. *Dorsal antebrachial interosseous membrane:* the posterior interosseous branch from the radial nerve containing fibers from the fifth to eighth cervical nerves (C5, C6, C7, C8) innervate the dorsal antebrachial interosseous membrane.

Functions

Clears and activates the channels and collaterals, and resolves Phlegm to relieve asthma.

Clinical indications

Deafness, tinnitus, bronchial asthma, cholecystitis, gallstones, muscular aches, ear pain, convulsions, arm pain.

36.

(PIENLI) PIANLI, LI 6, HAND YANG MING LARGE INTESTINE MERIDIAN, CONNECTING POINT

Location

With the elbow flexed and placing the forearm on its ulnar side, the point is located 3 inches above the skin crease of the dorsal wrist. Draw a line between Quchi [LI 11] and Yangxi [LI 5]. The point is located 3 inches above Yangxi [LI 5].

Needle and moxibustion method

Slightly oblique insertion towards the elbow 0.5–0.8 inch.
— *Needle sensation:* local soreness and distension.
— *Moxibustion dosage:* 3–5 cones; stick 15 minutes.

Cross-sectional anatomy of the needle passage

a. *Skin:* the branches from the lateral and posterior antebrachial cutaneous nerves from a branch of the sixth cervical nerve (C6) innervate the skin.
b. *Subcutaneous tissue:* includes the previously described skin nerve branches.
c. *Tendons of extensor carpi radialis longus and extensor pollicis brevis muscles:* the branches from the radial nerve containing fibers from the sixth and seventh

cervical nerves (C6, C7) innervate the extensor radialis longus muscle, and the posterior interosseous branches from the radial nerve containing fibers from the sixth and seventh cervical nerves (C6, C7) innervate the extensor pollicis brevis muscle. The needle passes on the dorsal side of the tendon of the extensor carpi radialis brevis muscle.

d. *Tendon of the abductor pollicis longus muscle:* the posterior interosseous branches from the radial nerve containing fibers from the sixth and seventh cervical nerves (C6, C7) innervate the abductor pollicis longus muscle.

Functions
Clears and activates the channels and collaterals, expels Wind and removes Dampness.

Clinical indications
Facial palsy, epistaxis, deafness, tinnitus, toothache, epilepsy, elbow pain, edema, tonsillitis, sore throat.

37.

(NEIKUAN) NEIGUAN, PC 6, HAND JUE YIN PERICARDIUM MERIDIAN, CONNECTING POINT

Location
In a seated or supine position with the palm open, the point is located on the palmar side of the forearm 2 inches above the transverse crease of the wrist, and between the tendons of the flexor carpi radialis and palmaris longus muscles. Alternative method: find Daling [PC 7] first, and the point is then located 2 inches above Daling [PC 7].

Needle and moxibustion method
Perpendicular insertion 0.5–1.0 inch penetrating to Waiguan [TB 5].
— *Needle sensation:* local soreness and distension, or an electrical sensation radiating to the fingertips.
   Oblique insertion proximally 1.0–2.0 inches (treating disease of the trunk).
— *Needle sensation:* local distension and soreness radiating to the elbow, axilla and chest.
   Oblique insertion to the radial side 0.3–0.5 inch (treating finger numbness).
— *Needle sensation:* local electrical sensation radiating to the fingertips.
— *Moxibustion dosage:* 3–7 cones; stick 5–15 minutes.

Cross-sectional anatomy of the needle passage
(Fig. 1.9)
a. *Skin:* the branches from the lateral and medial antebrachial cutaneous nerve containing fibers from

the seventh cervical nerve (C7) innervate the skin.

b. *Subcutaneous tissue:* includes the previously described cutaneous skin nerve branches.

c. The needle is passed between the tendons of the flexor carpi radialis and palmaris longus muscles: the median nerve innervates both muscles. The branches from the median nerve containing fibers from the sixth and seventh cervical nerves (C6, C7) innervate the flexor carpi radialis muscle, and the branches from the median nerve containing fibers from the seventh cervical to first thoracic nerves (C7, C8, T1) innervate the palmaris longus muscle.

d. *Flexor digitorum superficialis muscle:* the branches from the median nerve containing fibers from the seventh cervical to first thoracic nerves (C7, C8, T1) innervate the flexor digitorum superficialis muscle.

e. On the radial side of the needle is the median nerve and median artery: the median nerve lies deep to the flexor digitorum superficialis muscle, and passes between the flexor digitorum profundus muscle and the flexor pollicis longus muscle. If the needle is slightly directed to the radial side, it will be inserted into the median nerve, with an electrical sensation radiating to the fingertips. The median artery, a branch of the anterior interosseous artery which descends from the ulnar artery, supplies nutrient and accompanies the median nerve.

f. *Flexor digitorum profundus muscle:* the branches from the anterior interosseous nerve, a branch of the median nerve containing fibers from the seventh cervical to first thoracic nerves (C7, C8, T1), innervate the radial side of the flexor digitorum profundus muscle. The needle is inserted into this part. The branches from the ulnar nerve containing fibers from the eighth cervical and first thoracic nerves (C8, T1) innervate the ulnar side of the flexor digitorum profundus muscle.

g. *Pronator quadratus muscle:* the branches from the anterior interosseous nerve, a branch of the median nerve containing fibers from the seventh cervical to first thoracic nerves (C7, C8, T1), innervate the pronator quadratus muscle. The pronator quadratus muscle is strongly attached to the anterior interosseous membrane. If the needle is inserted deeply, it will pass through the anterior interosseous membrane and will penetrate into Waiguan [TB 5].

Functions
Regulates the flow of Qi to soothe chest oppression and gastrointestinal disturbances, and relieves mental stress.

Clinical indications
Rheumatic heart disease, pericarditis, shock, angina pectoris, tachycardia, hematemesis, chest pain, jaundice, stomach pain, abdominal pain, diaphragm cram-

ping, headache, hyperthyroidism, epilepsy, hysteria, asthma, throat pain and swelling, hand pain.

38.

(WAIKUAN) WAIGUAN, TB 5, HAND SHAO YANG TRIPLE BURNER MERIDIAN, CONNECTING POINT

Location
With the elbow flexed, the point is located on the dorsal side of the forearm, 2 inches above the skin crease of the dorsal wrist, at the midpoint between the radius and ulnar bone. Alternative method: find Yangchi [TB 4] first and the point is then located 2 inches above Yangchi [TB 4].

Needle and moxibustion method
Perpendicular insertion 0.5–1.5 inches or penetrating to Neiguan [PC 6].
—*Needle sensation:* local soreness and distension, sometimes radiating to the fingertips.
   Oblique insertion proximally 1.5–2.0 inches (treating disease of the trunk).

— *Needle sensation:* soreness and distension radiating proximally, and if the needle is twisted heavily several times, sometimes radiating to the elbow and shoulder.
— *Moxibustion dosage:* 3–5 cones; stick 5–15 minutes.

Cross-sectional anatomy of the needle passage
(Fig. 1.9)
a. *Skin:* the branches of the posterior antebrachial cutaneous nerve containing fibers from the seventh cervical nerve (C7) innervate the skin.
b. *Subcutaneous tissue:* includes the previously described skin nerve branches.
c. *Extensor digiti minimi and extensor digitorum communis muscles:* the extensor digiti minimi muscle is located at the ulnar side, and the extensor digitorum communis muscle is located at the radial side. These two muscles run parallel together. The needle is inserted between these two muscles. If the needle is inserted to the radial side, it will pass into the extensor digitorum communis muscle. The branches from the posterior interosseous nerve, a branch of the radial nerve containing fibers from the sixth to eighth cervical nerves (C6, C7, C8), innervate these muscles.

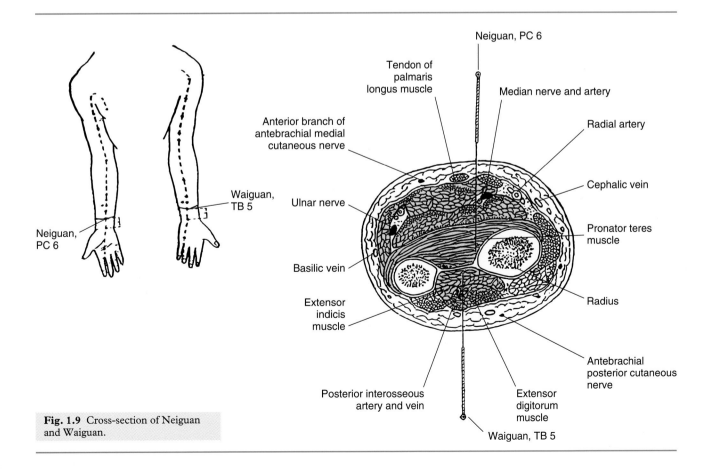

Fig. 1.9 Cross-section of Neiguan and Waiguan.

d. On the radial side of the needle is the posterior interosseous nerve, artery, and vein. If the needle is slightly inserted to the radial side, it will pass into the posterior interosseous nerve, with an electrical sensation radiating to the dorsal wrist and dorsal hand.

e. Extensor pollicis longus and extensor indicis muscles: the extensor pollicis longus muscle is located on the radial side, and the extensor indicis muscle is located on the ulnar side. The branches from the radial nerve containing fibers from the sixth to eighth cervical nerves (C6, C7, C8) innervate these two muscles. Sometimes the needle is inserted deeper, and it will then pass into Neiguan [PC 6].

Functions
Regulates the flow of Qi to promote Blood circulation, reduces fever, and dispels Wind.

Clinical indications
Common cold, high fever, pneumonia, mumps, tinnitus, deafness, migraine, hemiplegia, upper extremities joint pain, facial palsy, neck strain, enuresis.

39.
(LIENCHUEH) LIEQUE, LU 7, HAND TAI YIN LUNG MERIDIAN, CONNECTING POINT

Location
In a seated or supine position, the point is located on the lateral and inferior part of the forearm above the styloid process of the radius, 1.5 inches above the skin crease of the wrist. Alternative method: ask the patient to cross both thumbs and index fingers with one hand's index finger pressing just above the styloid process of the radius of the other hand. The point is then located in the fossa under the index fingertip.

Needle and moxibustion method
Perpendicular lateral insertion 0.3–0.5 inch (treating stenosing tendinitis). Superior oblique insertion 0.5–1.0 inch towards the elbow joint.
— *Needle sensation:* local soreness and distension, or radiating to the elbow, or down to the thumb and index finger.
— *Moxibustion dosage:* 3–5 cones; stick 5–15 minutes.

Cross-sectional anatomy of the needle passage
(Fig. 1.10)
a. Skin: the branches from the lateral antebrachial cutaneous nerve containing fibers from the sixth cervical nerve (C6) and superficial branches of the

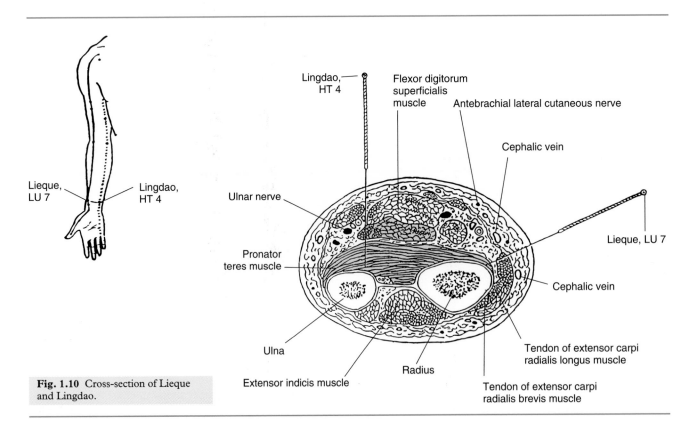

Fig. 1.10 Cross-section of Lieque and Lingdao.

radial nerve containing fibers from the sixth cervical nerve (C6) innervate the skin.

b. *Subcutaneous tissue:* includes the previously described skin nerve branches. The cephalic vein passes slightly posterior to the point.

c. *Tendon of extensor pollicis longus muscle:* the branches from the posterior interosseous nerve of the radial nerve containing fibers from the sixth and seventh cervical nerves (C6, C7) innervate the extensor pollicis muscle.

d. *Tendon of brachioradialis muscle:* the branches from the radial nerve containing fibers from the fifth and sixth cervical nerves (C5, C6) innervate the brachioradialis muscle.

e. *Pronator quadratus muscle:* the anterior interosseous nerve of the median nerve containing fibers from the seventh cervical to first thoracic nerves (C7, C8, T1) innervates the pronator quadratus muscle.

Functions
Ventilates the Lung to expel Wind, and clears and activates the channels and collaterals.

Clinical indications
Headache, cough, asthma, urticaria, facial palsy, facial spasm, neck and shoulder pain, wrist joint and surrounding soft tissue disease, trigeminal nerve pain, bronchial asthma, bronchitis, sore throat, rhinitis.

40.

(LINGTAO) LINGDAO, HT 4, HAND SHAO YIN HEART MERIDIAN, RIVER POINT

Location
In a seated or supine position with the palm facing up, the point is located 1.5 inches above the transverse crease of the wrist or 1.5 inches above Shenmen [HT 7], on the radial side of the tendon of the flexor carpi ulnaris muscle.

Needle and moxibustion method
Perpendicular insertion 0.3–0.5 inch.
— *Needle sensation:* local numbness and distension radiating to the hand.
— *Moxibustion dosage:* 3–5 cones; stick 10–15 minutes.

Cross-sectional anatomy of the needle passage
(Fig. 1.10)

a. *Skin:* the branches from the medial antebrachial cutaneous nerve containing fibers from the eighth cervical nerve (C8) innervate the skin.

b. *Subcutaneous tissue:* includes the previously described skin nerve branches.

c. The needle passes between the flexor carpi ulnaris

and flexor digitorum superficialis muscles. The branches from the ulnar nerve containing fibers from the eighth cervical and first thoracic nerves (C8, T1) innervate the flexor carpi ulnaris muscle. The branches from the median nerve containing fibers from the seventh cervical to first thoracic nerves (C7, C8, T1) innervate the flexor digitorum superficialis muscle. The needle passes on the ulnar side of the ulnar artery, vein and nerve.

d. *Ulnar side of the flexor digitorum profundus muscle:* the branches from the ulnar nerve containing fibers from the eighth cervical and first thoracic nerves (C8, T1) innervate the flexor digitorum profundus muscle.

e. *Pronator quadratus muscle:* the branches from the anterior interosseous nerve of the median nerve containing fibers from the seventh cervical to first thoracic nerves (C7, C8, T1) innervate the pronator quadratus muscle.

Functions
Nourishes the Heart and invigorates Qi, relieves mental stress and stops convulsions.

Clinical indications
Tachycardia, insomnia, nausea, loss of voice, hysteria, elbow joint pain.

41.

(YANGLAO) YANGLAO, SI 6, HAND TAI YANG SMALL INTESTINE MERIDIAN, CLEFT POINT

Location
With the elbow flexed and the palm facing the chest, the point is located on the radial side of the styloid process of the ulna, 1 inch above the dorsal skin crease of the wrist.

Needle and moxibustion method
Perpendicular insertion 0.5–1.0 inch. Superior oblique insertion 0.5–1.0 inch.
— *Needle sensation:* local soreness and numbness radiating to the elbow or the shoulder.
— *Moxibustion dosage:* 3–5 cones; stick 10 minutes.

Cross-sectionxal anatomy of the needle passage

a. *Skin:* the branches from the medial antebrachial cutaneous and dorsal ulnar nerves containing fibers from the eighth cervical nerve (C8) innervate the skin.

b. *Subcutaneous tissue:* includes the previously described skin nerve branches.

c. *Tendon of the extensor carpi ulnaris muscle:* The branches from the deep radial nerve containing fibers from the sixth, seventh and eighth cervical nerves (C6, C7, C8) innervate the extensor carpi ulnaris muscle.

Alternative method:

a and *b* same as the previously described insertion.

c. The needle is passed between the tendons of the extensor digiti minimi and extensor digitorum muscles; the branches from the radial nerve containing fibers from the sixth, seventh and eighth cervical nerves (C6, C7, C8) innervate both muscles.

d. Deep needling penetrates to posterior interosseous artery and vein, and the inferior bone space between the radius and ulna.

Functions

Reduces fever, expels Wind, and clears the channels to alleviate pain.

Clinical indications

Lower back pain, shoulder pain, elbow pain, arm pain, paralysis of the lower extremities, rheumatoid arthritis, optic neuritis, neck stiffness.

42.

(TUNGLI) TONGLI, HT 5, HAND SHAO YIN HEART MERIDIAN

Location

With the palm facing up, the point is located 1 inch above the transverse crease of the wrist or 1 inch above Shenmen [HT 7], on the radial side of the tendon of the flexor carpi ulnaris muscle.

Needle and moxibustion method

Perpendicular insertion 0.3–0.5 inch.

— *Needle sensation:* local soreness and numbness radiating down the ulnar side.

— *Moxibustion dosage:* 3–5 cones; stick 10 minutes.

Cross-sectional anatomy of the needle passage

a. *Skin:* the branches from the medial antebrachial cutaneous nerve containing fibers from the eighth cervical nerve (C8) innervate the skin.

b. *Subcutaneous tissue:* includes the previously described skin nerve branches.

c. The needle is passed between the tendon of the flexor carpi ulnaris and the flexor digitorum superficialis muscles. The branches from the ulnar nerve containing fibers from the eighth cervical and first thoracic nerves (C8, T1) innervate the flexor carpi ulnaris muscle. The branches from the median nerve containing fibers from the seventh cervical to first thoracic nerves (C7, C8, T1) innervate the flexor digitorum superficialis muscle. The needle is passed

on the ulnar side of the ulnar artery, vein and nerve.

d. *Flexor digitorum profundus muscle:* the needle is passed on the ulnar side of the flexor digitorum profundus muscle. The branches from the ulnar nerve containing fibers from the eighth cervical and first thoracic nerves (C8, T1) innervate the muscle.

e. *Posterior space of anterior flexor brachii muscle:* between the flexor digitorum profundus and pronator quadratus muscles.

f. *Pronator quadratus muscle:* the branches from the anterior interosseous nerve from the branches of the median nerve containing fibers from the seventh cervical to first thoracic nerves (C7, C8, T1) innervate the muscle.

g. *Anterior interosseous nerve, artery and vein:* the interosseous nerve is a branch of the median nerve, the interosseous artery is a division of the ulnar artery, and the interosseous vein joins the ulnar vein.

Functions

Relieves mental stress, calms down internal Wind and regulates the Yin Qi.

Clinical indications

Tachycardia, dizziness, headache, tonsillitis, hysteria, neurosis, schizophrenia, functional uterine bleeding, wrist arthritis.

43.

(CHINGCHU) JINGQU, LU 8, HAND TAI YIN LUNG MERIDIAN, RIVER POINT

Location

In a seated or supine position and with the palm facing up, the point is located 1 inch above the skin crease of the wrist, on the medial side of the styloid process of the radius and the lateral side of the radial artery, in the fossa between the tendons of the carpi radialis and abductor pollicis longus muscles, or 1 inch above Taiyuan [LU 9].

Needle and moxibustion method

Perpendicular insertion 0.3–0.5 inch. Superior oblique insertion 0.3–0.5 inch. WARNING: Avoid the radial artery.

— *Needle sensation:* local numbness and distension.

— *Moxibustion dosage:* 3–5 cones; stick 15 minutes.

Cross-sectional anatomy of the needle passage

a. *Skin:* the branches from the lateral antebrachial cutaneous nerve containing fibers from the sixth cervical nerve (C6) innervate the skin.

b. *Subcutaneous tissue:* includes the previously described skin nerve branches, the superficial branch of the radial cephalic vein and the superficial palmar branch of the radial artery. The needle passes on the radial side of the radial artery.

c. The needle passes between the tendons of the flexor carpi radialis and abductor pollicis longus muscles. The branches from the median nerve containing fibers from the sixth and seventh cervical nerves (C6, C7) innervate the flexor carpi radialis muscle. The branches from the posterior interosseous nerve of the radial nerve containing fibers from the sixth and seventh cervical nerves (C6, C7) innervate the abductor pollicis longus muscle. The radial artery is a branch of the brachial artery and the radial vein joins the brachial vein.

d. *Insertion of tendon of the brachioradialis muscle:* the branches from the radial nerve containing fibers from the fifth and sixth cervical nerves (C5, C6) innervate the muscle.

e. *Pronator quadratus muscle:* the branches from the volar interosseous nerve of the median nerve containing fibers from the seventh and eighth cervical and first thoracic nerves (C7, C8, T1) innervate the muscle.

Functions
Reduces fever and alleviates sore throat, and relieves cough and asthma.

Clinical indications
Asthma, nausea, wrist pain, sore throat, tonsillitis, bronchitis, fever, cough, radial nerve pain or palsy, esophageal spasm.

44.

(YINSHI) YINXI, HT 6, HAND SHAO YIN HEART MERIDIAN, CLEFT POINT

Location
With the palm facing up, the point is located 0.5 inch above the transverse crease of the wrist, on the radial side of the tendon of the flexor carpi ulnaris muscle, and 0.5 inch above Shenmen [HT 7].

Needle and moxibustion method
Perpendicular insertion 0.3–0.5 inch.
— *Needle sensation:* local soreness and numbness radiating to the hand.
— *Moxibustion dosage:* 3–5 cones; stick 15 minutes.

Cross-sectional anatomy of the needle passage
a. *Skin:* the branches from the medial antebrachial cutaneous nerve containing fibers from the eighth cervical nerve (C8) innervate the skin.

b. *Subcutaneous tissue:* includes the previously described skin nerve branches.

c. The needle passes between the tendons of the flexor carpi ulnaris and flexor digitorum superficialis muscles. The branches from the ulnar nerve containing fibers from the eighth cervical and first thoracic nerves (C8, T1) innervate the flexor carpi ulnaris muscle. The branches from the median nerve containing fibers from the seventh cervical to first thoracic nerves (C7, C8, T1) innervate the flexor digitorum superficialis muscle. The needle is passed on the radial side of the ulnar artery, vein and nerve.

d. *Ulnar nerve:* one of the largest branches of the brachial plexus containing the seventh and eighth cervical and first thoracic nerves (C7, C8, T1).

e. The needle is passed on the radial side of the ulnar artery and veins. The ulnar artery is a branch of the brachial artery and the ulnar vein joins the cephalic vein.

Functions
Clears and activates the channels and collaterals, and relieves mental stress.

Clinical indications
Headache, dizziness, angina pectoris, tachycardia, tuberculosis, epistaxis, tonsillitis, hysteria, nausea, chillness.

45.

(YANGSHI) YANGXI, LI 5, HAND YANG MING LARGE INTESTINE MERIDIAN, RIVER POINT

Location
The point is located on the radial side of the dorsal wrist joint, in the fossa between the tendons of the extensor pollicis brevis and longus muscles. By fully extending the thumb, the fossa can be seen more clearly.

Needle and moxibustion method
Perpendicular insertion 0.3–0.5 inch.
— *Needle sensation:* local soreness and distension.
— *Moxibustion dosage:* 3 cones (WARNING: No direct moxibustion on the joint); stick 10–15 minutes.

Cross-sectional anatomy of the needle passage
(Fig. 1.11)
a. *Skin:* the superficial branches from the radial nerve containing fibers from the sixth cervical nerve (C6) innervate the skin.

b. *Subcutaneous tissue:* includes the previously described skin nerve branches.

c. The needle passes between the tendons of the extensor pollicis brevis and longus muscles. The branches from the posterior interosseous nerve from the deep branches of the radial nerve containing fibers from the sixth and seventh cervical nerves (C6, C7) innervate these two muscles.

d. *Anterior tendon of the extensor carpi radialis longus muscle:* the branches from the radial nerve containing fibers from the sixth and seventh cervical nerves (C6, C7) innervate the extensor carpi radialis longus muscle.

Functions

Expels Wind and purges pathogenic Fire, relaxes the muscles and tendons and relieves rigidity of the local joints.

Clinical indications

Headache, eye pain, conjunctivitis, tinnitus, deafness, toothache, tonsillitis, hysteria, schizophrenia, childhood indigestion, wrist joint and surrounding soft tissue disease, facial palsy.

46.

(YANGCHIH) YANGCHI, TB 4, HAND SHAO YANG TRIPLE BURNER MERIDIAN, SOURCE POINT

Location

The point is located in the skin crease of the dorsum of the wrist, directly proximal to the junction of the third and fourth metacarpals, in the fossa between the tendons of the extensor digitorum communis and extensor digiti minimi muscles.

Needle and moxibustion method

Perpendicular insertion 0.3–0.5 inch.
— *Needle sensation:* local soreness and distension, or radiating to the middle finger.

Horizontal insertion to either side 0.5–1.0 inch (treating arthritis of wrist).
— *Needle sensation:* local distension and soreness radiating to the whole wrist.
— *Moxibustion dosage:* 3–5 cones; stick 10 minutes.

Cross-sectional anatomy of the needle passage
(Fig. 1.11)

a. *Skin:* the dorsal branches from the ulnar nerve containing fibers from the seventh and eighth cervical nerves (C7, C8) and the branches from the posterior antebrachial cutaneous nerve containing fibers from the seventh and eighth cervical nerves (C7, C8) innervate the skin.

b. *Subcutaneous tissue:* includes the previously described skin nerve branches and cephalic vein.

c. The needle passes between the tendons of the extensor digitorum and the extensor digiti minimi muscles. The extensor digitorum muscle is located on the radial side, and the extensor digiti minimi muscle on the ulnar side. The branches from the posterior interosseous nerve from the branch of the radial nerve containing fibers from the sixth to eighth cervical nerves (C6, C7, C8) innervate these two muscles.

Functions

Dispels Wind to relieve Exterior syndromes, and clears and activates the channels and collaterals.

Clinical indications

Common cold, tonsillitis, malaria, wrist joint and surrounding soft tissue disease, diabetes mellitus, conjunctivitis, deafness.

47.

(TAIYUAN) TAIYUAN, LU 9, HAND TAI YIN LUNG MERIDIAN, STREAM AND SOURCE POINT

Location

With the palm facing up, the point is located on the skin crease of the wrist, in the fossa between the tendons of the flexor carpi radialis and abductor pollicis longus muscles. Alternative method: find the skin crease of the wrist first, then the point is located on the lateral side of the radial artery.

Needle and moxibustion method

Perpendicular insertion 0.3–0.5 inch.
— *Needle sensation:* local soreness and distension.
— *Moxibustion dosage:* 1–3 cones (WARNING: No direct moxibustion on the joint); stick 3–5 minutes.

Cross-sectional anatomy of the needle passage
(Fig. 1.11)

a. *Skin:* the branches from the lateral antebrachial cutaneous nerve containing fibers from the sixth cervical nerve (C6) innervate the skin.

b. *Subcutaneous tissue:* includes the previously described skin nerve branches, the superficial branch of the radial nerve, the cephalic vein, and the superficial palmar branch of the radial artery. The superficial branch of the radial nerve is one of the two terminal branches of the radial nerve. The cephalic vein, supplied by the radial side of the dorsal palmar vein, drains to the axillary vein. The superficial palmar branch of the radial artery arises from the radial artery, providing a contribution to the superficial palmar arch.

c. The needle passes between the tendons of the flexor carpi radialis and the abductor pollicis longus muscles. The branches from the median nerve containing fibers from the sixth and seventh cervical nerves (C6, C7) innervate the flexor carpi radialis muscle. The branches from the posterior interosseous nerve of the radial nerve containing fibers from the sixth and seventh cervical nerves (C6, C7) innervate the abductor pollicis longus muscle.

d. *Radial artery and vein:* the radial artery and vein are located at the ulnar side of the needle. The radial artery, together with the ulnar artery, is one of the two terminal branches of the brachial artery.

Functions

Expels Wind, resolves Phlegm, and regulates the function of the Lung to relieve cough.

Clinical indications

Bronchitis, pertussis, influenza, bronchial asthma, emphysema, lung tuberculosis, tonsillitis, chest pain, wrist joint and surrounding soft tissue disease, conjunctivitis, toothache.

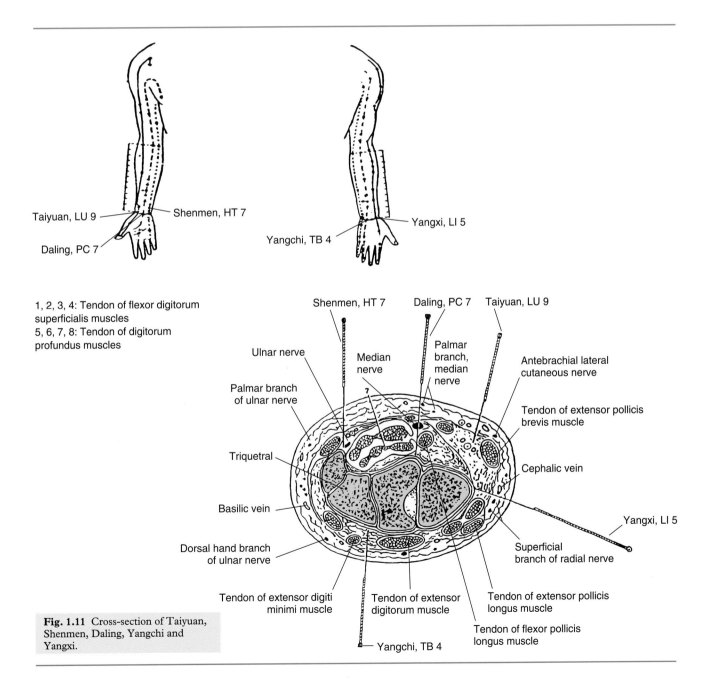

1, 2, 3, 4: Tendon of flexor digitorum superficialis muscles
5, 6, 7, 8: Tendon of digitorum profundus muscles

Fig. 1.11 Cross-section of Taiyuan, Shenmen, Daling, Yangchi and Yangxi.

48.

(TALING) DALING, PC 7, HAND JUE YIN PERICARDIUM MERIDIAN, STREAM AND SOURCE POINT

Location
Clenching the hand firmly and flexing the wrist, three tendon sheaths show on the wrist. The medial one is the tendon of the flexor carpi ulnaris muscle, the lateral one the tendon of the flexor carpi radialis muscle, and the middle one the tendon of the palmaris longus muscle. The point is located on the transverse crease of the wrist, between the tendons of the flexor carpi radialis and the palmaris longus muscles.

Needle and moxibustion method
Perpendicular insertion 0.3–0.5 inch.
— *Needle sensation:* local soreness and distension, or sometimes an electrical sensation radiating to the finger tips.

Oblique insertion to the carpal tunnel (treating carpal tunnel syndrome).
— *Needle sensation:* local distension and soreness, sometimes electrical sensation radiating to the finger tips.
— *Moxibustion dosage:* 1–2 cones (WARNING: No direct moxibustion on the joint); stick 5–15 minutes.

Cross-sectional anatomy of the needle passage
(Fig. 1.11)
a. *Skin:* the branches from the median nerve containing fibers from the seventh cervical nerve (C7) innervate the skin.
b. *Subcutaneous tissue:* includes the previously described skin nerve branches.
c. The needle is passed between the tendons of the flexor carpi radialis and the palmaris longus muscles. The branches from the median nerve containing fibers from the sixth and seventh cervical nerves (C6, C7) innervate the anterior part of the muscles. The branches from the median nerve containing fibers from the seventh and eighth cervical nerves (C7, C8) innervate the posterior part of the muscles.
d. *Median nerve:* the median nerve lies on the superficial part of the wrist. If the needle is inserted into the median nerve, a strong electrical sensation radiates to the radial side of the palm and finger tips.
e. The needle is passed between the tendons of the flexor pollicis longus, the flexor digitorum superficialis, and flexor digitorum profundus muscles. The branches from the anterior interosseous nerve of the median nerve containing fibers from the eighth cervical and first thoracic nerves (C8, T1) innervate the flexor pollicis longus muscle. The needle is inserted on the ulnar side of the tendons of the flexor digitorum superficialis and profundus muscles. The branches from the median nerve containing fibers from the seventh cervical to first thoracic nerves (C7, C8, T1) innervate the radial side of these two muscles. The branches from the ulnar nerve containing fibers from the eighth cervical and first thoracic nerves (C8, T1) innervate the ulnar side of the flexor digitorum profundus muscle.

Functions
Clears away Heart Fire and tranquilizes the mind, soothes chest oppression and regulates the function of the stomach.

Clinical indications
Myocarditis, tachycardia, angina pectoris, gastritis, tonsillitis, insomnia, pleurisy, schizophrenia, shock, convulsions, heat stroke, wrist joint and surrounding soft tissue disease, headache.

49.

(SHENMEN) SHENMEN, HT 7, HAND SHAO YIN HEART MERIDIAN, STREAM AND SOURCE POINT

Location
The point is located on the skin crease of the wrist, in the fossa on the lateral side of the tendon of the flexor carpi ulnaris muscle.

Needle and moxibustion method
Perpendicular insertion 0.3–0.5 inch.
— *Needle sensation:* local soreness and distension, or sometimes an electrical sensation radiating to the finger tips.
— *Moxibustion dosage:* 1–3 cones (WARNING: No direct moxibustion on the joint); stick 5–15 minutes.

Cross-sectional anatomy of the needle passage
(Fig. 1.11)
a. *Skin:* the branches from the medial antebrachial cutaneous nerve containing fibers from the eighth cervical nerve (C8) and the palmar branches of the ulnar nerve containing fibers from the eighth cervical nerve (C8) innervate the skin.
b. *Subcutaneous nerve:* the previously described skin nerve branches.
c. On the medial side of the point is the tendon of the flexor carpi ulnaris muscle. The branches from the median nerve containing fibers from the eighth cervical and first thoracic nerves (C8, T1) innervate the flexor carpi ulnaris muscle.
d. On the lateral side of the point are the ulnar nerve,

artery and vein. The ulnar nerve is located at the superficial layer. If the needle is inserted slightly to the radial side, it will puncture the ulnar nerve. The electric sensation radiates to the ulnar side of the hand and fingertips. The ulnar artery, together with the ulnar vein, is one of two branches of the brachial artery.

Functions
Reduces fever and clears away Heart Fire, tranquilizes and reduces anxiety.

Clinical indications
Tachycardia, insomnia, angina pectoris, psychosis, neurosis, hysteria, convulsions, tongue muscle numbness, nightmares.

50.
(YANGKU) YANGGU, SI 5, HAND TAI YANG SMALL INTESTINE MERIDIAN, RIVER POINT

Location
The point is located on the ulnar side of the transverse crease of the wrist, in the fossa between the styloid process of the ulna and the pisiform bone.

Needle and moxibustion method
Perpendicular insertion 0.3–0.5 inch.
— *Needle sensation:* local soreness and distension.
— *Moxibustion dosage:* 3–5 cones; stick 15 minutes.

Cross-sectional anatomy of the needle passage
a. *Skin:* the branches from the dorsal ulnar nerve containing fibers from the eighth cervical nerve (C8) innervate the skin.
b. *Subcutaneous tissue:* includes the previously described skin nerve branches.
c. *Extensor reticulum:* the antebrachial fascia reinforced by circular fibers at the wrist. The needle is passed through the extensor reticulum.
d. *Tendon of the extensor carpi ulnaris muscle:* the branches from the deep radial nerve containing fibers from the sixth, seventh and eighth cervical nerves (C6, C7, C8) innervate the muscle. The needle is passed on the dorsal side of the muscle.

Functions
Reduces fever, expels Wind, and clears the channels to alleviate pain.

Clinical indications
Caries, sore throat, common cold, hysteria, schizophrenia, infantile convulsion, wrist pain, fever, deafness, dizziness.

51.
(WANKU) WANGU, SI 4, HAND TAI YANG SMALL INTESTINE MERIDIAN, SOURCE POINT

Location
With the hand half clenched, the point is located on the medial side of the palm in the fossa between the base of the fifth metacarpal and the pisiform bone.

Needle and moxibustion method
Perpendicular insertion 0.3–0.5 inch.
— *Needle sensation:* local distension and soreness, sometimes radiating to the palm.
— *Moxibustion dosage:* 3–5 cones; stick 15 minutes.

Cross-sectional anatomy of the needle passage
a. *Skin:* the branches from the medial antebrachial cutaneous nerve, the palmar branch of the ulnar nerve, and the dorsal ulnar nerve containing fibers from the eighth cervical nerve (C8) innervate the skin.
b. *Subcutaneous tissue:* includes the previously described skin nerve branches and the dorsal venous rete.
c. *Abductor digiti minimi muscle:* the branches from the profundus branch of the ulnar nerve containing fibers from the eighth cervical and first thoracic nerves (C8, T1) innervate the muscle.
d. *Pisometacarpal ligament:* the ligament from the pisiform bone to the palmar side of the base of the fourth and fifth metacarpals.
e. The needle is passed between the tendon of the extensor carpi ulnaris muscle and the base of the fifth metacarpal.

Functions
Reduces fever, removes Dampness, and expels Wind to relieve rigidity of the muscles and tendons.

Clinical indications
Fever, headache, common cold, neck stiffness, jaundice, wrist weakness, pleurisy, pterygium, vomiting, hysteria, schizophrenia, diabetes mellitus, hepatitis, cholecystitis.

52.
(HOKU) HEGU, LI 4, HAND YANG MING LARGE INTESTINE MERIDIAN, SOURCE POINT

Location
The point is located on the dorsum of the hand, between the first and second metacarpals at the

midpoint of the radial margin of the second metacarpal bone. Alternative method: ask the patient to adduct the thumb and the index finger; the point is located at the highest spot of the first and second metacarpal muscles.

Needle and moxibustion method

Perpendicular insertion 0.5–1.0 inch.
— *Needle sensation:* local distension and soreness radiating to the shoulder or the elbow.

Oblique insertion: obliquely insert the needle at 20° angle in the palmar carpal joint direction 1.0–1.5 inch (treating facial disease).
— *Needle sensation:* local soreness, distension, and numbness radiating to the fingertips.

Deep insertion: penetrating the needle to Laogong [PC 8] or Houxi [SI 3] 2.0–3.0 inches (treating finger spasm or muscular paralysis).
— *Needle sensation:* numbness of palmar side of hand, or radiating to the fingertips (treating finger spasm and numbness).
— *Moxibustion dosage:* 3–5 cones; stick 5–15 minutes.
WARNING: No acupuncture or moxibustion on pregnant women.

Cross-sectional anatomy of the needle passage
(Fig. 1.12)
Perpendicular insertion:
a. *Skin:* the branches from the superficial radial nerve containing fibers from the sixth cervical nerve (C6) innervate the skin.
b. *Subcutaneous tissue:* includes the previously described skin nerve branches. The point is surrounded by the dorsal venous plexus, which drains to the cephalic vein.
c. *First dorsal interosseous muscle:* the muscle originates from the first metacarpal bone, and inserts on the radial side of the base of the proximal phalanges. The muscle abducts the index finger, flexes the metacarpophalangeal joint, and extends the interphalangeal joint. The branches from the deep branch of the ulnar nerve containing fibers from the eighth cervical and first thoracic nerves (C8, T1) innervate the first dorsal interosseous muscle.
d. *Adductor pollicis muscle:* the branches from the deep branch of the ulnar nerve containing fibers from the eighth cervical and first thoracic nerves (C8, T1) innervate the adductor pollicis muscle.
Oblique insertion:
a–c same as the perpendicular insertion.

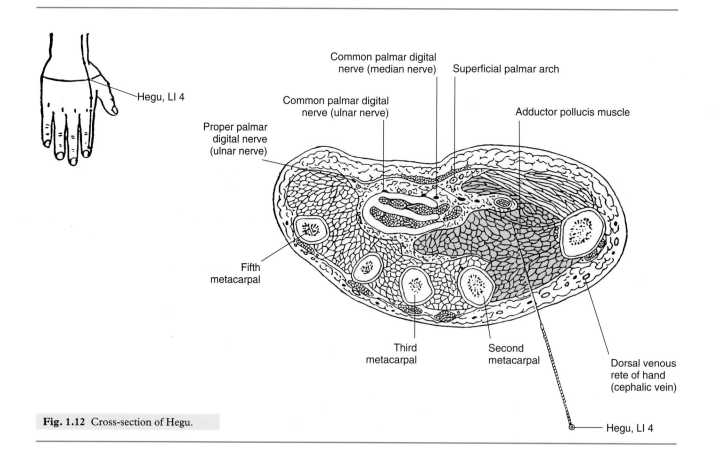

Fig. 1.12 Cross-section of Hegu.

d. The needle superficially passes beside the extensor pollicis longus muscle tendon (dorsal side). The posterior interosseous branches of the radial nerve containing fibers from the sixth and seventh cervical nerves (C6, C7) innervate the extensor pollicis longus muscle. The deep part of the point is the adductor pollicis muscle (palmar side). The radial artery and vein pass the dorsal side of the proximal adductor pollicis muscle.

Functions
Reduces fever, expels Wind, and tranquilizes the mind to stop convulsions.

Clinical indications
Common cold, facial palsy and spasm, hemiplegia, acupuncture anesthesia of head and neck, infantile convulsions, pain, hysteria, schizophrenia, neuroses, mumps, constipation, sweating.

53.

(YUCHI) YUJI, LU 10, HAND TAI YIN LUNG MERIDIAN

Location
The point is located on the thenar eminence 1 inch distal to Taiyuan [LU 9], medial to the midpoint of the first metacarpal on the palmar side of the hand.

Needle and moxibustion method
Perpendicular insertion 0.5–0.8 inch.
— *Needle sensation:* local soreness and distension.
— *Moxibustion dosage:* 3–5 cones; stick 15 minutes.

Cross-sectional anatomy of the needle passage
a. *Skin:* the branches from the superficial radial nerve and lateral antebrachial cutaneous nerve containing fibers from the sixth cervical nerve (C6) innervate the skin.
b. *Subcutaneous tissue:* includes the previously described skin nerve branches and the cephalic vein of the thumb.
c. *Abductor pollicis brevis muscle:* the branches from the median nerve containing fibers from the sixth and seventh cervical nerves (C6, C7) innervate the muscle.
d. *Opponens pollicis muscle:* the branches from the median nerve containing fibers from the sixth and seventh cervical nerves (C6, C7) innervate the muscle.
e. *Flexor pollicis brevis muscle:* consists of superficial and profundus heads. The superficial portion is innervated by a branch of the median nerve and the

profundus portion by a branch of ulnar nerve. Both contain fibers from the sixth and seventh cervical nerves (C6, C7).

Functions
Ventilates the Lung to relieve Exterior syndromes, and reduces fever to relieve sore throat.

Clinical indications
Cough, bronchitis, pneumonia, tonsillitis, tuberculosis, bronchial asthma, hematemesis, hoarseness of voice, dizziness, abdominal pain, chest pain, back pain, fever and chills.

54.

(LAOKUNG) LAOGONG, PC 8, HAND JUE YIN PERICARDIUM MERIDIAN, SPRING POINT

Location
The point is located on the proximal transverse skin crease of the palm, between the second and third metacarpals, and close to the lateral side of the third metacarpal. Alternative method: when a loose fist is made the point is located in the space between the middle and the ring fingertips.

Needle and moxibustion method
Perpendicular insertion 0.3–0.5 inch.
— *Needle sensation:* local soreness and distension.
— *Moxibustion dosage:* 1–3 cones, (WARNING: No direct moxibustion on the palm); stick 5–10 minutes.

Cross-sectional anatomy of the needle passage
(Fig. 1.13)
a. *Skin:* the branches from the palmar cutaneous nerve, a branch of the median nerve containing fibers from the sixth and seventh cervical nerves (C6, C7), innervate the skin. The palmar skin layer is thickened, lacks elasticity, and contains sweat glands but no hair and sebaceous glands.
b. *Subcutaneous tissue:* the fibrous fasciculi strongly connect the palmar skin to the palmar aponeurosis, which separates the subcutaneous adipose tissue into several chambers. The previously described skin nerve branches tranverse the area.
c. *Palmar aponeurosis:* the deeper fascial layer is thickened prominently to form a dense connective tissue layer. Proximally, the palmar aponeurosis is connected to the tendon of the palmaris longus muscle and the bands of the flexor muscle. Distally, the palmar aponeurosis is split into the four tendon sheaths of the fingers and the metacarpal ligaments at the ulnar side. The median nerve innervates the palmar aponeurosis.

d. On the radial side of the needle are the flexor digitorum superficialis and profundus muscles. The branches from the median nerve containing fibers from the seventh and eighth cervical nerves (C7, C8) innervate the flexor digitorum superficialis muscle. The branches from the median nerve containing fibers from the eighth cervical and first thoracic nerves (C8, T1) innervate the flexor digitorum profundus muscle. On the ulnar side of the needle is the second lumbrical muscle, first common digital artery, and second common digital nerve. The branches from the median nerve containing fibers from the sixth and seventh cervical nerves (C6, C7) innervate the second lumbrical muscle. The first common digital artery arises from the superficial palmar arch and bifurcates into two phalangeal arteries, which run on the medial side of the index and the lateral side of the middle finger. The second common digital nerve is a branch of the median nerve.

e. Palmar interosseous muscle and dorsal interosseous muscle: the branches from the profundus branch of the ulnar nerve containing fibers from the eighth cervical and first thoracic nerves (C8, T1) innervate these two muscles. If the needle is inserted deeply, it will penetrate into Wailaogong [EX-UE 8].

WARNING: Due to the many peripheral nerves in this area, directly puncturing the skin of the palm is very painful. Alternatively, access this point by penetrating through from Wailoagong (EX-UE 8).

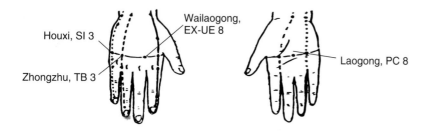

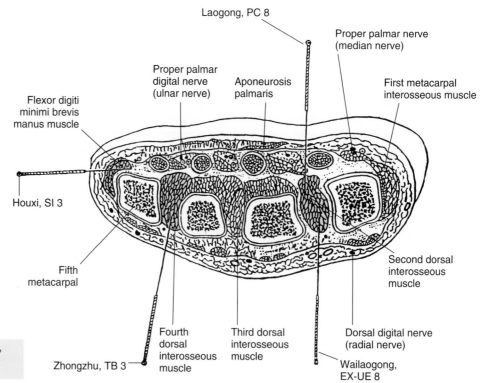

Fig. 1.13 Cross-section of Houxi, Zhongzhu, Wailaogong and Laogong.

Functions

Removes Heat from the Blood to prevent convulsions, relieves mental stress and regulates the function of the Stomach.

Clinical indications

Coma due to cerebrovascular disease, angina pectoris, stomatitis, infantile convulsions, hysteria, psychosis, finger numbness, sweating, stroke, nausea, hemorrhoids.

55.

(WAILAOKUNG) WAILAOGONG, EX-UE 8, EXTRA POINT OF THE UPPER EXTREMITIES

Location

The point is located on the dorsum of the hand in the fossa 0.5 inch proximal to the metacarpophalangeal joint, and between the second and third metacarpals. Alternative method: find Laogong [PC 8] first, then Wailaogong [EX-UE 8] is located directly opposite to Laogong [PC 8] on the dorsum of the hand.

Needle and moxibustion method

Perpendicular insertion 0.5–0.8 inches.
— *Needle sensation:* local soreness and distension, or sometimes numbness radiating to the fingertips.

Cross-sectional anatomy of the needle passage

(Fig. 1.13)

a. *Skin:* the branches from the posterior palmar radial nerve containing fibers from the sixth and seventh cervical nerves (C6, C7) innervate the skin.
b. *Subcutaneous tissue:* includes the previously described skin nerve branches and the dorsal venous plexus.
c. The needle passes on the ulnar side of the dorsal metacarpal artery. The dorsal carpal radial artery gives rise to the the dorsal metacarpal artery.
d. *Second dorsal interosseous muscle:* the branches from the profundus branch of the ulnar nerve containing fibers from the eighth cervical and first thoracic nerves (C8, T1) innervate the second dorsal interosseous muscle.
If the needle is inserted deeply, it will pass into Laogong [PC 8].

Clinical indications

Migraine, sore throat, shoulder pain, neck strain, numbness and itching of the palm.

56.

(CHUNGCHU) ZHONGZHU, TB 3, HAND SHAO YANG TRIPLE BURNER MERIDIAN, STREAM POINT

Location

With the hand slightly clenched, the point is located on the dorsum of the hand, in the fossa proximal to the metacarpophalangeal joint between the heads of the fourth and fifth metacarpals, or 1 inch above Yemen [TB 2].

Needle and moxibustion method

Perpendicular insertion 0.4 inch. WARNING: Avoid the subcutaneous vessels.
— *Needle sensation:* local soreness and distension radiating proximally or distally.
— *Moxibustion dosage:* 3–5 cones; stick 5–10 minutes.

Cross-sectional anatomy of the needle passage

(Fig. 1.13)

a. *Skin:* the branches from the dorsal digital nerve of the branch of the dorsal ulnar nerve containing fibers from the eighth cervical nerve (C8) innervate the skin.
b. *Subcutaneous tissue:* includes the previously described skin nerve branches and the dorsal venous plexus.
c. The needle is inserted radial to the dorsal metacarpal artery. The dorsal carpal radial artery gives rise to the dorsal metacarpal artery.
d. *Fourth dorsal interosseous muscle:* the branches from the profundus branches of the ulnar nerve containing fibers from the eighth cervical and first thoracic nerves (C8, T1) innervate the fourth dorsal interosseous muscle.

Functions

Reduces fever and regulates the flow of Qi, improves visual and auditory acuity.

Clinical indications

Deafness, tinnitus, headache, common cold, conjunctivitis, optic neuritis, shoulder pain, pleurisy, sore throat, fever.

57.

(HOUSHI) HOUXI, SI 3, HAND TAI YANG SMALL INTESTINE MERIDIAN, STREAM POINT

Location

With the hand half clenched, the point is located on the medial edge of the palm proximal to the head of the fifth metacarpal bone, at the junction of the skin of the palm and the skin of the dorsum of the hand.

Needle and moxibustion method
Perpendicular insertion 0.5–1.0 inch.
— *Needle sensation:* local soreness and distension radiating to the whole palm.

Penetrating to Hegu [LI 4] 1.5–2.0 inches (treating finger spasm).
— *Needle sensation:* local distension and soreness radiating to the whole palm.
— *Moxibustion dosage:* 1–3 cones; stick 5–15 minutes.

Cross-sectional anatomy of the needle passage
(Fig. 1.13)
a. *Skin:* the branches from the dorsal ulnar nerve containing fibers from the eighth cervical nerve (C8) and the palmar cutaneous ulnar nerve containing fibers from the eighth cervical nerve (C8) innervate the skin.
b. *Subcutaneous tissue:* the previously described skin nerve branches.
c. *Extensor digiti minimi muscle:* the branches from the profundus branches of the ulnar nerve containing fibers from the eighth cervical and first thoracic nerves (C8, T1) innervate the extensor digiti minimi muscle.
d. *Flexor digiti minimi brevis muscle:* the branches from the profundus branch of the ulnar nerve containing fibers from the eighth cervical and first thoracic nerves (C8, T1) innervate the flexor digiti minimi muscle.
e. On the palmar side of the needle is the palmar digital nerve at the ulnar side of the small finger and the palmar proper artery. The palmar digital nerve is the branch of the ulnar nerve, and the palmar proper artery is the branch of the superficial palmar arch.

Functions
Reduces fever and expels Wind, and refreshes and invigorates the mind.

Clinical indications
Malaria, epilepsy, psychosis, hysteria, pleurisy, cold sweats, neck strain, deafness, back pain, conjunctivitis, pterygium, tonsillitis.

58.
(SANCHIAN) SANJIAN, LI 3, HAND YANG MING LARGE INTESTINE MERIDIAN, STREAM POINT

Location
With the hand half clenched, the point is located on the radial side of the index finger in the fossa proximal to the head of the second metacarpal bone.

Needle and moxibustion method
Perpendicular insertion 0.5–0.8 inch.
— *Needle sensation:* local soreness and distension radiating to the dorsum of the hand.
— *Moxibustion dosage:* 3–5 cones; stick 15 minutes.

Cross-sectional anatomy of the needle passage
a. *Skin:* the branches from the dorsal digital branch of the radial nerve and the proper palmar digital branch of the median nerve containing fibers from the sixth cervical nerve (C6) innervate the skin.
b. *Subcutaneous tissue:* includes the previously described skin nerve branches and the radial artery of the index finger.
c. *First dorsal interosseous muscle:* the branches from the ulnar nerve containing fibers from the eighth cervical and first thoracic nerves (C8, T1) innervate the muscle.
d. The needle is inserted between the first lumbrical muscle and second metacarpal bone. The branches from the median nerve containing fibers from the sixth and seventh cervical nerves (C6, C7) innervate the muscle.
e. The needle is passed between the tendons of the flexor digitorum superficialis and profundus muscles and the first interosseous muscle. The branches from the median nerve containing fibers from the seventh cervical to first thoracic nerves (C7, C8, T1) innervate the flexor digitorum superficialis and profundus muscles. The branches from the ulnar nerve containing fibers from the eighth cervical and first thoracic nerves (C8, T1) innervate the first interosseous muscle.

Functions
Reduces fever and expels Wind, and clears the channels to relieve rigidity of the joints.

Clinical indications
Shoulder pain, elbow pain, tonsillitis, toothache, eye pain, bronchial asthma, fever, erythema of hand.

59.

(SHAOFU) SHAOFU, HT 8, HAND SHAO YIN HEART MERIDIAN, SPRING POINT

Location
With the hand clenched, the point is located on the palm directly at the tip of the little finger, between the fourth and fifth metacarpals.

Needle and moxibustion method
Perpendicular insertion 0.3–0.5 inch.
— *Needle sensation:* local distension and pain radiating to the little finger.
— *Moxibustion dosage:* 3–5 cones; stick 10 minutes.

Cross-sectional anatomy of the needle passage
a. *Skin:* the branches from the common and proper palmar digital nerve from the ulnar nerve containing fibers from the eighth cervical and first thoracic nerves (C8, T1) innervate the skin. The palmar skin is thickened, lacks elasticity, and contains sweat glands but no hair and sebaceous glands.
b. *Subcutaneous tissue:* the fibrous fasciculi are strongly attached to the palmar skin and palmar aponeurosis, separating the subcutaneous adipose tissue into several chambers. The previously described skin nerve branches pass through the tissue.
c. *Palmar aponeurosis:* the deep fascia layer is thickened like connective tissue. Proximally, the palmar aponeurosis connects the tendons of the palmaris longus and flexor muscles. Distally, the palmar aponeurosis splits into four tendon sheaths in the fingers and forms the metacarpal ligament on the ulnar side. The branches from the median nerve containing fibers from the seventh cervical to first thoracic nerves (C7, C8, T1) innervate the palmar aponeurosis.
d. On the ulnar side of the needle is the flexor digitorum superficialis and the profundus muscles. The branches from the median nerve containing fibers from the seventh and eighth cervical nerves (C7, C8) innervate the flexor digitorum superficialis muscle. The branches from the ulnar nerve containing fibers from the eighth cervical and first thoracic nerves (C8, T1) innervate the flexor digitorum profundus muscle.
e. *Fourth lumbrical muscle:* the needle is passed into the lumbrical muscle. The branches from the deep ulnar nerve containing fibers from the eighth cervical nerve (C8) innervate the muscle.
f. On the radial side of the needle is the third common digital artery and fourth common digital nerve. The needle is inserted into the fourth lumbrical muscle. The branches from the ulnar nerve innervate the fourth lumbrical muscle. The third common digital artery arises from the superficial palmar arch. The fourth common digital nerve is a branch of the ulnar nerve.
g. *Fourth palmar interosseous and dorsal interosseous muscles:* the profundus branches from the ulnar nerve containing fibers from the eighth cervical and first thoracic nerves (C8, T1) innervate these two muscles.

Functions
Removes Blood Stasis and clears the collaterals, and reduces fever to relieve mental stress.

Clinical indications
Hysteria, neurosis, chronic tonsillitis, angina pectoris, tachycardia, chest pain, arm and forearm numbness, arthritis of the elbow and wrist.

60.

(CHIENKU) QIANGU, SI 2, HAND TAI YANG SMALL INTESTINE MERIDIAN, SPRING POINT

Location
With the hand half clenched, the point is located on the ulnar side of the hand distal to the metacarpopha-langeal joint of the little finger.

Needle and moxibustion method
Perpendicular insertion 0.3–0.5 inch.
— *Needle sensation:* local soreness and distension.
— *Moxibustion dosage:* 1–3 cones; stick 10 minutes.

Cross-sectional anatomy of the needle passage
a. *Skin:* the branches from the dorsal digital and proper palmar digital branches of the ulnar nerve containing fibers from the eighth cervical nerve (C8) innervate the skin.
b. *Subcutaneous tissue:* includes the previously described skin nerve branches and the proper palmar digital artery.
c. *Dorsal digital artery and proper palmar digital nerve:* the ulnar artery gives rise to the dorsal digital artery. The proper palmar nerve is a branch of the ulnar nerve.

Functions
Reduces fever and expels Wind, clears the channels to regulate Qi, and alleviates mental stress.

Clinical indications
Headache, epistaxis, tonsillitis, sore throat, shoulder pain, fever, epilepsy, malaria, mastitis.

61.

(YENMEN) YEMEN, TB 2, HAND SHAO YANG TRIPLE BURNER MERIDIAN, SPRING POINT

Location
With the hand slightly clenched, the point is located in the fossa between the metacarpophalangeal joints of the ring and little fingers, proximal to the margin of the web.

Needle and moxibustion method
Proximal oblique insertion 0.2–0.3 inch.
— *Needle sensation:* local numbness and distension.
— *Moxibustion dosage:* 3–5 cones; stick 5–10 minutes.

Cross-sectional anatomy of the needle passage
a. *Skin:* the branches from the dorsal digital nerve of the ulnar nerve containing fibers from the eighth cervical and first thoracic nerves (C8, T1) innervate the skin.
b. *Subcutaneous tissue:* includes the previously described skin nerve branches and the dorsal digital artery and vein.
c. *Tendon of the fourth lumbrical and third interosseous muscle:* the branches from the deep palmar ulnar nerve containing fibers from the eighth cervical and first thoracic nerves (C8, T1) innervate both muscles.
d. *Dorsal digital artery and vein:* the dorsal digital artery, together with the dorsal digital vein, is a branch of the ulnar artery.

Functions
Reduces fever and expels Wind, and improves auditory and visual acuity.

Clinical indications
Headache, common cold, hysteria, conjunctivitis, tinnitus, sudden deafness, sore throat, malaria, arm pain, dizziness, gingivitis.

62.

(ERHCHIEN) ERJIAN, LI 2, HAND YANG MING LARGE INTESTINE MERIDIAN, SPRING POINT

Location
With the hand half clenched, the point is located on the radial side of the index finger, distal to the metacarpophalangeal joint; or clenching the hand firmly, the point is located in the fossa at the palmar crease of the index finger.

Needle and moxibustion method
Perpendicular insertion 0.2–0.3 inch.
— *Needle sensation:* local numbness and distension.
— *Moxibustion dosage:* 3–5 cones; stick 15 minutes.

Cross-sectional anatomy of the needle passage
a. *Skin:* the branches from the dorsal proper digitalis of the median nerve and the proper palmar digitalis nerves of the radial nerve innervate the skin. The nerve of the point is supplied from the sixth cervical nerve (C6).
b. *Subcutaneous tissue:* the previously described skin nerve branches.
c. *Tendons of the extensor digitorum, extensor indicis, first interosseous dorsalis and first lumbrical muscles:* the branches from the deep radial nerve containing fibers from the sixth, seventh and eighth cervical nerves (C6, C7, C8) innervate the extensor digitorum muscle. The branches from the deep radial nerve containing fibers from the sixth, seventh and eighth cervical nerves (C6, C7, C8) innervate the flexor digitorum profundus muscle. The branches from the deep palmar branch of the ulnar nerve containing fibers from the eighth cervical and first thoracic nerves (C8, T1) innervate the first interosseous dorsalis muscle. The branches from the third and fourth digital branches of the median nerve containing fibers from the sixth and seventh cervical nerves (C6, C7) innervate the first lumbrical muscle.
d. *Dorsal digital artery and vein, and proper palmar digital artery and vein:* the dorsal digital artery and proper palmar digital artery, together with their respective veins, are branches of the radial artery.

Functions
Reduces fever to relieve Exterior syndromes, and clears the collaterals to relieve sore throat.

Clinical indications
Headache, epistaxis, toothache, tonsillitis, gingivitis, facial palsy, facial muscle spasm, shoulder and elbow pain, fever.

63.

(SZUFENG) SIFENG, EX-UE 10, EXTRA POINT OF THE UPPER EXTREMITIES

Location
The points are located in the midpoint of the palmar side of the skin crease of the second, third, fourth and fifth proximal phalangeal joints.

Needle and moxibustion method
Using a triangular needle, puncture the skin and

squeeze out a small amount of yellow colored mucus. Perpendicular insertion 0.1–0.2 inch.
— *Needle sensation:* local distension and pain.
— *Moxibustion dosage:* no moxibustion permitted.

Cross-sectional anatomy of the needle passage
(e.g. the point of the index finger)

a. *Skin:* the branches from the proper palmar pollicis digitorum nerve of the median nerve containing fibers from the sixth cervical nerve (C6) innervate the skin. (NOTE: The nerve distribution of the middle finger is the same as the index finger. The branches from the median nerve and the proper palmar pollicis digitorum nerve from the ulnar nerve innervate the skin of the ring finger. The branches from the proper palmar pollicis digitorum nerve from the ulnar nerve innervate the little finger.)

b. *Subcutaneous tissue:* includes the previously described skin nerve branches, the proper palmar digital arteries, and the subcutaneous digital vein.

c. *Flexor digitorum profundus muscle tendon:* the branches from the median nerve containing fibers from the seventh cervical to first thoracic nerves (C7, C8, T1) innervate the flexor digitorum profundus muscle of the index and middle fingers. The branches from the ulnar nerve containing fibers from the eighth cervical and first thoracic nerves (C8, T1) innervate the flexor digitorum profundus muscle of the ring and small fingers.

Clinical indications
Pertussis, infantile indigestion, infantile malnutrition, arthritis of the finger, ascariasis.

64.

(PAHSIEH) BAXIE, EX-UE 9, EXTRA POINT OF THE UPPER EXTREMITIES

Location
When a loose fist is made, the points are located on the dorsum of the hand between the metacarpophalangeal joints and proximal to the margin of the web. There are thus a total of eight points on the right and left hands. (NOTE: From lateral to medial are Tadu, Shangdu, Zhondu, Xiadu.)

Needle and moxibustion method
Perpendicular insertion about 0.5–1.0 inch in the direction of the metacarpals, or using a triangular needle to induce bleeding.
— *Needle sensation:* local soreness and distension, or electrical sensation radiating to the fingertips.
— *Moxibustion dosage:* 7 cones; stick 10 minutes.

Cross-sectional anatomy of the needle passage
(e.g. Tadu)

a. *Skin:* the branches from the dorsal branch of the palmar digital nerve of the radial nerve containing fibers from the sixth cervical nerve (C6) innervate the skin. (NOTE: The nerve distribution of Shangdu is the same as Tadu, whereas the dorsal branches of the palmar digital nerve of the ulnar nerve innervate the skin of Zhondu and Xiadu.)

b. *Subcutaneous tissue:* includes the previously described skin nerve branches and the dorsal venous rete.

c. *First lateral dorsal interosseous muscle:* the deep branches of the ulnar nerve containing fibers from the eighth cervical and first thoracic nerves (C8, T1) innervate the dorsal interosseous muscle.

d. *Adductor pollicis muscle:* the branches from the deep ulnar nerve containing fibers from the eighth cervical and first thoracic nerves (C8, T1) innervate the adductor pollicis muscle.

Clinical indications
Joint diseases of the fingers, numbness of the fingers, headache, toothache, sore throat, snake bite.

65.

(SHAOSHANG) SHAOSHANG, LU 11, HAND TAI YIN LUNG MERIDIAN, WELL POINT

Location
With the palm facing up and the hand half clenched, the point is located on the radial side of the thumb 0.1 inch lateral and proximal to the nail base of the thumb.

Needle and moxibustion method
Superior perpendicular insertion 0.1–0.2 inch, perpendicular insertion 0.1–0.2 inch or use a triangular needle to induce bleeding.
— *Needle sensation:* local pain.
— *Moxibustion dosage:* 1–3 cones; stick 15 minutes.

Cross-sectional anatomy of the needle passage

a. *Skin:* the proper palmar digital branches of the median nerve containing fibers from the sixth cervical nerve (C6) innervate the skin.

b. *Subcutaneous tissue:* many dense connective tissue septa, which connect the skin and periosteum of the distal phalanges, separate the subcutaneous tissue into many small chambers. The previously described skin nerve branches and the dorsal digital branches of the proper palmar digital artery and vein supply the tissue.

c. *Finger nail root:* at the deep level of the nail bed.

Functions

Reduces fever and relieves sore throat, restores consciousness and induces resuscitation.

Clinical indications

Tonsillitis, mumps, jaundice, asthma, fever, common cold, cough, pneumonia, cerebrovascular disease, coma, childhood indigestion, psychosis.

66.

(SHAOTSE) SHAOZE, SI 1, HAND TAI YANG SMALL INTESTINE MERIDIAN, WELL POINT

Location

With the palm prone and the fingers outstretched, the point is located on the ulnar side of the little finger about 0.1 inch lateral and inferior to the nail root, or at the intersection of the lines drawn from the lateral edge of the finger nail and the nail root.

Needle and moxibustion method

Slightly superior oblique insertion 0.1 inch or use a triangular needle to induce bleeding.
— *Needle sensation:* local distension and soreness.
— *Moxibustion dosage:* 1–3 cones; stick 5–15 minutes.

Cross-sectional anatomy of the needle passage

a. *Skin:* the dorsal branches of the proper palmar digital nerve of the ulnar nerve containing fibers from the eighth cervical nerve (C8) innervate the skin.
b. *Subcutaneous tissue:* many dense connective tissue septa, which connect the skin and the periosteum of the distal phalanges, separate the subcutaneous tissue into many small chambers. The previously described skin nerve branches and dorsal digital branch of the palmar ulnar artery of the small finger supply the area.
c. *Finger nail root:* at the deep level of the nail bed.

Functions

Clears the channels to induce resuscitation, and activates the collaterals to promote lactation.

Clinical indications

Headache, mumps, insufficient milk, mastitis, hepatitis, pterygium, conjunctivitis, coma, cerebrovascular disease, convulsions, pleurisy.

67.

(SHIHHSUAN) SHIXUAN, EX-UE 11, EXTRA POINT OF THE UPPER EXTREMITIES

Location

The points are located on the fingertips of all 10 fingers, and about 0.1 inch distal to the nail.

Needle and moxibustion method

Shallow insertion 0.1–0.2 inch or use a triangular needle to induce bleeding.
— *Needle sensation:* local soreness and distension.
— *Moxibustion dosage:* 3 cones.

Cross-sectional anatomy of the needle passage

a. *Skin:* the branches from the median nerve containing fibers from the sixth cervical nerve (C6) innervate the thumb and index finger. The branches from the median nerve containing fibers from the seventh cervical nerve (C7) innervate the middle finger. The branches from the median and ulnar nerves containing fibers from the eighth cervical nerve (C8) innervate the ring finger. The branches from the ulnar nerve containing fibers from the eighth cervical nerve (C8) innervate the small finger.
b. *Subcutaneous tissue:* many dense connective tissue septa, which connect the skin and the periosteum of the distal phalanges, separate the subcutaneous tissue into many small chambers. The adipose tissue contains many small nerves and vessels.

Clinical indications

Shock, coma, high fever, stroke, epilepsy, hysteria, infantile convulsions, numbness of the fingers.

68.

(KUANCHUNG) GUANCHONG, TB 1, HAND SHAO YANG TRIPLE BURNER MERIDIAN, WELL POINT

Location

With the palm prone, the point is located on the ulnar side of the ring finger 0.1 inch lateral and proximal to the nail base.

Needle and moxibustion method

Shallow or oblique insertion 0.1 inch or use a triangular needle to induce bleeding.
— *Needle sensation:* local soreness.
— *Moxibustion dosage:* 1–3 cones; stick 5–10 minutes.

Cross-sectional anatomy of the needle passage

a. *Skin:* the proper palmar digital branches from the

ulnar nerve containing fibers from the eighth cervical nerve (C8) innervate the skin.

b. *Subcutaneous tissue:* many dense connective tissue septa, which connect the skin and periosteum of the distal phalanges, separate the subcutaneous tissue into many small chambers. The previously described skin nerve branches and the dorsal digital branch of the proper palmar digital artery supply the area.

c. *Finger nail root:* the needle reaches the deep nail root.

Functions

Refreshes the mind and relieves mental stress, and regulates and promotes the function of Triple Jiao (Triple Warmer).

Clinical indications

Headache, sore throat, fever, shoulder pain, pterygium, nausea.

69.

(CHUNGCHUNG) ZHONGCHONG, PC 9, HAND JUE YIN PERICARDIUM MERIDIAN, WELL POINT

Location

The point is located on the radial side of the middle finger 0.1 inch lateral and proximal to the nail base.

Needle and moxibustion method

Superior oblique insertion 0.1–0.2 inch, perpendicular insertion 0.1–0.2 inch or use a triangular needle to induce bleeding.
— *Needle sensation:* local soreness.
— *Moxibustion dosage:* 1–3 cones; stick 5–10 minutes.

Cross-sectional anatomy of the needle passage

a. *Skin:* the proper palmar digital branches from the median nerve containing fibers from the seventh cervical nerve (C7) innervate the skin.

b. *Subcutaneous tissue:* many dense connective tissue septa, which connect the skin and periosteum of the distal phalanges, separate the subcutaneous tissue into many small chambers. The previously described skin nerve branches and the dorsal digital branch of the proper palmar digital artery supply the area.

c. *Finger nail root:* the needle reaches the deep nail root.

Functions

Relieves syncope, clears away Heart Fire, and reduces fever.

Clinical indications

Precordial pain, angina pectoris, myocarditis, hysteria,

heat stroke, coma, shock, cerebrovascular disease, infantile convulsions.

70.

(SHANGYANG) SHANGYANG, LI 1, HAND YANG MING LARGE INTESTINE MERIDIAN, WELL POINT

Location

With the fingers extended and the palm prone, the point is located on the radial side of the index finger 0.1 inch proximal to the nail base.

Needle and moxibustion method

Superior oblique insertion 0.1–0.2 inch, perpendicular insertion 0.1–0.2 inch or use a triangular needle to induce bleeding.
— *Needle sensation:* local distension and soreness.
— *Moxibustion dosage:* 1–3 cones; stick 15 minutes.

Cross-sectional anatomy of the needle passage

a. *Skin:* the proper palmar digital branches from the median nerve containing fibers from the sixth cervical nerve (C 6) innervate the skin.

b. *Subcutaneous tissue:* many dense connective tissue septa, which connect the skin and periosteum of the distal phalanges, separate the subcutaneous tissue into many small chambers. The previously described skin nerve branches and the dorsal digital branch of the proper palmar digital artery supply the area.

c. *Finger nail root:* the needle reaches the deep nail root.

Functions

Reduces fever, relieves swelling around the jaw and throat, and clears the channels to relieve sore throat.

Clinical indications

Fever, glaucoma, deafness, dizziness, toothache, shoulder pain, tonsillitis.

71.

(SHAOCHUNG) SHAOCHONG, HT 9, HAND SHAO YIN HEART MERIDIAN, WELL POINT

Location

With the palm facing up and half flexing the little finger, the point is located on the radial side of the little finger 0.1 inch lateral and proximal to the nail base.

Needle and moxibustion method

Superior insertion 0.1 inch or use a triangular needle to induce bleeding.

— *Needle sensation:* local soreness.
— *Moxibustion dosage:* 3–5 cones; stick 10 minutes.

Cross-sectional anatomy of the needle passage

a. *Skin:* the the proper palmar digital branches from the ulnar nerve containing fibers from the eighth cervical and first thoracic nerves (C8, T1) innervate the skin.

b. *Subcutaneous tissue:* many dense connective tissue septa, which connect the skin and periosteum of the distal phalanges, separate the subcutaneous tissue into many small chambers. The previously described skin nerve branches and the dorsal digital branch of the proper palmar digital artery supply the area.

c. *Finger nail root:* the needle reaches the deep nail root.

Functions

Revives depleted Yang, rescues the patient from collapse, and relieves mental stress.

Clinical indications

Precordial pain, tachycardia, angina pectoris, myocarditis, hepatitis, jaundice, hysteria, epilepsy, schizophrenia, shock, coma, heat stroke.

Cross-sectional anatomy of the lower extremities

The lower extremities consist of the buttock, the thigh, the knee, the leg, the ankle, and the foot. The lower extremities are attached to the lower part of the trunk with the upper border as the inguinal ligament anteriorly and the iliac crest posteriorly.

For superficial measurement during acupuncture treatment, the distance from the superior margin of the pubic symphysis to the medial epicondyle of the femur is 18 inches, from the greater trochanter of the femur to the horizontal crease of the popliteal is 19 inches, from the horizontal crease of the popliteal to the lateral malleolus is 16 inches, from the lateral malleolus to the sole is 3 inches, and from the posterior crease of the buttock to the horizontal crease of the popliteal is 14 inches.

1.

(CHULIAO) JULIAO, GB 29, FOOT SHAO YANG GALLBLADDER MERIDIAN

Location
At the midpoint of the anterior superior iliac spine and the greater trochanter of the femur, 3 inches posterior to Weidao [GB 28], in the anterior fossa of the greater trochanter of the femur. Locate in the lateral recumbent position with the thigh flexed.

Needle and moxibustion method
Oblique insertion into the hip joint 2.0–3.0 inches.
— *Needle sensation:* soreness and distension radiating to the hip joint.
— *Moxibustion dosage:* 5–7 cones; stick 5–20 minutes.

Cross-sectional anatomy of the needle passage
(Fig. 2.1)
a. *Skin:* the lateral cutaneous branches of the iliohypogastric nerve containing fibers from the first lumbar nerve (L1) innervate the skin.
b. *Subcutaneous tissue:* the previously described skin nerve branches supply the area.
c. *Tensor fasciae latae muscle:* the superficial layer of the fascia lata and the thickest fascia of the body. When the needle is punctured through the fascia, a strong resistance is felt.
d. *Gluteus medius muscle:* the inner layer of the gluteus maximus and tensor fasciae latae muscles. The branches from the superior gluteus nerve containing fibers from the fourth lumbar to first sacral nerves (L4, L5, S1) innervate the gluteus medius muscle.
e. *Gluteus minimus muscle:* the inner layer of the gluteus medius muscle. The branches from the superior gluteus nerve containing fibers from the fourth lumbar to first sacral nerves (L4, L5, S1) innervate the muscle.

Functions
Removes Heat from the Liver and strengthens the function of the Spleen, and removes Dampness.

Clinical indications
Stomach pain, lower abdominal pain, orchitis, endometritis, cystitis, hip joint and surrounding soft tissue disease.

2.

(CHUNGMEN) CHONGMEN, SP 12, FOOT TAI YIN SPLEEN MERIDIAN

Location
In a supine position, draw a line between the anterior superior iliac spine and the upper border of the pubic symphysis. The point is located on this line, on the lateral side of the femoral artery or at the midpoint of the inguinal ligament, 3.5 inches lateral to Qugu [CV 2].

Needle and moxibustion method
Perpendicular insertion 1.0–2.0 inches, avoiding the femoral artery.
— *Needle sensation:* numbness and heaviness radiating to the anterior thigh and medial leg.
— *Moxibustion dosage:* 3–5 cones; stick 10 minutes.

Cross-sectional anatomy of the needle passage

a. *Skin:* the branches from the iliohypogastric nerve containing fibers from the first lumbar nerve (L1) innervate the skin.

b. *Subcutaneous tissue:* the previously described skin nerve branches.

c. *Inguinal ligament:* the needle is passed lateral and superior to the midpoint of the inguinal ligament.

d. The needle is passed to the lateral side of the femoral nerve, artery and vein. The femoral artery is a branch of the external iliac artery. The femoral nerve is derived from the lumbar plexus containing fibers from the twelfth thoracic to fourth lumbar nerves (T12–L4).

e. *Iliopsoas muscle:* the branches from the femoral nerve containing fibers from the second to fourth lumbar nerves (L2, L3, L4) innervate the iliacus muscle, and the branches from the lumbar nerve containing fibers from the second to fifth lumbar nerves (L2, L3, L4, L5) innervate the psoas muscle.

f. *Tendons of the exterior and interior abdominal oblique muscles:* the branches from the ilioinguinal nerve innervate both muscles.

Functions

Regulates the function of the Spleen, strengthens the function of the Kidney, and regulates the flow of Qi to remove Dampness.

Clinical indications

Abdominal pain, hernia, femoral nerve palsy, orchitis, pelvic inflammatory disease, vaginal inflammation, stomach spasm, hemorrhoids.

3.

(HUANTIAO) HUANTIAO, GB 30, FOOT SHAO YANG GALLBLADDER MERIDIAN

Location

Located in a lateral recumbent or prone position. In a lateral position, extending the lower leg and flexing the thigh, the point is located superior and posterior to the greater trochanter of the femur. Draw a line connecting the high point of the greater trochanter of the femur with the sacral hiatus and the point is located at the lateral third of this line; or in the middle of the triangle made by the greater trochanter, the ischial tuberosity and the posterior superior iliac spine.

Needle and moxibustion method

Perpendicular insertion towards the external genital organ 2.0–3.5 inches (treating sciatica).

— *Needle sensation:* local soreness and distension, or an electrical sensation radiating to the lower extremities.

Perpendicular insertion in the hip joint direction or

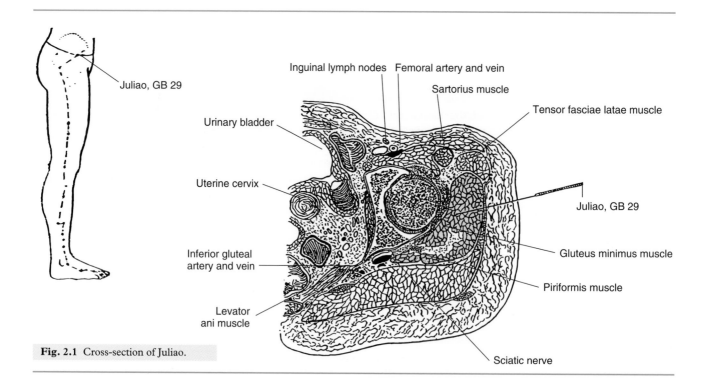

Fig. 2.1 Cross-section of Juliao.

bilateral lifting 2.0–3.0 inches (treating hip joint and surrounding tissue disease).
— *Needle sensation:* local soreness and distension radiating to the hip joint.
— *Moxibustion dosage:* 10–20 cones; stick 20 minutes.

Cross-sectional anatomy of the needle passage
(Fig. 2.2)

a. *Skin:* the branches from the superior cluneal nerve from the cutaneous branch of the posterior division of the second lumbar nerve (L2) innervate the skin. The skin of the buttock contains many sebaceous glands and sweat glands.

b. *Subcutaneous tissue:* innervated by the previously described skin nerve branches. The subcutaneous tissue contains much adipose tissue.

c. *Gluteus maximus muscle:* the largest and thickest muscle of the human body, which makes up the greater part of the buttock. The inferior cluneal nerve from the branches of fifth lumbar to second sacral nerves (L5, S1, S2) innervate the muscle.

d. *Sciatic nerve:* the largest and longest peripheral nerve of the human body. The sciatic nerve consists of the anterior branch from the fourth lumbar to third sacral nerves (L4, L5, S1, S2, S3). If the needle is inserted directly into the sciatic nerve, a strong electrical sensation radiates to the thigh, lower leg and foot.

e. *Posterior gluteal nerve, and inferior gluteal artery and vein:* If the needle is directed slightly medially 0.5 centimeter (one fifth inch) it will be inserted into the previously described structure. If the needle is passed into the posterior gluteal nerve, the electrical sensation radiates to the posterior and anterior thigh, but not to the foot. We use this differentiation to discover if the needle has punctured the sciatic nerve or not.

f. *Quadratus femoris muscle:* the branches from the quadratus femoris nerve containing fibers from the fourth lumbar to first sacral nerves (L4, L5, S1) innervate this muscle. The sciatic nerve passes through the superficial part of this muscle.

Functions
Dispels Wind and removes Dampness, and relieves rigidity of the muscles, tendons and joints of the leg and buttock.

Clinical indications
Sciatic pain, back and leg pain, knee and ankle pain, hemiplegia, palsy of the lower extremities, urticaria, psoriasis, hip joint and surrounding soft tissue disease, beriberi.

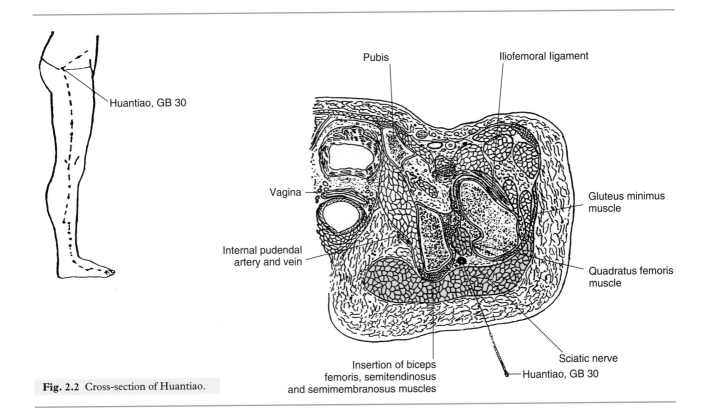

Fig. 2.2 Cross-section of Huantiao.

4.

(YINLIEN) YINLIAN, LIV 11, FOOT JUE YIN LIVER MERIDIAN

Location
In a supine position with the leg extended, the point is located 2 inches below the inguinal Qichong [ST 30], or 2 inches lateral and 2 inches inferior to Qugu [CV 2] lateral to the adductor muscle and medial to the femoral artery.

Needle and moxibustion method
Perpendicular insertion slightly directed to the medial side 1.0–1.5 inches.
— *Needle sensation:* local soreness and distension, or radiating to the medial side of the lower extremity.
— *Moxibustion dosage:* 3 cones; stick 5–10 minutes.
WARNING: In order to prevent the needle puncturing the femoral artery, don't direct the needle to the lateral side.

Cross-sectional anatomy of the needle passage
(Fig. 2.3)
a. *Skin:* the branches from the anterior cutaneous femoral nerve containing fibers from the second lumbar nerve (L2) innervate the skin.

b. *Subcutaneous tissue:* includes the previously described skin nerve branches, the greater saphenous vein, and the inguinal superficial lymph nodes. The greater saphenous vein is at the lateral side of the needle.

c. *Adductor longus muscle:* the branches from the obturator nerve containing fibers from the second and third lumbar nerves (L2, L3) innervate the muscle.

d. *Adductor brevis muscle:* the inner layer of the adductor longus muscle. The branches from the obturator nerve containing fibers from the third and fourth lumbar nerves (L3, L4) innervate the muscle.

e. *Adductor magnus muscle:* the inner layer of the adductor brevis muscle. The branches from the obturator nerve containing fibers from the third and fourth lumbar nerves (L3, L4) innervate the muscle.

Functions
Removes Heat from the Liver, regulates the flow of Qi, reduces fever and removes Dampness.

Clinical indications
Cramp of the lower extremities, dysmenorrhea, leukorrhea, pelvic pain, pelvic itching, female infertility.

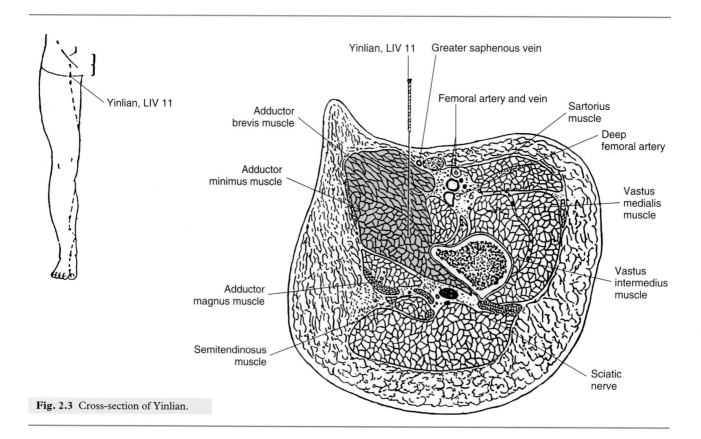

Fig. 2.3 Cross-section of Yinlian.

5.

(CHENGFU) CHENGFU, BL 36, FOOT TAI YANG BLADDER MERIDIAN

Location
In a prone position, the point is located on the midline of the posterior thigh, at the inferior margin of the gluteus maximus muscle, and at the midpoint of the skin crease of the buttock; or at the intersection of a line joining Weizhong [BL 40] with Zhibian [BL 54] and the skin crease of the buttock.

Needle and moxibustion method
Perpendicular insertion 1.5–2.5 inches.
— *Needle sensation:* local soreness and distension, or sometimes an electrical sensation radiating to the distal leg or the heel.
— *Moxibustion dosage:* 3 cones; stick 5–20 minutes.

Cross-sectional anatomy of the needle passage
(Fig. 2.4)
a. *Skin:* the branches from the posterior femoral cutaneous nerve containing fibers from the second sacral nerve (S2) innervate the skin.

b. *Subcutaneous tissue:* the branches from the posterior femoral cutaneous and inferior cluneal nerves.
c. *Gluteus maximus muscle:* the needle is passed through the lowest part of the gluteus maximus muscle. The branches from the inferior gluteal nerve containing fibers from the fifth lumbar to second sacral nerves (L5, S1, S2) innervate the muscle.
d. *Posterior femoral nerve:* the nerve is located at the inner layer of the gluteus maximus muscle and the superficial layer of the sciatic nerve.
e. *Long head of biceps femoris muscle and semitendinosus muscle:* these two muscles originate from the ischial tuberosity. The branches from the tibial nerve containing fibers from the fifth lumbar to second sacral nerves (L5, S1, S2) innervate these two muscles.
f. *Sciatic nerve and its accompanying artery:* the nerve is located at the deeper layer of the biceps femoris muscle and semitendinosus muscle. The points are located in the superficial layer of the adductor magnus. The needle is inserted at the medial side of the sciatic nerve.

Functions
Clears and activates the channels and collaterals, and regulates the flow of Qi and Blood circulation.

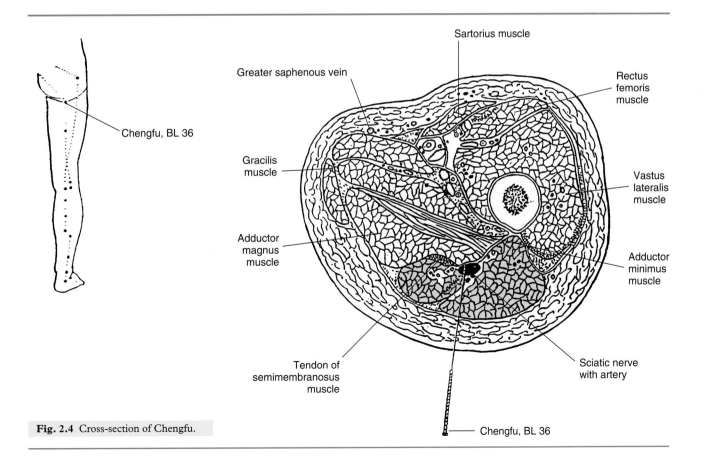

Fig. 2.4 Cross-section of Chengfu.

Clinical indications

Sciatic pain, paralysis and weakness of the lower extremities, numbness, hemorrhoids, constipation, buttock tumors and inflammation, oliguria, endometritis.

6.

(PIKUAN) BIGUAN, ST 31, FOOT YANG MING STOMACH MERIDIAN

Location

In a supine position, draw a vertical line on the anterior thigh from the anterior superior iliac spine and another horizontal line from the inferior pubic symphysis, the point is located at the intersection of the two lines, in the fossa lateral to the sartorius muscle.

Needle and moxibustion method

Perpendicular insertion 1.0–1.5 inches.
— *Needle sensation:* local soreness and numbness, sometimes radiating to the knee.
— *Moxibustion dosage:* 3–7 cones; stick 20 minutes.

Cross-sectional anatomy of the needle passage

a. *Skin:* the branches from the lateral femoral cutaneous nerve containing fibers from the third lumbar nerve (L3) innervate the skin.
b. *Subcutaneous tissue:* the previously described skin nerve branches.
c. *Sartorius and tensor fasciae latae muscle:* the needle passes between these two muscles. The branches from the femoral nerve containing fibers from the second and third lumbar nerves (L2, L3) innervate the sartorius muscle. The branches from the superior gluteal nerve containing fibers from the fourth lumbar to first sacral nerves (L4, L5, S1) innervate the tensor fasciae latae muscle.
d. *Lateral femoral circumflex artery and vein:* the lateral femoral circumflex artery and vein, are connected to the profunda femoris artery.

Functions

Relaxes muscles and tendons and activates the collaterals, and regulates the flow of Qi to relieve rigidity of the joints.

Clinical indications

Paralysis of the lower extremities, abdominal pain, beri-beri, lower back pain, pelvic pain.

7.

(TSUWULI) ZUWULI, LIV 10, FOOT JUE YIN LIVER MERIDIAN

Location

In a supine position with the leg extended, the point is located 3 inches below Qichong [ST 30], at the lateral margin of the adductor longus muscle and the medial margin of the femoral artery.

Needle and moxibustion method

Perpendicular insertion 0.5–1.0 inch.
— *Needle sensation:* local soreness and distension.
— *Moxibustion dosage:* 3–5 cones; stick 5–10 minutes.
WARNING: To avoid the femoral artery, the needle should not be directed laterally.

Cross-sectional anatomy of the needle passage

a. *Skin:* the branches from the anterior cutaneous femoral nerve containing fibers from the second lumbar nerve (L2) innervate the skin.
b. *Subcutaneous tissue:* includes the previously described skin nerve branches and the greater saphenous vein.
c. *Adductor longus muscle:* the branches from the obturator nerve containing fibers from the second and third lumbar nerves (L2, L3) innervate the muscle.
d. *Adductor brevis muscle:* the deep layer of the adductor longus muscle. The branches from the obturator nerve containing fibers from the third and fourth lumbar nerves (L3, L4) innervate the muscle.
e. *Adductor magnus muscle:* the deeper layer of the adductor brevis muscle. The branches from the obturator nerve containing fibers from the third and fourth lumbar nerves (L3, L4) innervate the muscle.

Functions

Reduces Heat and removes Dampness, and reinforces the function of the Bladder to arrest enuresis.

Clinical indications

Sweating, intestinal obstruction, lower abdominal distention, enuresis, seminal emission, urinary tract infection, eczema in the external genital region.

8.

(YINMEN) YINMEN, BL 37, FOOT TAI YANG BLADDER MERIDIAN

Location

In a prone position, the point is located in between the biceps femoris and semitendinosus muscle, 6 inches below Chengfu [BL 36] on the line connecting Chengfu [BL 36] with Weizhong [BL 40].

Needle and moxibustion method
Perpendicular insertion 1.5–2.5 inches.
— *Needle sensation:* local soreness and distension, or electrical sensation radiating to the foot.
— *Moxibustion dosage:* 3–5 cones; stick 5–20 minutes.

Cross-sectional anatomy of the needle passage
(Fig. 2.5)
a. *Skin:* the branches from the posterior femoral cutaneous nerve containing fibers from the second sacral nerve (S2) innervate the skin.
b. *Subcutaneous tissue:* includes the previously described skin nerve branches.
c. *Long head of biceps femoris and semitendinosus muscles:* the branches from the tibial nerve containing fibers from the fifth lumbar to second sacral nerves (L5, S1, S2) innervate these two muscles.
d. *Sciatic nerve and accompanying artery:* the sciatic nerve innervates part of the adductor magnus superficially and at a deeper level it supplies the biceps femoris and semitendinosus muscles. If the needle is inserted into the sciatic nerve, a strong electrical sensation radiates to the foot.

Functions
Warms the channels and clears the collaterals, dispels Cold and alleviates pain.

Clinical indications
Sciatic pain, lower back pain, herniation of an intervertebral disk, lower extremity numbness and paralysis, hip joint pain and inflammation.

9.

(CHIMEN) JIMEN, SP 11, FOOT TAI YIN SPLEEN MERIDIAN

Location
In a seated position and flexing the knee, draw a line between Xuehai [SP 10] and Chongmen [SP 12], the point is located 6 inches above Xuehai [SP 10], and medial to the sartorius muscle; or on the medial thigh 8 inches above the patella.

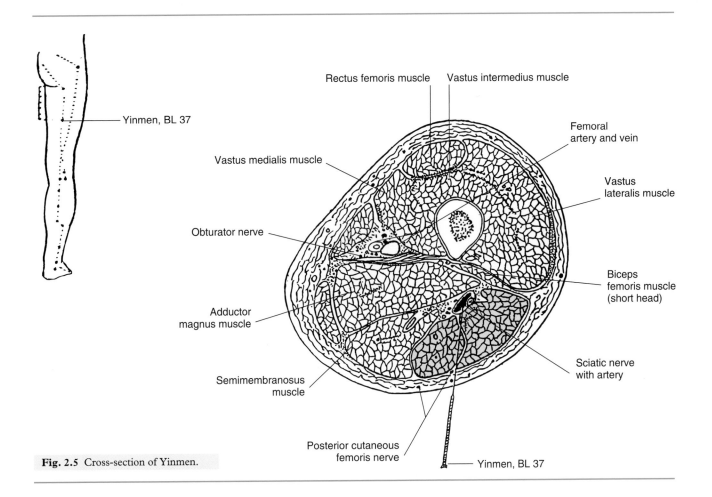

Rectus femoris muscle
Vastus intermedius muscle
Yinmen, BL 37
Vastus medialis muscle
Femoral artery and vein
Vastus lateralis muscle
Obturator nerve
Biceps femoris muscle (short head)
Adductor magnus muscle
Sciatic nerve with artery
Semimembranosus muscle
Posterior cutaneous femoris nerve
Yinmen, BL 37

Fig. 2.5 Cross-section of Yinmen.

Needle and moxibustion method

Perpendicular insertion 0.5–1.0 inch. To avoid the femoral artery, deep insertion should be avoided.
— *Needle sensation:* Soreness and numbness radiating to the distal lower extremities.
— *Moxibustion dosage:* 3–5 cones; stick 10 minutes.

Cross-sectional anatomy of the needle passage

a. *Skin:* the branches from the anterior femoral cutaneous nerve containing fibers from the second lumbar nerve (L2) innervate the skin.
b. *Subcutaneous tissue:* includes the previously described skin nerve branches and the greater saphenous vein.
c. *Sartorius muscle:* the needle is passed medial to the sartorius muscle. The branches from the femoral nerve containing fibers from the second and third lumbar nerves (L2, L3) innervate the muscle.
d. The needle is passed anterior and lateral to the femoral nerve, artery and vein. The external iliac artery gives rise to the femoral artery.
e. *Adductor magnus muscle:* the deep layer of the sartorius muscle. The branches from the tibial nerve containing fibers from the fourth and fifth lumbar nerves (L4, L5) innervate the muscle.

Functions

Strengthens the function of the Spleen and removes Dampness, and clears the Water passages.

Clinical indications

Hemorrhoids, beriberi, lower abdominal pain, gonorrhea, urethral obstruction, premature ejaculation, orchitis, inguinal pain.

10.

(FENGSHIH) FENGSHI, GB 31, FOOT SHAO YANG GALLBLADDER MERIDIAN

Location

On the lateral thigh, on a line drawn between the greater trochanter of the femur and the head of the fibula, the point is located 7 inches above the skin crease of the knee, or 2 inches above Zhongdu [GB 32]. Or when the arm is straightened against the lateral thigh the point is located at the tip of the middle finger.

Needle and moxibustion method

Perpendicular insertion 1.5–2.5 inches.
— *Needle sensation:* local soreness and distension, or sometimes radiating distally.
— *Moxibustion dosage:* 5–7 cones; stick 5–20 minutes.

Cross-sectional anatomy of the needle passage
(Fig. 2.6)

a. *Skin:* the branches from the lateral femoral cutaneous nerve containing fibers from the second lumbar nerve (L2) innervate the skin.

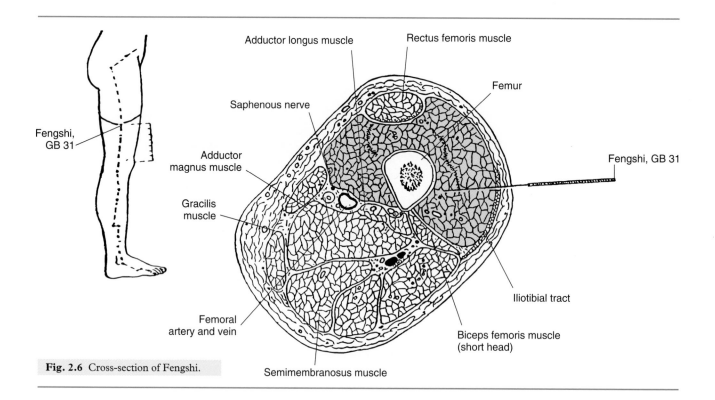

Fengshi, GB 31

Adductor longus muscle
Rectus femoris muscle
Saphenous nerve
Femur
Adductor magnus muscle
Gracilis muscle
Fengshi, GB 31
Femoral artery and vein
Iliotibial tract
Biceps femoris muscle (short head)
Semimembranosus muscle

Fig. 2.6 Cross-section of Fengshi.

b. *Subcutaneous tissue:* includes the previously described skin nerve branches.

c. *Iliotibial tract:* the lateral part of the fascia lata of the thigh. The tensor fasciae latae muscle joins together with the iliotibial tract, becoming a thickened fascia.

d. *Vastus lateralis of quadriceps muscle:* one of the quadriceps muscles located at the lateral thigh. The branches from the femoral nerve containing fibers from the second to fourth lumbar nerves (L2, L3, L4) innervate this muscle.

e. *Vastus medius of quadriceps muscle:* one of the quadriceps muscles. The branches from the femoral nerve containing fibers from the second to fourth lumbar nerves (L2, L3, L4) innervate this muscle.

Functions
Promotes the Blood circulation, clears the collaterals, dispels Wind and expels Cold.

Clinical indications
Paralysis of the lower extremities, back pain, leg pain, lateral femoral cutaneous neuritis, urticaria, beriberi, uterine adnexa inflammation, itching.

11.
(FUTU) FUTU, ST 32, FOOT YANG MING STOMACH MERIDIAN

Location
In a seated or supine position, the point is located on the anterior thigh on a line between the anterior superior spine of the ilium and the lateral patellar bone, 6 inches above the lateral superior margin of the patella; or put the proximal skin crease of the palm on the middle of the patella and put the fingers together on the front thigh and the points are then located at the tip of the middle finger.

Needle and moxibustion method
Perpendicular insertion along the lateral femur 2.0–3.0 inches. If the patient has weak needle response, select a new location 0.5 inch lateral to the previous point.
— *Needle sensation:* local soreness and distension, and radiating to the lateral knee.
— *Moxibustion dosage:* 5–7 cones; stick 5–20 minutes.

Cross-sectional anatomy of the needle passage
(Fig. 2.7)
a. *Skin:* the branches from the anterior femoral cutaneous and lateral femoral cutaneous nerves

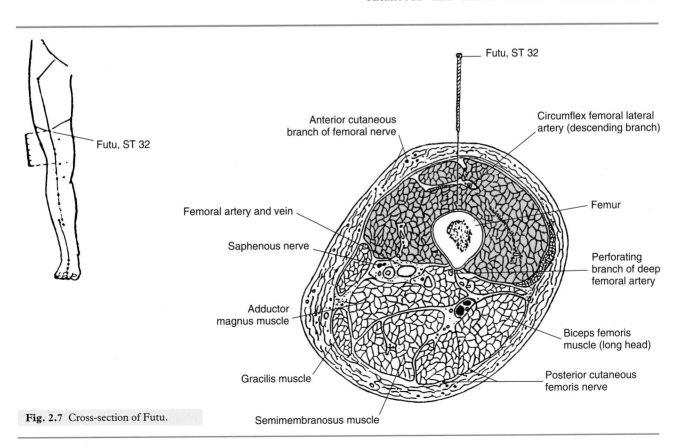

Fig. 2.7 Cross-section of Futu.

containing fibers from the third lumbar nerve (L3) innervate the skin.

b. *Subcutaneous tissue:* includes the previously described skin nerve branches.

c. *Rectus femoris muscle:* one of the quadriceps muscles, the muscle is located at the front thigh. The branches from the femoral nerve containing fibers from the second to fourth lumbar nerves (L2, L3, L4) innervate the muscle. The needle is inserted at the lateral part of the muscle.

d. The needle is passed medial to the lateral circumflex artery descending branch and the muscular branch of the femoral nerve. The lateral femoral circumflex artery and vein, are branches of the profundus femoris artery. The femoral nerve is a major branch of the lumbar plexus containing fibers from the second to fourth lumbar nerves (L2, L3, L4). If the needle is passed in a slightly lateral direction, it will penetrate into the nerve.

e. *Vastus intermedius muscle:* one of the quadriceps muscles. The muscle is a deep layer of the rectus femoris, in front of the femur, and between the vastus medialis and vastus lateralis muscles. The branches from the femoral nerve containing fibers from the second to fourth lumbar nerves (L2, L3, L4) innervate the muscle.

f. *Femur:* the needle inserted about 2 inches may reach the femur. A strong resistance may be felt. Don't continue to insert the needle. If the needle has reached the femur, slightly change the direction laterally along the femur and continue the insertion.

Functions
Regulates the flow of Qi to promote Blood circulation, and removes Blood Stasis to activate the collaterals.

Clinical indications
Paralysis of the lower extremities, numbness, knee joint inflammation, cramp, beriberi, rheumatoid arthritis, urticaria, pelvic pain.

12.

(CHUNGTU) ZHONGDU, GB 32, FOOT SHAO YANG GALLBLADDER MERIDIAN

Location
In seated or lateral recumbent position, draw a line between the greater trochanter of the femur and the head of the fibula. The point is located 5 inches above the skin crease of the knee or 2 inches below Fengshi [GB 31].

Needle and moxibustion method
Perpendicular insertion 0.7–1.2 inches.
— *Needle sensation:* local soreness and distension radiating locally and distally.
— *Moxibustion dosage:* 5–7 cones; stick 10 minutes.

Cross-sectional anatomy of the needle passage
a. *Skin:* the branches from the lateral femoral cutaneous nerve containing fibers from the second lumbar nerve (L2) innervate the skin.

b. *Subcutaneous tissue:* includes the previously described skin nerve branches.

c. *Iliotibial tract:* the lateral part of the fascia lata of the thigh. The tensor fasciae latae muscle joins together with the iliotibial tract to become this thickened fascia.

d. *Vastus lateralis muscle:* one of the quadriceps muscles located at the lateral thigh. The branches from the femoral nerve containing fibers from the second lumbar to fourth lumbar nerves (L2, L3, L4) innervate the muscle.

e. *Vastus medius muscle:* one of the quadriceps muscles. The branches from the femoral nerve containing fibers from the second to fourth lumbar nerves (L2, L3, L4) innervate the muscle.

Functions
Dispels Wind and clears the collaterals, and warms the channels to dispel Cold.

Clinical indications
Beriberi, knee joint arthritis, leg pain, sciatic nerve pain, paralysis and spasm of the lower extremities.

13.

(YINPAO) YINBAO, LIV 9, FOOT JUE YIN LIVER MERIDIAN

Location
With the knee flexed, the point is located on the medial thigh 4 inches above the medial epicondyle of the femur, and in the fossa between the posterior margin of the sartorius muscle and the gracilis muscle.

Needle and moxibustion method
Perpendicular insertion 0.5–0.7 inch.
— *Needle sensation:* local numbness and distension.
— *Moxibustion dosage:* 3–7 cones; stick 10 minutes.

Cross-sectional anatomy of the needle passage
a. *Skin:* the branches from the anterior femoral cutaneous nerve containing fibers from the third lumbar nerve (L3) innervate the skin.

b. Subcutaneous tissue: includes the previously described skin nerve branches and the greater saphenous vein.

c. Sartorius and gracilis muscles: the needle is passed between the sartorius and gracilis muscles. The branches from the femoral nerve containing fibers from the second and third lumbar nerves (L2, L3) innervate the sartorius muscle. The branches from the obturator nerve containing fibers from the third and fourth lumbar nerves (L3, L4) innervate the gracilis muscle. The needle is passed between the posterior margin of the sartorius muscle and the gracilis muscle.

d. Adductor magnus muscle: the muscle is located lateral to the sartorius and gracilis muscles. The branches from the tibial nerve containing fibers from the fourth and fifth lumbar nerves (L4, L5) innervate the muscle.

e. Saphenous nerve and femoral artery and vein: the femoral nerve gives rise to the saphenous nerve. The femoral artery is a branch of the external iliac artery.

Functions

Removes Heat from the Liver, tonifies the function of the Kidney, reduces fever and clears the channels.

Clinical indications

Lower back, shoulder and lower extremities spasm and numbness, dysmenorrhea, irregular menstruation, endometritis, vaginal inflammation, eczema of the external genital region, infertility, nocturnal emission, enuresis, impotence.

14.

(HSIYANGKUAN) XIYANGGUAN, GB 33, FOOT SHAO YANG GALLBLADDER MERIDIAN

Location

In a seated position with the knee flexed, the point is located on the lateral thigh between the iliotibial tract and the tendon of the biceps femoris 3 inches above Yanglingquan [GB 34] and lateral to Dubi [ST 35]; or at the same height of the superior margin of the patella, the point is located in the fossa of the lateral epicondyle of the femur.

Needle and moxibustion method

Perpendicular insertion 0.8–1.2 inches.
— *Needle sensation:* local soreness and distension radiating to the medial thigh.
— *Moxibustion dosage:* 3–5 cones; stick 10 minutes.

Cross-sectional anatomy of the needle passage

a. Skin: the branches from the lateral femoral cutaneous nerve containing fibers from the third lumbar nerve (L3) innervate the skin.

b. Subcutaneous tissue: includes the previously described skin nerve branches.

c. Iliotibial tract and the tendon of the biceps muscles: the needle is passed between the iliotibial tract and the tendon of the biceps muscles. The branches from the tibial nerve containing fibers from the fifth lumbar to second sacral nerves (L5, S1, S2) and the common peroneal nerve containing fibers from the fifth lumbar to second sacral nerves (L5, S1, S2) innervate the long and short head of the biceps femoris muscle.

d. Lateral superior genicular artery and vein: the lateral superior genicular artery, together with the lateral superior genicular vein, is a branch of the descending branch of the lateral femoral circumflex artery.

Functions

Reduces fever and dispels Wind, and activates the collaterals to alleviate pain.

Clinical indications

Knee joint pain and swelling, leg numbness, rheumatoid arthritis, sciatic nerve pain, vomiting.

15.

(YINSHIH) YINSHI, ST 33, FOOT YANG MING STOMACH MERIDIAN

Location

In a seated position with the knee flexed, the point is located on the anterior thigh 3 inches above the lateral superior margin of the patella, or at the midpoint between Futu [ST 32] and the lateral superior patella, on the line connecting the anterior superior iliac spine and the lateral patella.

Needle and moxibustion method

Perpendicular insertion 0.7–1.0 inch.
— *Needle sensation:* local soreness and distension.
— *Moxibustion dosage:* 3–5 cones; stick 15 minutes.

Cross-sectional anatomy of the needle passage

a. Skin: the branches from the anterior femoral cutaneous nerve containing fibers from the third lumbar nerve (L3) and the lateral femoral cutaneous nerve containing fibers from the third lumbar nerve (L3) innervate the skin.

b. Subcutaneous tissue: includes the previously described skin nerve branches.

c. *Vastus lateralis and vastus femoris muscles:* both muscles are part of the quadriceps muscle. The branches from the femoral nerve containing fibers from the second to fourth lumbar nerves (L2, L3, L4) innervate both muscles. The needle is passed between the vastus lateralis and vastus femoris muscles.

d. *Descending branch of the lateral circumflex artery:* the artery is a branch of the lateral femoral circumflex artery.

Functions

Expels Wind and removes Dampness, and strengthens the function of the Stomach to nourish Yin.

Clinical indications

Atrophy and palsy of the lower extremities, pelvic pain, beriberi, edema, ascites, diabetes mellitus.

16.

(XUEHAI) XUEHAI, SP 10, FOOT TAI YIN SPLEEN MERIDIAN

Location

In a seated position with the knee flexed, the point is located on the anterior inferior medial thigh, at the protrusion of the vastus medialis muscle, and 2 inches above the medial superior margin of the patella; or put the palm on the patient's knee, the middle finger on the lateral thigh and the thumb on the medial thigh at about 45°. The point is located at the tip of the thumb.

Needle and moxibustion method

Perpendicular insertion 1.0–2.0 inches.
— *Needle sensation:* local soreness and distension, sometimes radiating to the knee region.
— *Moxibustion dosage:* 3–5 cones; stick 5–15 minutes.

Cross-sectional anatomy of the needle passage
(Fig. 2.8)

a. *Skin:* the branches from the anterior femoral cutaneous nerve containing fibers from the third lumbar nerve (L3) innervate the skin.

b. *Subcutaneous tissue:* includes the previously described skin nerve branches.

c. *Vastus medialis muscle:* one of the quadriceps muscles. The branches from the femoral nerve containing fibers from the second to fourth lumbar nerves (L2, L3, L4) innervate the muscle.

d. The needle is inserted anterior and medial to the femur.

Functions

Regulates the flow of Qi and Blood circulation, and regulates the function of the Lower Jiao (Lower Burner).

Clinical indications

Urticaria, skin itching, endometritis, orchitis, neuritis, anemia, uterine bleeding, dysmenorrhea.

17.

(LIANGCHIU) LIANGQIU, ST 34, FOOT YANG MING STOMACH MERIDIAN, CLEFT POINT

Location

In a supine or seated position with the knee flexed, the point is located 2 inches above the lateral superior margin of the patella, between the rectus femoris and vastus lateralis muscles, directly above Dubi [ST 35].

Needle and moxibustion method

Perpendicular insertion 1.0–1.5 inches.
— *Needle sensation:* local soreness and distension, radiating to the knee joint.
— *Moxibustion dosage:* 3–5 cones; stick 5–15 minutes.

Cross-sectional anatomy of the needle passage
(Fig. 2.8)

a. *Skin:* the branches from the anterior and lateral femoral cutaneous nerves containing fibers from the second lumbar nerve (L2) innervate the skin.

b. *Subcutaneous tissue:* includes the previously described skin nerve branches.

c. The needle is passed between the rectus femoris and vastus lateralis muscles. The branches from the femoral nerve containing fibers from the second to fourth lumbar nerves (L2, L3, L4) innervate both muscles.

d. *The descending branch of the lateral femoral circumflex artery, together with the lateral femoral circumflex vein, and the femoral nerve:* the needle is inserted between these structures to the deeper layers.

e. *Tendon of vastus medialis muscle:* one of the quadriceps muscles. The branches from the femoral nerve containing fibers from the second to fourth lumbar nerves (L2, L3, L4) innervate the muscle. This muscle is located at the deeper layer of the rectus femoris muscle.

f. *Lateral collateral tendon of knee joint:* the vastus intermedialis muscular branches of the femoral nerve containing fibers from the second to fourth lumbar nerves (L2, L3, L4) innervate the tendon.

g. *Femur:* the major component of this area is tendon, which is a thin connective tissue. The needle is inserted about 1 inch anterior and lateral to the distal femur.

Functions

Regulates the function of the Stomach Qi, relaxes the muscles and activates the collaterals.

Clinical indications

Mastitis, numbness of the lower extremities, arthritis of the knee joint, gastritis.

18.

(FUSHI) FUXI, BL 38, FOOT TAI YANG BLADDER MERIDIAN

Location

In a prone position, the point is located in the lateral popliteal fossa 1 inch above Weiyang [BL 39] (Weiyang is located 1 inch lateral to Weichong [BL 40], and medial to the tendon of the biceps femoris muscle).

Needle and moxibustion method

Perpendicular insertion 0.5–1.0 inch.
— *Needle sensation:* local numbness and distension radiating distally.
— *Moxibustion dosage:* 3–7 cones; stick 10 minutes.

Cross-sectional anatomy of the needle passage

a. *Skin:* the branches from the posterior femoral cutaneous nerve containing fibers from the second sacral nerve (S2) innervate the skin.
b. *Subcutaneous tissue:* includes the previously described skin nerve branches.
c. *Tendon of biceps femoris muscle:* the needle is passed medial to the tendon of the biceps femoris muscle. The branches from the tibial nerve containing fibers from the fifth lumbar to second sacral nerves (L5,

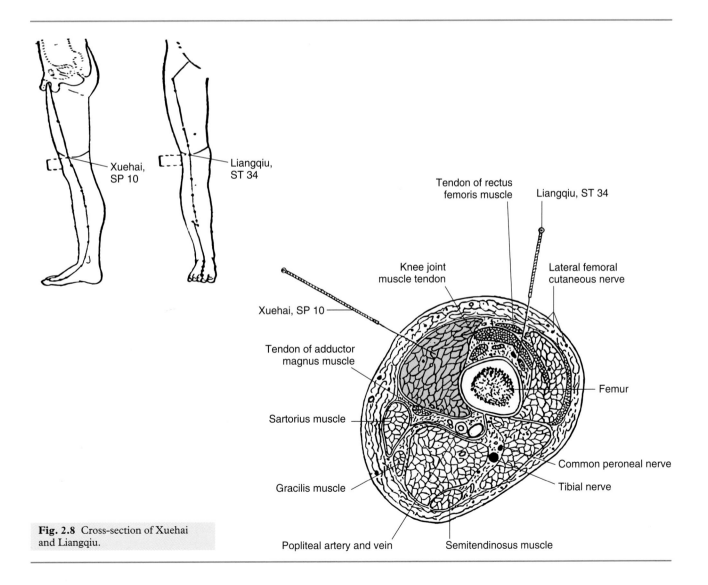

Fig. 2.8 Cross-section of Xuehai and Liangqiu.

S1, S2) and the common peroneal nerve containing fibers from the fifth lumbar to second sacral nerves (L5, S1, S2) innervate the long head and short head of the biceps femoris muscles, respectively.

d. *Common peroneal nerve:* the needle is passed medial to the common peroneal nerve, which is a branch of the sciatic nerve.

e. *Lateral superior genicular artery:* the femoral artery gives rise to the lateral superior genicular artery.

Functions
Clears and activates the channels and collaterals, and relieves rigidity of the muscles, tendons and joints.

Clinical indications
Constipation, acute gastritis, thigh numbness, cystitis, numbness of the lower extremities, sciatic nerve pain, local spasm.

19.
(CHUCHUAN) QUQUAN, LIV 8, FOOT JUE YIN LIVER MERIDIAN, CONVERGING POINT

Location
In a seated or prone position with the knee flexed, the point is located on the medial aspect of the thigh in the fossa on the medial side of the popliteal skin crease, between the medial epicondyle of the femur and the tendon of the semimembranosus.

Needle and moxibustion method
Perpendicular insertion 1.0–1.5 inches.
— *Needle sensation:* local soreness and distension.
— *Moxibustion dosage:* 3–5 cones; stick 5–15 minutes.

Cross-sectional anatomy of the needle passage
(Fig. 2.9)
a. *Skin:* the branches from the obturator cutaneous nerve and the saphenous nerve containing fibers

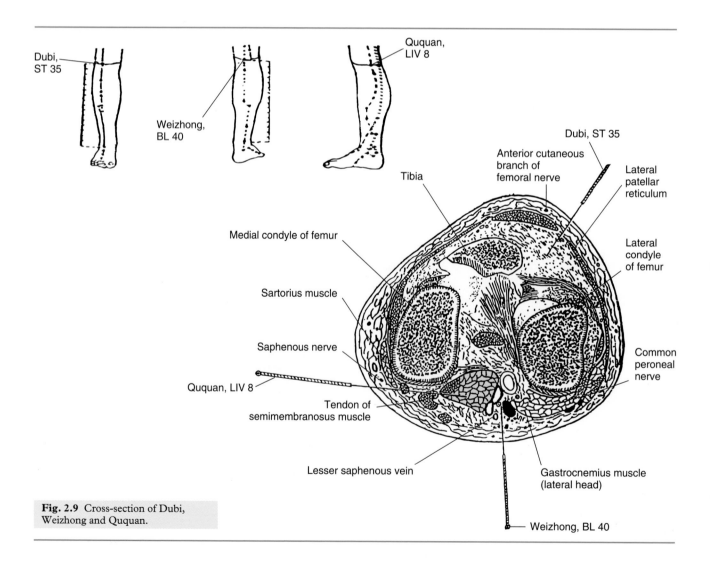

Fig. 2.9 Cross-section of Dubi, Weizhong and Ququan.

from the fourth lumbar nerve (L4) innervate the skin.

b. *Subcutaneous tissue:* includes the previously described skin nerve branches and the greater saphenous vein.

c. *Sartorius muscle:* the needle is passed posterior to the sartorius muscle. The branches from the femoral nerve containing fibers from the second and third lumbar nerves (L2, L3) innervate the muscle.

d. *Tendon of the gracilis muscle:* the tendon is located in the inner layer of the sartorius muscle. The needle is passed posterior to the tendon of the gracilis muscle. The branches from the obturator nerve containing fibers from the third and fourth lumbar nerves (L3, L4) innervate the muscle.

e. *Semimembranosus muscle:* the muscle is located medial and posterior to the tendon of the gracilis muscle. The needle is passed anterior to the semimembranosus muscle. The branches from the tibial nerve containing fibers from the fifth lumbar to second sacral nerves (L5, S1, S2) innervate the muscle.

f. *Medial head of gastrocnemius muscle:* the muscle originates from the medial condyle of the femur. The needle is inserted into the muscle. The branches from the tibial nerve containing fibers from the first and second sacral nerves (S1, S2) innervate the muscle.

g. The needle is inserted 2 inches into the medial head of the gastrocnemius muscle. The needle may contact the popliteal artery, popliteal vein and the tibial nerve at the popliteal fossa.

Functions
Reinforces the function of the Liver, tonifies the function of the Kidney, reduces Heat and removes Dampness.

Clinical indications
Uterine prolapse, dysmenorrhea, irregular menstruation, infertility, pelvic pain, hernia pain, hemorrhoids, prostate inflammation, knee joint pain, schizophrenia, hysteria, liver cirrhosis, enteritis, dysentery.

20.
(TUPI) DUBI, ST 35, FOOT YANG MING STOMACH MERIDIAN

Location
With the knee flexed at 90°, the point is located at the inferior margin of the patella in the fossa lateral to the tendon of the patella.

Needle and moxibustion method
Perpendicular insertion: in a slightly medial direction, 1.5–2.0 inches.
— *Needle sensation:* local soreness and distension, sometimes radiating inferiorly.

Oblique insertion: from the lateral fossa to the medial fossa of the patella 2.0–2.5 inches.
— *Needle sensation:* local soreness and distension.
— *Moxibustion dosage:* 3–5 cones; stick 5–15 minutes.

Cross-sectional anatomy of the needle passage
(Fig. 2.9)

a. *Skin:* the branches from the lateral sural cutaneous nerve and the lateral femoral cutaneous nerve containing fibers from the third lumbar nerve (L3) innervate the skin.

b. *Subcutaneous tissue:* includes the previously described skin nerve branches.

c. The needle is passed between the patellar ligament and the lateral patellar retinaculum, through the knee joint bursa, into the lateral meniscus.

d. If the needle is passed through the lateral meniscus and synovial membrane, it may puncture the knee joint. WARNING: A carefully sterilized needle is necessary, or it may cause knee joint infection.

e. If the needle is inserted from the lateral fossa to the medial fossa, it may be passed posterior to the patellar ligament. It is very easy to penetrate, because the structures consist of the loose connective tissue, the adipose tissue and the suprapatellar skin follicles.

Functions
Clears and activates the channels and collaterals, dispels Cold and relieves pain.

Clinical indications
Beriberi, edema, knee joint pain and numbness, rheumatoid arthritis, jaundice, Achilles tendon pain, vomiting.

21.
(WEICHUNG) WEIZHONG, BL 40, FOOT TAI YANG BLADDER MERIDIAN, CONVERGING POINT

Location
In a prone position, the point is located in the middle of the skin crease of the popliteal fossa, at the midpoint between the tendons of the biceps femoris and the semitendinosus muscles.

Needle and moxibustion method

Perpendicular insertion 0.5–1.0 inch.
— *Needle sensation:* local soreness and distension, and electrical sensation radiating to the foot.

Use a triangular needle to induce bleeding (treating acute lumbar sprain).
— *Moxibustion dosage:* 3–5 cones; stick 3–5 minutes.

Cross-sectional anatomy of the needle passage

(Fig. 2.9)

a. *Skin:* the branches from the posterior cutaneous nerve containing fibers from the second sacral nerve (S2) innervate the skin.
b. *Subcutaneous tissue:* includes the previously described skin nerve branches and the lesser saphenous vein.
c. The needle is passed between the medial head and lateral head of the gastrocnemius muscle. The branches from the femoral nerve containing fibers from the first and second sacral nerves (S1, S2) innervate the muscle.
d. *Proximal part of the medial sural cutaneous nerve:* the tibial nerve gives rise to the medial sural cutaneous nerve, together with the small saphenous vein, to the posterior part of the leg.
e. *Tibial nerve:* the tibial nerve contains fibers from the fourth lumbar to third sacral nerves (L4, L5, S1, S2, S3) and is one of the two branches of the sciatic nerve. The points are located on the medial side of the tibial nerve. If the needle is inserted into the point, a strong electrical sensation will radiate to the foot.
f. Deep needling can contact the popliteal artery and vein. The popliteal vein is at the superficial part of the popliteal artery. The popliteal vein joins the femoral vein at the adductor hiatus. Both popliteal artery and vein are medium size vessels. To avoid possible laceration of the vessels, don't insert the needle deeply without proper care.

Functions

Relaxes rigidity and pain of the lumbar and knee joints, and removes pathogenic Heat from the Blood.

Clinical indications

Common cold, lower back pain, acute lumbar sprain, sciatic nerve pain, knee joint pain, heat stroke, cerebro-vascular accident, convulsions, erysipelas.

22.

(WEIYANG) WEIYANG, BL 39, FOOT TAI YANG BLADDER MERIDIAN

Location

In a prone position, the point is located on the lateral side of the skin crease of the popliteal fossa, 1 inch lateral to Weizhong [BL 40], and medial to the tendon of the biceps femoris muscle.

Needle and moxibustion method

Perpendicular insertion 0.5–1.0 inch.
— *Needle sensation:* local soreness and distension radiating to the upper thigh.
— *Moxibustion dosage:* 3–7 cones; stick 10 minutes.

Cross-sectional anatomy of the needle passage

a. *Skin:* the branches from the medial sural cutaneous nerve containing fibers from the second sacral nerve (S2) innervate the skin.
b. *Subcutaneous tissue:* includes the previously described skin nerve branches.
c. *Tendon of biceps femoris muscle:* the needle is passed medial to the tendon of the biceps femoris muscle. The branches from the tibial nerve containing fibers from the fifth lumbar to second sacral nerves (L5, S1, S2) and the common peroneal containing fibers from the fifth lumbar to second sacral nerves (L5, S1, S2) innervate the long head and short head respectively of the biceps femoris muscle.
d. *Common peroneal nerve:* the needle is passed medial to the common peroneal nerve, which is a branch of the sciatic nerve.
e. *Lateral superior genicular artery and vein:* the femoral artery gives rise to the lateral superior genicular artery.

Functions

Dredges the channels and regulates the Blood circulation, reduces Heat and removes Dampness.

Clinical indications

Abdominal distension, ascites, hemorrhoids, lower back pain, convulsions.

23.

(YINKU) YINGU, KI 10, FOOT SHAO YIN KIDNEY MERIDIAN, CONVERGING POINT

Location

In a seated or prone position with the knee flexed, the point is located at the medial end of the skin crease of the popliteal fossa between the tendons of the semimembranosus and semitendinosus muscles, or at the midpoint between Ququan [LIV 8] and Weizhong [BL 40].

Needle and moxibustion method
Perpendicular insertion 0.8–1.0 inch.
— *Needle sensation:* local soreness and distension.
— *Moxibustion dosage:* 3–5 cones; stick 10 minutes.

Cross-sectional anatomy of the needle passage
a. *Skin:* the branches from the obturator cutaneous nerve containing fibers from the third lumbar nerve (L3) innervate the skin.
b. *Subcutaneous tissue:* includes the previously described skin nerve branches and the greater saphenous vein.
c. *Tendon of semimembranosus and semitendinosus muscles:* the branches from the tibial nerve containing fibers from the fifth lumbar and first sacral nerves (L5, S1) innervate both muscles.
d. *Gastrocnemius muscle, medial head:* the needle is inserted into the muscle. The branches from the tibial nerve containing fibers from the first and second sacral nerves (S1, S2) innervate the muscle.
e. *Posterior cruciate ligament:* the needle may be inserted to the posterior part of the cruciate ligament and a strong resistance will be felt.

Functions
Tonifies the function of the Kidney, reduces Heat, and regulates the flow of Qi to alleviate pain.

Clinical indications
Impotence, knee arthritis, gonorrhea, penile pain, vaginitis, inflammation of labia major, uterine bleeding, convulsion, schizophrenia.

24.
(YINLINGCHUAN) YINLINGQUAN, SP 9, FOOT TAI YIN SPLEEN MERIDIAN, CONVERGING POINT

Location
In a seated or prone position, the point is located on the medial side of the knee, in the fossa inferior to the medial condyle of the tibia, at the same height as the inferior margin of the tibial tuberosity, at the insertion of the sartorius muscle and opposite Yanglingquan [GB 34].

Needle and moxibustion method
Along the border posterior of the tibia, perpendicular insertion 1.0–3.0 inches.
— *Needle sensation:* local soreness and distension,

radiating to the sole of the foot.
— *Moxibustion dosage:* 3–5 cones; stick 5-15 minutes.

Cross-sectional anatomy of the needle passage
(Fig. 2.10)
a. *Skin:* the branches from the obturator cutaneous nerve containing fibers from the third lumbar nerve (L3) innervate the skin.
b. *Subcutaneous tissue:* includes the previously described skin nerve branches and the greater saphenous vein.
c. *Semitendinosus muscle:* the branches from the sciatic nerve containing fibers from the fifth lumbar and first sacral nerves (L5, S1) innervate the muscle.
d. *Gastrocnemius muscle medial head:* the muscle originates from the posterior medial condyle of the femur. The branches from the tibial nerve containing fibers from the first and second sacral nerves (S1, S2) innervate the muscle.
e. The needle is passed posterior to the tendon of the semimembranosus muscle. The insertion of the semimembranosus muscle is the posterior medial condyle of the tibia.
f. If the needle is inserted 2 inches deep into the popliteal fossa, it may contact the tibial nerve, popliteal artery and popliteal vein.

Functions
Reduces fever and removes Dampness, and regulates the function of San Jiao (Triple Warmer).

Clinical indications
Ascites, abdominal distension, urine retention, urinary tract infection, dysmenorrhea, nephritis, beriberi, impotence, rheumatic arthritis, rheumatoid arthritis, knee joint sprain, numbness of the lower extremities.

25.
(YANGLINGCHUAN) YANGLINGQUAN, GB 34, FOOT SHAO YANG GALLBLADDER MERIDIAN, CONVERGING POINT

Location
In a seated or prone position with the knee half flexed, the point is located in the fossa anterior and inferior to the head of the fibula.

Needle and moxibustion method
Perpendicular insertion along the posterior margin of the femur in an oblique inferior direction 1.0–3.0 inches.
— *Needle sensation:* local soreness and distension radiating inferiorly.
Perpendicular insertion along the posterior margin of the fibula in a horizontal direction penetrating to Yinglingquan [SP 9] 3 inches.

— *Needle sensation:* soreness and distension of the whole knee.

Oblique insertion in a posterior inferior oblique direction 1.0–2.0 inches.

— *Needle sensation:* electrical sensation radiating to the posterior leg.

— *Moxibustion dosage:* 3–5 cones; stick 5–15 minutes.

Cross-sectional anatomy of the needle passage
(Fig. 2.10)

a. *Skin:* the branches from the lateral sural cutaneous nerve containing fibers from the fifth lumbar nerve (L5) innervate the skin.

b. *Subcutaneous tissue:* includes the previously described skin nerve branches.

c. *Tibialis anterior muscle:* the branches from the deep peroneal nerve containing fibers from the fourth lumbar to first sacral nerves (L4, L5, S1) innervate the muscle.

d. *Extensor digitorum longus muscle:* at the medial side of the tibialis anterior muscle. The branches from the deep peroneal nerve containing fibers from the fourth lumbar to first sacral nerves (L4, L5, S1) innervate the muscle.

f. *Fibulotibial joint:* the needle is horizontally inserted to the fibulotibial joint, and a strong needle resistance is felt. The needle is directed inferiorly to penetrate through the interosseous membrane into Yinglingquan [SP 9].

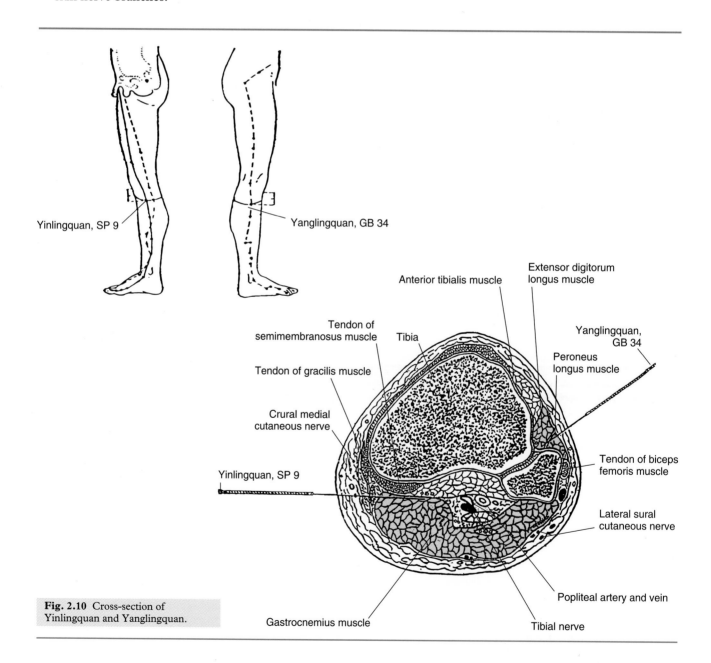

Fig. 2.10 Cross-section of Yinlingquan and Yanglingquan.

Functions

Dispels Wind and removes Dampness, strengthens the bone and reinforces the muscles and tendons.

Clinical indications

Hepatitis, cholecystitis, vomiting, habitual constipation, beriberi, facial edema, hypertension, lower extremities paralysis and numbness, pleurisy, knee joint and surrounding tissue disease.

26.

(HSIKUAN) XIGUAN, LIV 7, FOOT JUE YIN LIVER MERIDIAN

Location

In a seated or supine position and flexing the knee, the point is located 2 inches below Xiyan [EX-LE 5], and 1 inch posterior and slightly superior to Yinlingquan [SP 9].

Needle and moxibustion method

Perpendicular insertion 0.5–0.8 inch.
— *Needle sensation:* local soreness and distension.
— *Moxibustion dosage:* 3–5 cones; stick 10 minutes.

Cross-sectional anatomy of the needle passage

a. *Skin:* the branches from the saphenous nerve containing fibers from the third and fourth lumbar nerves (L3, L4) innervate the skin.
b. *Subcutaneous tissue:* includes the previously described skin nerve branches and the greater saphenous vein.
c. *Soleus muscle:* the needle is passed into the medial head of the soleus muscle. The branches from the tibial nerve containing fibers from the fifth lumbar to second sacral nerves (L5, S1, S2) innervate the muscle.
d. *Flexor digitorum longus muscle:* the muscle is attached to the posterior tibia. The branches from the tibial nerve containing fibers from the fifth lumbar and first sacral nerves (L5, S1) innervate the muscle.
e. *Tibial nerve, posterior tibial artery and posterior tibial vein:* the deep layer of the point is the tibial nerve, posterior tibial artery and posterior tibial vein. The popliteal artery gives rise to the posterior tibial artery. The tibial nerve is a branch of the sciatic nerve.

Functions

Dispels Wind to remove numbness, and relieves stiffness and tension of the muscles, tendons and joints.

Clinical indications

Rheumatoid arthritis, gout, hemiplegia, sore throat, knee joint arthritis, tonsillitis.

27.

(HOYANG) HEYANG, BL 55, FOOT TAI YANG BLADDER MERIDIAN

Location

In a prone position, the point is located 2 inches below Weizhong [BL 40], and between the medial and lateral heads of the gastrocnemius muscle.

Needle and moxibustion method

Perpendicular insertion 1.0–1.5 inches.
— *Needle sensation:* local soreness and distension radiating to the foot.
— *Moxibustion dosage:* 3–5 cones; stick 15 minutes.

Cross-sectional anatomy of the needle passage

a. *Skin:* the branches from the medial sural cutaneous nerve containing fibers from the second sacral nerve (S2) innervate the skin.
b. *Subcutaneous tissue:* includes the previously described skin nerve branches and the lesser saphenous vein.
c. *Gastrocnemius muscle:* the needle is passed between the medial and lateral heads of the gastrocnemius muscle. The branches from the femoral nerve containing fibers from the first and second sacral nerves (S1, S2) innervate the muscle.
d. *Soleus muscle:* the branches from the tibial nerve containing fibers from the fifth lumbar to second sacral nerves (L5, S1, S2) innervate the muscle.
e. *Tibial nerve:* the tibial nerve contains fibers from the fourth lumbar to third sacral nerves (L4, L5, S1, S2, S3) and is one of two branches of the sciatic nerve. The point is located on the medial side of the tibial nerve. If the needle is punctured into the nerve, a strong electrical sensation radiates to the foot.
f. Deep needling may contact the popliteal artery and vein. To avoid lacerating the vessels, do not lift and thrust the needle without proper care.

Functions

Removes Heat and eliminates Dampness by diuresis, strengthens the function of the Kidney and regulates menstruation.

Clinical indications

Lower back pain, hemorrhoids, hernia pain, orchitis, emission, impotence, endometritis.

28.

(TSUSANLI) ZUSANLI, ST 36, FOOT YANG MING STOMACH MERIDIAN, CONVERGING POINT

Location

With a flexed knee or in a supine position, ask the patient put the thumb on the middle of the patella with the remaining four fingers closed together and placed on the lateral side of the patella. The point is located at the tip of the middle finger. Alternative method: the point is located in the fossa 1 finger breadth lateral to the anterior margin of the tibia, and 3 inches inferior to Dubi [ST 35].

Needle and moxibustion method

Perpendicular insertion slightly towards the tibia 1.0–2.0 inches.
—*Needle sensation:* electric sensation radiating to the dorsum of the foot.

Oblique insertion in an inferior direction 2.0–3.0 inches.
— *Needle sensation:* soreness and distension radiating to the dorsum of the foot, sometimes to the knee.
— *Moxibustion dosage:* 5–15 cones; stick 10-30 minutes.

Cross-sectional anatomy of the needle passage
(Fig. 2.11)

a. *Skin:* the lateral sural cutaneous branches of the common popliteal nerve containing fibers from the fifth lumbar nerve (L5) innervate the skin.
b. *Subcutaneous nerve:* includes the previously described skin nerve branches.
c. *Tibialis anterior muscle:* the muscle is the anterior compartment of the leg muscle. The branches from the deep peroneal nerve containing fibers of the fourth lumbar to first sacral nerves (L4, L5, S1) innervate the muscle.
d. If the needle is punctured slightly laterally, it will be inserted into the anterior tibial artery and vein.
e. *Interosseous membrane:* the strong fibrous tissue is connected to the medial crest of the fibula and the interosseous margin of the tibia. The branches from the deep peroneal nerve innervate the anterior part of the interosseous membrane. The branches from the tibial nerve innervate the posterior part of the interosseous membrane.
f. *Tibialis posterior muscle:* the muscle runs posterior to the interosseous membrane, and lies between flexor hallucis longus and flexor digitorum longus muscles. The branches from the tibial nerve containing fibers from the fifth lumbar and first sacral nerves (L5, S1) innervate the muscle.

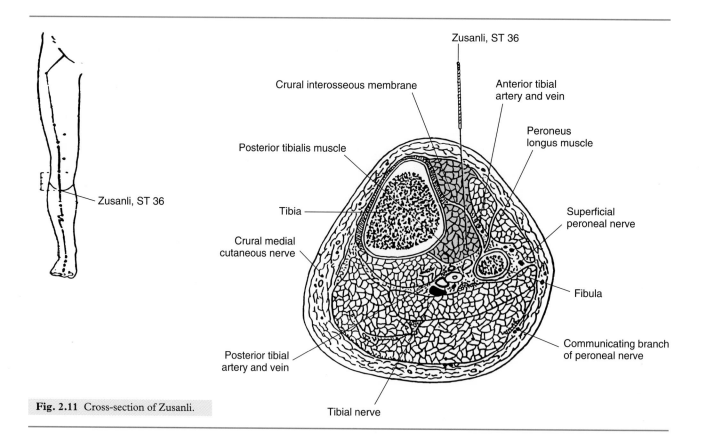

Fig. 2.11 Cross-section of Zusanli.

g. *Tibial nerve, posterior tibial artery and posterior tibial vein:* if the needle is inserted slightly medially 2 inches deep, it may penetrate into the previously described structures.

Functions

Strengthens and regulates the functions of the Spleen and Stomach, strengthens the body's resistance and restores the normal function of the body.

Clinical indications

Acute and chronic gastritis, stomach cramp, peptic ulcer, acute pancreatitis, hemiplegia, shock, anemia, allergic disease, jaundice, hypertension, epilepsy, asthma, neurosis, fever, beriberi, headache.

29.

(TANNANGXUE) DANNANGXUE, EX-LE 6, EXTRA POINT OF THE LOWER EXTREMITIES

Location

In a seated or lateral recumbent position, the point is located 1 inch below Yanglingquan [GB 34], or the point in the area of the most obvious pressure pain when cholecystitis is present.

Needle and moxibustion method

Perpendicular insertion 1.0–2.0 inches.
— *Needle sensation:* soreness and distension radiating down the leg.

Cross-sectional anatomy of the needle passage

(Fig. 2.12)
a. *Skin:* the branches from the lateral sural cutaneous nerve containing fibers from the fifth lumbar nerve (L5) innervate the skin.
b. *Subcutaneous tissue:* includes the previously described skin nerve branches.
c. *Peroneus longus muscle:* the branches from the superficial peroneal nerve containing fibers from the fourth lumbar to first sacral nerves (L4, L5, S1) innervate the muscle.
d. The needle is passed on the posterior side of the deep peroneal nerve, the anterior tibial artery and the anterior tibial vein. The deep peroneal nerve is one of the two branches of the common peroneal nerve. The needle may be inserted into these structures.
e. If the needle is inserted deeper, it may be passed through the interosseous membrane into the tibialis posterior muscle.

Clinical indications

Acute and chronic cholecystitis, gallstones, gallbladder ascariasis, pleurisy, atrophy of the lower extremities.

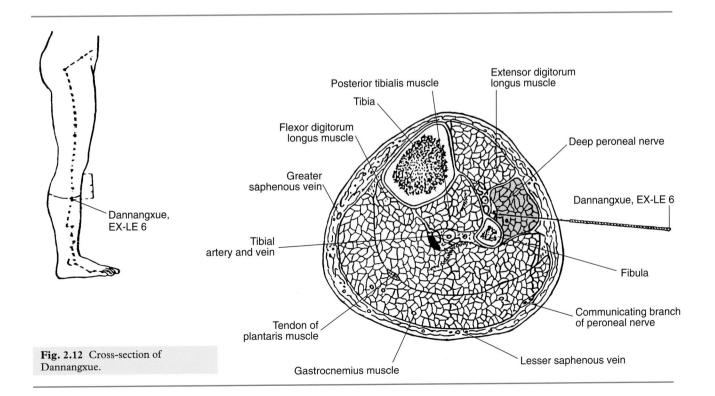

Fig. 2.12 Cross-section of Dannangxue.

30.

(LANWEIXUE) LANWEIXUE, EX-LE 7, EXTRA POINT OF THE LOWER EXTREMITIES

Location
In a seated or supine position with the knee flexed, the point is located 2 inches below Zusanli [ST 36], and at the point of the most obvious pressure pain when appendicitis occurs.

Needle and moxibustion method
Perpendicular insertion 1.5–2.0 inches.
— *Needle sensation:* distension and soreness radiating to the dorsal foot.

Cross-sectional anatomy of the needle passage
(Fig. 2.13)
a. *Skin:* the branches from the lateral sural cutaneous nerve containing fibers from the fifth lumbar nerve (L5) innervate the skin.
b. *Subcutaneous tissue:* includes the previously described skin nerve branches.
c. *Tibialis anterior muscle:* the branches from the deep peroneal nerve containing fibers from the fourth and fifth lumbar nerves (L4, L5) innervate the muscle. The needle is inserted at the lateral part of the muscle.
d. The needle is passed medial to the deep peroneal nerve, the anterior tibial artery and the anterior tibial vein. If the needle is inserted into the deep peroneal nerve, an electrical sensation radiates to the dorsal foot.
e. *Interosseous membrane:* the strong fibrous tissue is connected to the tibia and fibula. The branches from the deep peroneal nerve innervate the anterior part of the interosseous membrane. The branches from the tibial nerve innervate the posterior part.
f. *Tibialis posterior muscle:* the needle is passed through the interosseous membrane into the muscle. The branches from the tibial nerve containing fibers from the fifth lumbar and first sacral nerves (L5, S1) innervate the muscle.

Clinical indications
Acute and chronic appendicitis, epigastric pain, indigestion, paralysis of the lower extremities.

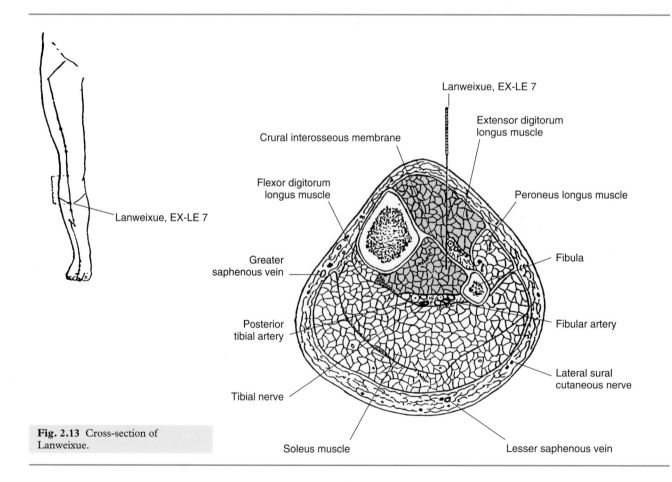

Lanweixue, EX-LE 7

Extensor digitorum longus muscle

Crural interosseous membrane

Flexor digitorum longus muscle

Peroneus longus muscle

Lanweixue, EX-LE 7

Greater saphenous vein

Fibula

Posterior tibial artery

Fibular artery

Lateral sural cutaneous nerve

Tibial nerve

Fig. 2.13 Cross-section of Lanweixue.

Soleus muscle

Lesser saphenous vein

31.

(CHENGCHIN) CHENGJIN, BL 56, FOOT TAI YANG BLADDER MERIDIAN

Location

In a prone position, the point is located 5 inches below the middle of the skin crease of the popliteal fossa, at the midpoint between Heyang [BL 55] and Chengshan [BL 57] 5 inches below Weizhong [BL 40].

Needle and moxibustion method

Perpendicular insertion 1.0–2.0 inches.
— *Needle sensation:* local soreness and distension radiating to the foot.
— *Moxibustion dosage:* 3–5 cones; stick 15 minutes.

Cross-sectional anatomy of the needle passage

a. *Skin:* the branches from the sural nerve containing fibers from the first and second sacral nerve (S1, S2) innervate the skin.
b. *Subcutaneous tissue:* includes the previously described skin nerve branches and the lesser saphenous vein.
c. *Gastrocnemius muscle:* the branches from the femoral nerve containing fibers from the first and second sacral nerves (S1, S2) innervate the muscle.
d. *Soleus muscle:* the branches from the tibial nerve containing fibers from the fifth lumbar to second sacral nerves (L5, S1, S2) innervate the muscle.
e. *Tibial nerve and posterior peroneal artery and vein:* the needle is passed to the medial side of the tibial nerve, the posterior peroneal artery and the posterior peroneal vein. If the needle is punctured into the nerve, a strong electrical sensation will radiate to the foot. The posterior peroneal artery is a branch of the popliteal artery. Avoid puncturing the needle into the artery.

Functions

Relieves rigidity of the muscles and tendons, promotes Blood circulation, and reduces Heat and resolves swelling.

Clinical indications

Lower back spasm, constipation, hemorrhoids, leg numbness, convulsion, dizziness, epistaxis, enteritis, constipation, hemorrhoids.

32.

(TICHI) DIJI, SP 8, FOOT TAI YIN SPLEEN MERIDIAN, CLEFT POINT

Location

In a seated or supine position, on the medial side of the leg on the posterior margin of the tibia. Draw a line between Yinlingquan [SP 9] and the medial malleolus of the tibia and the point is located 3 inches below Yinlingquan [SP 9], or 5 inches below the kneejoint.

Needle and moxibustion method

Perpendicular insertion 1.0–1.5 inches.
— *Needle sensation:* local soreness and distension radiating distally.
— *Moxibustion dosage:* 3–5 cones; stick 15 minutes.

Cross-sectional anatomy of the needle passage

a. *Skin:* the branches from the saphenous nerve containing fibers from the third and fourth lumbar nerves (L3, L4) innervate the skin.
b. *Subcutaneous tissue:* includes the previously described skin nerve branches and the greater saphenous vein.
c. *Soleus muscle:* the needle is passed between the soleus muscle and the posterior tibial nerve. The branches from the tibial nerve containing fibers from the fifth lumbar to second sacral nerves (L5, S1, S2) innervate the soleus muscle.
d. *Flexor digitorum longus muscle:* the branches from the tibial nerve containing fibers from the fifth lumbar to second sacral nerves (L5, S1, S2) innervate the muscle.
e. *Tibial nerve, posterior tibial artery and posterior tibial vein:* the popliteal artery gives rise to the posterior tibial artery. The tibial nerve is a branch of the sciatic nerve.

Functions

Regulates the functions of the Spleen, treats Blood disorders, and regulates the function of the uterus.

Clinical indications

Abdominal distension, lower back pain, ascites, hemorrhoids, hernia, dysmenorrhea, premature ejaculation.

33.

(SHANGSHUHSU) SHANGJUXU, ST 37, FOOT YANG MING STOMACH MERIDIAN

Location

In a seated or prone position, the point is located 6 inches below the knee, in the fossa one finger width lateral to the tibia on the tibialis anterior muscle between the tibia and fibula. Alternative method: the point is located 3 inches below Zusanli [ST 36].

Needle and moxibustion method
Perpendicular insertion 0.5–1.2 inches.
— *Needle sensation:* local soreness and distension, or electrical sensation radiating to the dorsum of the foot.
   Oblique insertion 0.5–1.2 inches.
— *Needle sensation:* soreness and numbness radiating to the dorsum of the foot or to the knee.
— *Moxibustion dosage:* 3–7 cones; stick 5–20 minutes.

Cross-sectional anatomy of the needle passage
(Fig. 2.14)
a. *Skin:* the branches of the lateral sural subcutaneous nerve containing fibers from the fifth lumbar nerve (L5) innervate the skin.
b. *Subcutaneous tissue:* includes the previously described skin nerve branches.
c. *Tibialis anterior muscle:* the muscle is in the anterior crural compartment. The branches from the deep peroneal nerve containing fibers from the fourth lumbar to first sacral nerves (L4, L5, S1) innervate the muscle.
d. The needle passes on the medial side of the deep peroneal nerve, the anterior tibial artery and the anterior tibial vein. The deep peroneal nerve is one of two branches of the common peroneal nerve, running along the anterior interosseous membrane together with the anterior tibial artery and vein to the dorsal foot. If the needle is inserted into the nerve, an electrical sensation radiates to the dorsum of the foot.
e. *Interosseous membrane:* the interosseous membrane is connected to the tibia and fibula. The branches from the deep peroneal nerve innervate the anterior part of the interosseous membrane and the branches from the tibial nerve innervate the posterior part.
f. *Tibialis posterior muscle:* the muscle is located posteriorly to the interosseous membrane. The branches from the tibial nerve containing fibers from the fifth lumbar and first sacral nerves (L5, S1) innervate the muscle.

Functions
Regulates the function of the Spleen and Stomach, dredges the channels and regulates the flow of Qi.

Clinical indications
Abdominal distension, abdominal pain, appendicitis, diarrhea, gastritis, beriberi, knee pain, back pain, hemiplegia.

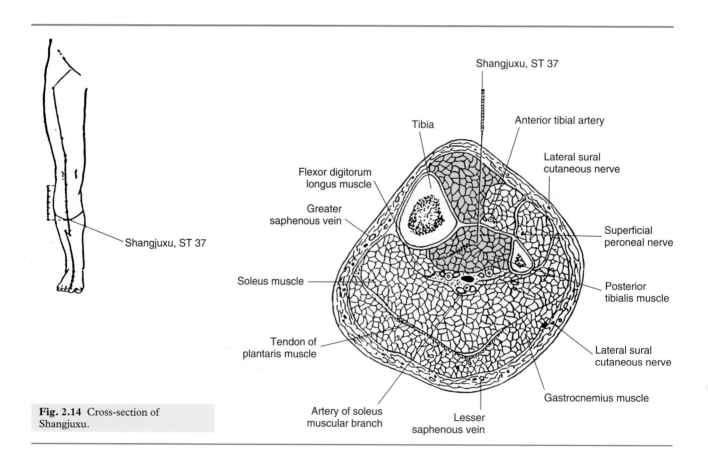

Fig. 2.14 Cross-section of Shangjuxu.

34.

(CHUNGTU) ZHONGDU, LIV 6, FOOT JUE YIN LIVER MERIDIAN, CLEFT POINT

Location

In a seated or supine position, the point is located on the medial aspect of the leg 7 inches above the medial malleolus, beside the medial border of the tibia.

Needle and moxibustion method

Perpendicular insertion 0.3–0.5 inch.
— *Needle sensation:* local soreness and distension radiating distally.
— *Moxibustion dosage:* 3 cones.

Cross-sectional anatomy of the needle passage

a. *Skin:* the branches from the saphenous nerve containing fibers from the third lumbar nerve (L3) innervate the skin.
b. *Subcutaneous tissue:* includes the previously described skin nerve branches and the greater saphenous vein.
c. *Soleus muscle:* the muscle is located posterior to the flexor digitorum longus and tibialis posterior muscles. The branches from the tibial nerve containing fibers from the fifth lumbar to second sacral nerves (L5, S1, S2) innervate the muscle.
d. *Flexor digitorum longus muscle:* the muscle is attached to the medial posterior part of the tibia. The branches from the tibial nerve containing fibers from the fifth lumbar and first sacral nerves (L5, S1) innervate the muscle.
e. *Tibialis posterior muscle:* the muscle is located at the medial side of the flexor digitorum longus muscle, posterior tibial muscle and interosseous membrane. The branches from the tibial nerve containing fibers from the fifth lumbar and first sacral nerves (L5, S1) innervate the muscle.

Functions

Reinforces the function of the Liver, strengthens the function of the Kidney, and reduces Heat and Dampness.

Clinical indications

Abdominal pain, pelvic pain, poliomyelitis, uterine prolapse, hernia.

35.

(FENGLUNG) FENGLONG, ST 40, FOOT YANG MING STOMACH MERIDIAN, CONNECTING POINT

Location

The point is located at the midpoint between the inferior margin of the patella and the skin crease of the ankle joint, 1.5 inches lateral to the anterior margin of the tibia, and between the tibia and fibula; or 8 inches above the lateral malleolus and one finger's breadth lateral to Tiaokuo [ST 38].

Needle and moxibustion method

Perpendicular insertion 1.0–1.5 inches.
— *Needle sensation:* soreness and distension radiating up to the thigh and down to the lateral malleolus.
— *Moxibustion dosage:* 5–7 cones; stick 5–10 minutes.

Cross-sectional anatomy of the needle passage

(Fig. 2.15)
a. *Skin:* the branches from the lateral sural cutaneous nerve containing fibers from the fifth lumbar nerve (L5) innervate the skin.
b. *Subcutaneous tissue:* includes the previously described skin nerve branches.
c. *Extensor digitorum longus muscle:* the branches from the deep peroneal nerve containing fibers from the fourth lumbar to first sacral nerves (L4, L5, S1) innervate the muscle.
d. *Extensor hallucis longus muscle:* the branches from the deep peroneal nerve containing fibers from the fourth lumbar to first sacral nerves (L4, L5, S1) innervate the muscle.
e. *Interosseous membrane:* the needle is passed from the anterior compartment muscles through the interosseous membrane to the posterior compartment muscles.
f. *Tibialis posterior muscle:* the branches from the tibial nerve containing fibers from the fifth lumbar to first sacral nerves (L5, S1) innervate the muscle.

Functions

Regulates the function of the Spleen to remove Dampness, and regulates the function of the Stomach to resolve Phlegm.

Clinical indications

Cough, sputum, headache, dizziness, beriberi, edema of the extremities, menopause, postpartum hemorrhage, shoulder tendinitis, hysteria, schizophrenia, convulsions.

36.

(CHENGSHAN) CHENGSHAN, BL 57, FOOT TAI YANG BLADDER MERIDIAN

Location

In a seated or prone position, the point is located directly below the belly of the gastrocnemius muscle which produces a reverse V shape when fully extending the foot. Or 8 inches below Weizhong [BL 40] on the line connecting Weizhong with the tendon calcaneus.

Needle and moxibustion method

Perpendicular insertion 1.0–2.5 inches.
— *Needle sensation:* local soreness or radiating to the popliteal fossa. On deep insertion an electric sensation radiates to the sole of the foot.
— *Moxibustion dosage:* 3–5 cones; stick 5–15 minutes.

Cross-sectional anatomy of the needle passage (Fig. 2.15)

a. *Skin:* the branches from the medial sural cutaneous nerve containing fibers from the fourth lumbar nerve (L4) innervate the skin.
b. *Subcutaneous tissue:* includes the previously described skin nerve branches and the lesser saphenous vein.
c. *Gastrocnemius muscle:* the branches from the tibial nerve from the first and second sacral nerves (S1, S2) innervate the muscle.
d. *Soleus muscle:* the muscle, together with the gastrocnemius muscle, forms the triceps muscle of the leg, located at the deep layer of the gastrocnemius muscle. The branches of the tibial nerve containing fibers from the first and second sacral nerves (S1, S2) innervate the muscle.
e. *Tibial nerve:* the nerve is located at the deep layer of the point. If the needle is inserted into the nerve, an electrical sensation will radiate to the heel of the foot.

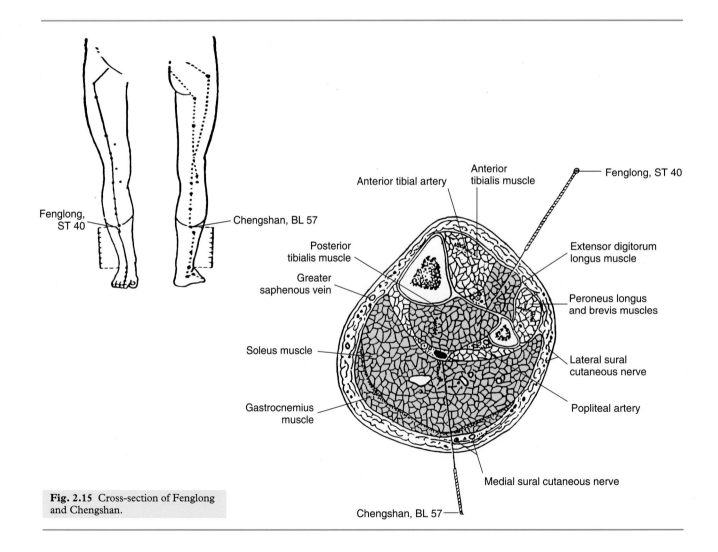

Fig. 2.15 Cross-section of Fenglong and Chengshan.

Functions

Relieves rigidity of the muscles and tendons, removes Heat from the Blood, and regulates the function of the Intestine to treat hemorrhoids.

Clinical indications

Back pain, sciatic pain, gastrocnemius muscle spasm, paralysis of the lower extremities, hemorrhoids, anal prolapse, infantile convulsions, epistaxis, tonsillitis, constipation.

37.

(TIAOKOU) TIAOKOU, ST 38, FOOT YANG MING STOMACH MERIDIAN

Location

In a seated or supine position, the point is located 8 inches below Dubi [ST 35], at the midpoint between Dubi [ST 35] and Jiexi [ST 41] between the tibia and fibula, one finger breadth lateral to the anterior tibial crest.

Needle and moxibustion method

Perpendicular insertion 0.7–1.0 inch.
— *Needle sensation:* local soreness and distension, or an electrical sensation radiating to the dorsum of the foot.
— *Moxibustion dosage:* 3–5 cones; stick 15 minutes.

Cross-sectional anatomy of the needle passage

a. *Skin:* the branches from the lateral sural cutaneous nerve containing fibers from the fifth lumbar nerve (L5) innervate the skin.
b. *Subcutaneous nerve:* includes the previously described skin nerve branches.
c. *Tibialis anterior muscle:* the muscle is in the anterior crural compartment. The branches from the deep peroneal nerve containing fibers from the fourth lumbar to first sacral nerves (L4, L5, S1) innervate the muscle.
d. The needle is passed to the medial side of the deep peroneal nerve, the anterior tibial artery and the anterior tibial vein. The deep peroneal nerve running along the anterior interosseous membrane and passing together with the anterior tibial artery and vein to the dorsum of the foot, is one of two branches of the common peroneal nerve. If the needle punctures the nerve, an electrical sensation will radiate to the dorsum of the foot.
e. *Interosseous membrane:* the membrane is connected to the tibia and fibula. The branches from the deep peroneal nerve innervate the anterior part of the interosseous membrane, and branches from the tibial nerve innervate the posterior part.

Functions

Promotes the Blood circulation to dredge the channels, and regulates the flow of Qi to alleviate pain.

Clinical indications

Palsy of the lower extremities, knee arthritis, beriberi, tonsillitis, convulsions, schizophrenia, hysteria, gastritis, enteritis, hepatitis, shoulder pain.

38.

(FEIYANG) FEIYANG, BL 58, FOOT TAI YANG BLADDER MERIDIAN, CONNECTING POINT

Location

In a seated or prone position, the point is located 7 inches above Kunlun [BL 60], or 1 inch lateral and inferior to Chengshan [BL 57].

Needle and moxibustion method

Perpendicular insertion 0.7–1.0 inch.
— *Needle sensation:* local soreness and distension radiating to the foot.
— *Moxibustion dosage:* 3–7 cones; stick 10 minutes.

Cross-sectional anatomy of the needle passage

a. *Skin:* the branches from the lateral sural cutaneous nerve containing fibers from the first sacral nerve (S1) innervate the skin.
b. *Subcutaneous tissue:* includes the previously described skin nerve branches.
c. *Gastrocnemius muscle:* the branches of the tibial nerve from the first and second sacral nerves (S1, S2) innervate the muscle.
d. *Soleus muscle:* the muscle is located at the deep layer of the gastrocnemius muscle. The branches from the tibial nerve containing fibers from the first and second sacral nerves (S1, S2) innervate the muscle.
e. *Peroneal artery and vein:* the popliteal artery gives rise to the peroneal artery.

Functions

Clears the collaterals to alleviate pain, removes Heat and expels Wind.

Clinical indications

Convulsions, schizophrenia, headache, dizziness, nasal obstruction, epistaxis, gout, edema and pain of the lower extremities, rheumatoid arthritis, hemorrhoids.

39.

(HSIACHUSHU) XIAJUXU, ST 39, FOOT YANG MING STOMACH MERIDIAN

Location
In a seated or supine position, the point is located 9 inches below Dubi [ST 35], 1 inch below Tiaokou [ST 38] one finger breadth lateral to the anterior tibial crest.

Needle and moxibustion method
Perpendicular insertion 0.5–1.5 inches.
— *Needle sensation:* local soreness and distension radiating to the dorsum of the foot.
— *Moxibustion dosage:* 7–15 cones; stick 15 minutes.

Cross-sectional anatomy of the needle passage
a. *Skin:* the branches from the lateral sural cutaneous nerve containing fibers from the fifth lumbar nerve (L5) innervate the skin.
b. *Subcutaneous tissue:* includes the previously described skin nerve branches.
c. *Tibialis anterior and extensor digitorum muscles:* the needle is inserted between the tibialis anterior and extensor digitorum longus muscles. The branches from the deep peroneal nerve containing fibers from the fourth and fifth lumbar nerves (L4, L5) innervate both muscles.
d. *Extensor hallucis longus muscle:* the branches from the deep peroneal nerve containing fibers from the fourth lumbar to first sacral nerves (L4, L5, S1) innervate the muscle.
e. *Deep peroneal nerve, anterior tibial artery and anterior tibial vein:* the needle is inserted to the lateral side of the deep peroneal nerve, the anterior tibial artery and the anterior tibial vein. The common peroneal nerve gives rise to the deep peroneal nerve.
f. *Interosseous membrane:* the membrane is connected to the tibia and fibula. The branches from the peroneal nerve innervate the anterior part of the interosseous membrane.

Functions
Regulates the function of the Intestines and Stomach, reduces Heat and removes Dampness.

Clinical indications
Pelvic pain, mastitis, palsy of the lower extremities, knee joint arthritis, anemia, beriberi, rheumatoid arthritis, diarrhea, convulsions.

40.

(WAICHIU) WAIQIU, GB 36, FOOT SHAO YANG GALLBLADDER MERIDIAN, CLEFT POINT

Location
In a seated position with the knee flexed, the point is located on the lateral aspect of the leg 7 inches above the lateral malleolus of the fibula and on the anterior margin of the fibula.

Needle and moxibustion method
Perpendicular insertion 0.7–1.0 inch.
— *Needle sensation:* local soreness and distension radiating to the dorsum of the foot.
— *Moxibustion dosage:* 3–7 cones; stick 15 minutes.

Cross-sectional anatomy of the needle passage
a. *Skin:* the branches from the lateral sural cutaneous nerve containing fibers from the first sacral nerve (S1) innervate the skin.
b. *Subcutaneous tissue:* includes the previously described skin nerve branches.
c. *Peroneus longus and brevis muscles:* the branches from the superficial peroneal nerve containing fibers from the fifth lumbar and first sacral nerves (L5, S1) innervate both muscles.
d. *Superficial peroneal nerve:* the common peroneal nerve gives rise to the superficial peroneal nerve.
e. *Extensor digitorum longus and extensor hallucis longus muscles:* the branches from the deep peroneal nerve containing fibers from the fourth lumbar to first sacral nerves (L4, L5, S1) innervate both muscles.
f. *Deep peroneal nerve, anterior tibial artery and anterior tibial vein:* the deep peroneal nerve is a branch of the common peroneal nerve. The popliteal artery gives rise to the anterior tibial artery.

Functions
Removes Heat from the Liver, regulates the flow of Qi, and dispels Wind to activate the collaterals.

Clinical indications
Neck stiffness, leg pain, chest pain, beriberi, convulsions, common cold.

41.

(YANGCHIAO) YANGJIAO, GB 35, FOOT SHAO YANG GALLBLADDER MERIDIAN

Location
In a seated position with the knee flexed, the point is located on the lateral aspect of the leg 7 inches above

the lateral malleolus of the fibula, on the posterior margin of the fibula.

Needle and moxibustion method

Perpendicular insertion 0.5–0.8 inch.
— *Needle sensation:* local soreness and distension radiating distally.
— *Moxibustion dosage:* 5–7 cones; stick 15 minutes.

Cross-sectional anatomy of the needle passage

a. *Skin:* the branches from the lateral sural cutaneous nerve containing fibers from the fifth lumbar nerve (L5) innervate the skin.
b. *Subcutaneous tissue:* includes the previously described skin nerve branches.
c. *Peroneus longus muscle:* the needle is passed posterior to the peroneus longus muscle. The branches of the superficial peroneal nerve from the fourth lumbar to first sacral nerves (L4, L5, S1) innervate the muscle.
d. *Soleus muscle:* the branches from the tibial nerve containing fibers from the fifth lumbar to first sacral nerves (L5, S1) innervate the muscle.
e. *Flexor hallucis longus muscle:* the branches from the tibial nerve containing fibers from the fifth lumbar to first sacral nerves (L5, S1) innervate the muscle.
f. *Peroneal artery and vein:* the popliteal artery gives rise to the peroneal artery.

Functions

Relieves rigidity of the muscles, tendons and joints, prevents convulsions and relieves mental anxiety.

Clinical indications

Palsy of the lower extremities, pleurisy, beriberi, facial edema, knee joint pain and numbness, convulsions, hysteria, schizophrenia.

42.

(LOUKU) LOUGU, SP 7, FOOT TAI YIN SPLEEN MERIDIAN

Location

In a seated or supine position, the point is located 6 inches above the medial malleolus of the tibia, 3 inches above Sanyinjiao [SP 6], at the posterior to the medial margin of the tibia.

Needle and moxibustion method

Perpendicular insertion 0.5–1.0 inch.
— *Needle sensation:* local soreness and distension radiating distally.
— *Moxibustion dosage:* 3–5 cones; stick 10 minutes.

Cross-sectional anatomy of the needle passage

a. *Skin:* the branches from the saphenous nerve containing fibers from the fourth lumbar nerve (L4) innervate the skin.
b. *Subcutaneous tissue:* includes the previously described skin nerve branches and the greater saphenous vein.
c. *Soleus muscle and tibia:* the needle is passed between the soleus muscle and the tibia. The branches from the tibial nerve containing fibers from the fifth lumbar to second sacral nerves (L5, S1, S2) innervate the soleus muscle.
d. *Flexor digitorum longus muscle:* the muscle is located at the deep layer of the soleus muscle. The branches from the tibial nerve containing fibers from the fifth lumbar to second sacral nerves (L5, S1, S2) innervate the muscle.
e. *Tibial nerve and posterior tibial artery and vein:* the popliteal artery gives rise to the posterior tibial artery. The tibial nerve is a branch of the sciatic nerve.

Functions

Regulates the function of the Liver and Kidney, and strengthens the function of the Spleen to remove Dampness.

Clinical indications

Abdominal distension, hysteria, cystitis, nephritis, enuresis, nocturnal emission, beriberi, leg palsy, ankle distension and pain.

43.

(LIKOU) LIGOU, LIV 5, FOOT JUE YIN LIVER MERIDIAN, CONNECTING POINT

Location

In a seated or supine position, the point is located 5 inches above the medial malleolus. Using the hand to push the medial gastrocnemius muscle, a fossa at the posterior margin of the tibia will appear, within which is Ligou [LIV 5].

Needle and moxibustion method

Perpendicular insertion along the posterior margin of the tibia 0.5–1.0 inch.
— *Needle sensation:* local soreness and distension.
   Oblique insertion in a superior oblique direction along the posterior margin of the tibia 1.5–2.5 inches (treating diseases of the trunk).
— *Needle sensation:* soreness and distension radiating proximally or, with vigorous twisting of the needle, a

strong numbness and swollen sensation radiating to the knee or the external genital region.
— *Moxibustion dosage:* 1–3 cones; stick 3–5 minutes.

Cross-sectional anatomy of the needle passage
(Fig. 2.16)

a. *Skin:* the branches from the saphenous nerve containing fibers from the fourth lumbar nerve (L4) innervate the skin.
b. *Subcutaneous tissue:* includes the previously described skin nerve branches and the greater saphenous vein.
c. *Flexor digitorum longus muscle:* the muscle is attached to the medial posterior margin of the tibia. The branches from the tibial nerve containing fibers from the fifth lumbar and first sacral nerves (L5, S1) innervate the muscle.
d. If the needle is inserted posteriorly into the tibia, a strong resistance will be felt.
e. *Tibialis posterior muscle:* the muscle is located at the medial side of the flexor digitorum longus muscle, and the posterior side of the tibia and interosseous membrane. The branches from the tibial nerve containing fibers from the fifth lumbar and first sacral nerves (L5, S1) innervate the muscle.
f. If the needle is inserted in an oblique superior direction, it will pass through the flexor digitorum longus muscle and penetrate to Lougu [SP 7].

Functions
Removes Heat from the Liver and regulates the flow of Qi, regulates menstruation and stops leukorrhea.

Clinical indications
Pelvic inflammatory disease, dysmenorrhea, premature ejaculation, impotence, orchitis.

44.

(CHUPIN) ZHUBIN, KI 9, FOOT SHAO YIN KIDNEY MERIDIAN

Location
In a seated or supine position, the point is located 5 inches above the medial malleolus of the tibia, on the line between Taixi [KI 3] and Yingu [KI 10], at the inferior part of the medial side of the gastrocnemius muscle; or 5 inches above Taixi (KI 3).

Needle and moxibustion method
Perpendicular insertion 0.5–1.0 inch.
— *Needle sensation:* local soreness and distension, or electrical sensation radiating to the sole of the foot.
— *Moxibustion dosage:* 3–5 cones; stick 10–15 minutes.

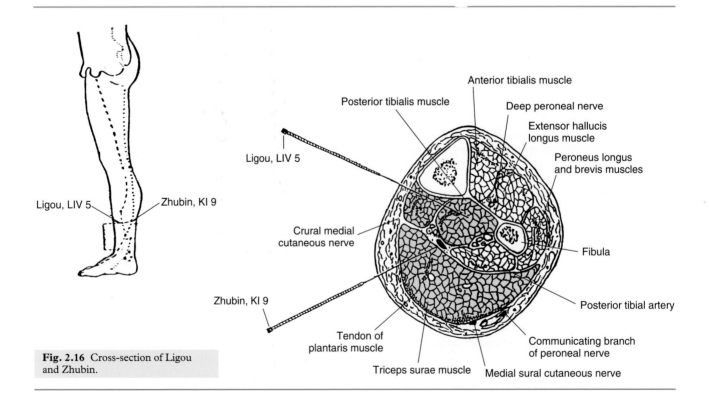

Fig. 2.16 Cross-section of Ligou and Zhubin.

Ligou, LIV 5

Zhubin, KI 9

Ligou, LIV 5

Zhubin, KI 9

Anterior tibialis muscle

Posterior tibialis muscle

Deep peroneal nerve

Extensor hallucis longus muscle

Peroneus longus and brevis muscles

Crural medial cutaneous nerve

Fibula

Posterior tibial artery

Tendon of plantaris muscle

Communicating branch of peroneal nerve

Triceps surae muscle

Medial sural cutaneous nerve

Cross-sectional anatomy of the needle passage
(Fig. 2.16)

a. *Skin:* the branches from the saphenous nerve containing fibers from the fourth lumbar nerve (L4) innervate the skin.

b. *Subcutaneous tissue:* includes the previously described skin nerve branches.

c. *Triceps muscle of calf:* consists of the gastrocnemius and soleus muscles. The branches from the tibial nerve containing fibers from the first and second sacral nerves (S1, S2) innervate these muscles.

d. *Tibial nerve:* one of two branches of the sciatic nerve. The posterior tibial artery and vein are located anterior to the tibial nerve. The posterior tibial artery is a branch of the popliteal artery. The posterior tibial vein joins the popliteal vein.

Functions
Strengthens the function of the Liver, tonifies the function of the Kidney, reduces Heat and induces diuresis.

Clinical indications
Epilepsy, convulsions, schizophrenia, gastritis, enteritis, cystitis, hernia pain, orchitis, medial leg pain.

d. *Superficial peroneal nerve:* the common peroneal nerve gives rise to the superficial peroneal nerve.

e. *Extensor digitorum longus and extensor hallucis longus muscles:* the branches from the deep peroneal nerve containing fibers from the fourth lumbar to first sacral nerves (L4, L5, S1) innervate both muscles.

f. *Interosseous membrane:* the branches from the deep peroneal nerve innervate the anterior part of the interosseous membrane, and the branches from the tibial nerve innervate the posterior part.

g. *Posterior tibialis muscle:* the branches from the tibial nerve containing fibers from the fifth lumbar and first sacral nerves (L5, S1) innervate the muscle.

h. *Tibial nerve and posterior tibial artery and vein:* if the needle is punctured through the interosseous membrane and the tibialis muscle, it will reach the tibial nerve and the posterior tibial artery and vein.

Functions
Clears away Heat from the Gallbladder to improve visual acuity, and dispels Wind and removes Dampness.

Clinical indications
Beriberi, knee joint pain, atrophy and numbness of the lower extremities, eye pain, convulsions, common cold, night blindness, myopia, optic neuritis, glaucoma.

45.

(KUANGMING) GUANGMING, GB 37, FOOT SHAO YANG GALLBLADDER MERIDIAN, CONNECTING POINT

Location
In a seated position, the point is located on the lateral side of the leg, on the anterior margin of the fibula 5 inches above the lateral malleolus of the fibula and 2 inches below Waiqiu [GB 36].

Needle and moxibustion method
Perpendicular insertion 0.7–1.0 inch.
— *Needle sensation:* local soreness and distension, radiating to the lateral aspect of the dorsum of the foot.
— *Moxibustion dosage:* 3–5 cones; stick 15 minutes.

Cross-sectional anatomy of the needle passage
a. *Skin:* the branches from the lateral sural cutaneous nerve containing fibers from the first sacral nerve (S1) innervate the skin.

b. *Subcutaneous tissue:* includes the previously described skin nerve branches.

c. *Peroneus longus and brevis muscles:* the branches from the superficial peroneal nerve containing fibers from the fifth lumbar and first sacral nerves (L5, S1) innervate both muscles.

46.

(YANGFU) YANGFU, GB 38, FOOT SHAO YANG GALLBLADDER MERIDIAN, RIVER POINT

Location
In a seated position, the point is located 4 inches above the lateral malleolus, at the anterior margin of the fibula.

Needle and moxibustion method
Perpendicular insertion 0.3–0.5 inch.
— *Needle sensation:* local soreness and distension radiating distally.
— *Moxibustion dosage:* 3–7 cones; stick 15 minutes.

Cross-sectional anatomy of the needle passage
(Fig. 2.17)

a. *Skin:* the branches from the lateral sural cutaneous nerve containing fibers from the first sacral nerve (S1) innervate the skin.

b. *Subcutaneous tissue:* includes the previously described skin nerve branches.

c. *Superficial peroneal nerve:* the common peroneal nerve gives rise to the superficial peroneal nerve.

d. *Extensor digitorum longus and extensor hallucis longus*

muscles: the branches from the deep peroneal nerve containing fibers from the fourth lumbar to second sacral nerves (L4, L5, S1, S2) innervate both muscles.

e. *Interosseous membrane:* the branches from the deep peroneal nerve innervate the anterior part of the interosseous membrane and the branches from the tibial nerve innervate the posterior part.

f. *Peroneal artery and vein:* located between the interosseous membrane and the extensor digitorum longus muscle. The peroneal artery, together with the peroneal vein, are branches of the posterior tibial artery.

Functions
Strengthens the muscles and tendons and activates the collaterals, reduces fever and dispels Wind.

Clinical indications
Migraine, axillary pain, knee joint pain, sciatic nerve pain, beriberi, tonsillitis, glaucoma.

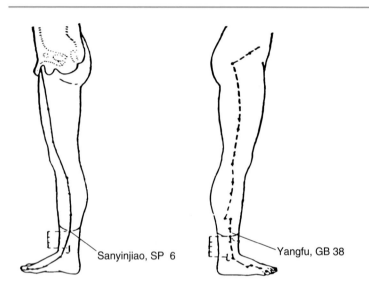

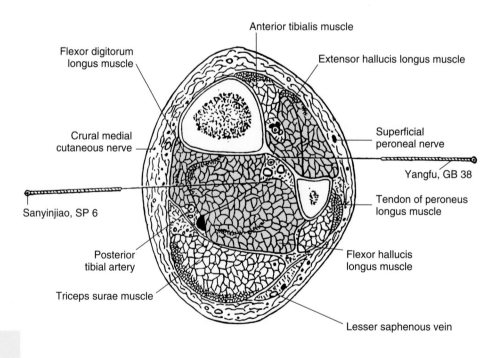

Fig. 2.17 Cross-section of Sanyinjiao and Yangfu.

47.

(SANYINJIAO) SANYINJIAO, SP 6, FOOT TAI YIN SPLEEN MERIDIAN

Location
In a seated or supine position, the point is located 3 inches or four finger widths above the medial malleolus, in the fossa posterior to the medial margin of the tibia, on a line drawn from the medial malleolus to Yinglingquan (SP 9).

Needle and moxibustion method
Perpendicular insertion: penetration to Xuanzhong [GB 39] 1.5–2.0 inches.
— *Needle sensation:* local soreness and distension.
   Perpendicular insertion: slightly posterior oblique direction 1.0–1.5 inches (treating foot disease).
— *Needle sensation:* an electrical sensation radiating to the sole of the foot.
   Oblique insertion: superior direction along the posterior tibia 1.5–2.5 inches (treating trunk disease).
— *Needle sensation:* local soreness and distension radiating proximally; with vigorous twisting of the needle, the numbness and distension radiate to the knee joint and the medial thigh.
— *Moxibustion dosage:* 3–7 cones; stick 10–20 minutes.

Cross-sectional anatomy of the needle passage
(Fig. 2.17)
a. *Skin:* the branches from the saphenous nerve containing fibers from the fourth lumbar nerve (L4) innervate the skin.
b. *Subcutaneous tissue:* includes the previously described skin nerve branches and the greater saphenous vein.
c. *Flexor digitorum longus muscle:* the branches from the tibial nerve containing fibers from the fifth lumbar and first sacral nerves (L5, S1) innervate the muscle.
d. *Posterior tibialis muscle:* the branches from the tibial nerve containing fibers from the fifth lumbar and first sacral nerves (L5, S1) innervate the muscle.
e. *Flexor hallucis longus muscle:* the muscle is located posterior and lateral to the posterior tibialis muscle. The branches from the tibial nerve containing fibers from the fifth lumbar and first sacral nerves (L5, S1) innervate the muscle.
f. If the needle is inserted perpendicularly, it will be passed through the flexor digitorum longus, flexor hallucis longus and soleus muscles, tibial artery and tibial vein, then through the interosseous membrane to the extensor hallucis longus and extensor digitorum longus muscles, and anterior tibial bone to the subcutaneous tissue.
g. If the needle is inserted in a posterior oblique direction, it can puncture the posterior tibial artery and vein, and the tibial nerve.
h. If the needle is inserted in an inferior oblique direction, it will be passed into the flexor digitorum longus and posterior tibialis muscles.

Functions
Regulates the functions of the Intestines and Stomach, removes Dampness and reduces Heat.

Clinical indications
Male and female genital organ disease, uterine bleeding, menopause, premature ejaculation, cystitis, prostatitis, urethritis, gonorrhea, pain and numbness of the lower extremities, gout, hemorrhoids, intestinal inflammatory disorder, amnesia hypochondria, hepatitis, jaundice.

48.

(FUYANG) FUYANG, BL 59, FOOT TAI YANG BLADDER MERIDIAN

Location
In a seated or prone position, the point is located 3 inches above Kunlun [BL 60] or 3 inches above the lateral malleolus of the fibula.

Needle and moxibustion method
Perpendicular insertion 0.7–1.0 inch.
— *Needle sensation:* local soreness and distension radiating to the foot.
— *Moxibustion dosage:* 3–5 cones; stick 10 minutes.

Cross-sectional anatomy of the needle passage
a. *Skin:* the branches from the lateral sural cutaneous nerve containing fibers from the first sacral nerve (S1) innervate the skin.
b. *Subcutaneous tissue:* includes the previously described skin nerve branches, the lesser saphenous vein and the peroneal nerve.
c. *Tendon calcaneus:* the needle is passed through the lateral tendon calcaneus. The branches from the tibial nerve containing fibers from the first and second sacral nerves (S1, S2) innervate the tendon.
d. *Flexor hallucis longus muscle:* the branches from the tibial nerve containing fibers from the fifth lumbar to second sacral nerves (L5, S1, S2) innervate the muscle.
e. *Peroneal artery and vein:* the popliteal artery gives rise to the peroneal artery.

Functions
Clears the collaterals to relieve rigidity of the joints, and clears away Wind Heat.

Clinical indications

Headache, lower back pain, pelvic pain, ankle pain, palsy of the lower extremities, facial neuralgia, hemorrhoids, epistaxis, hypertension, infantile convulsions.

49.

(FULIU) FULIU, KI 7, FOOT SHAO YIN KIDNEY MERIDIAN, RIVER POINT

Location

In a seated or supine position, the point is located 2 inches above Taixi [KI 3] or 2 inches above the medial malleolus of the tibia, at the anterior margin of the tendon calcaneus.

Needle and moxibustion method

Perpendicular insertion 1.0–1.5 inches.
— *Needle sensation:* local soreness and distension, or electrical sensation radiating to the foot.
— *Moxibustion dosage:* 3–7 cones; stick 5–20 minutes.

Cross-sectional anatomy of the needle passage
(Fig. 2.18)

a. *Skin:* the branches from the saphenous nerve containing fibers from the fourth lumbar nerve (L4) innervate the skin.

b. *Subcutaneous tissue:* includes the previously described skin nerve branches.

c. The needle is passed anterior to the tendon calcaneus and the plantaris tendon. The branches from the tibial nerve innervate the plantaris muscle. The tendon calcaneus is a tendon of the triceps muscle of the calf. The branches from the tibial nerve containing fibers from the first and second sacral nerves (S1, S2) innervate the triceps muscle of the calf.

d. The needle is passed posterior to the tibial nerve, artery and vein. If the needle is punctured in a slightly anterior direction, it will be inserted into the tibial nerve and an electrical sensation will radiate to the foot.

e. *Flexor hallucis longus muscle:* the branches from the tibial nerve containing fibers from the fifth lumbar to

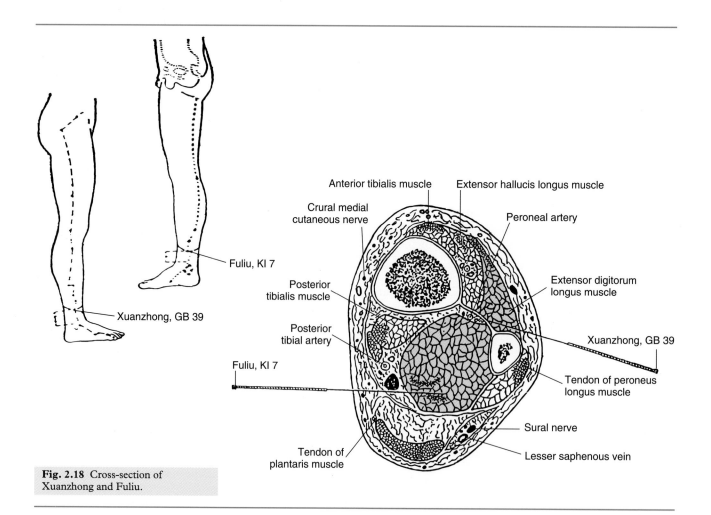

Fig. 2.18 Cross-section of Xuanzhong and Fuliu.

second sacral nerves (L5, S1, S2) innervate the muscle.

Functions
Reduces Heat and removes Dampness, tonifies the function of the Kidney and moistens dryness.

Clinical indications
Edema, cold sweating, poliomyelitis, peritonitis, gonorrhea, orchitis, lower extremities numbness, back pain, toothache, hemorrhoids.

50.
(CHIAOHSIN) JIAOXING, KI 8, FOOT SHAO YIN KIDNEY MERIDIAN

Location
In a seated or supine position, the point is located 2 inches above Taixi [KI 3], posterior to the medial margin of the tibia at the posterior margin of the flexor hallucis longus muscle; or 0.5 inch anterior to Fuliu [KI 7].

Needle and moxibustion method
Perpendicular insertion 0.5–0.7 inch.
— *Needle sensation:* local soreness and distension.
— *Moxibustion dosage:* 3–5 cones; stick 10 minutes.

Cross-sectional anatomy of the needle passage
a. *Skin:* the branches from the saphenous nerve containing fibers from the fourth lumbar nerve (L4) innervate the skin.
b. *Subcutaneous tissue:* includes the previously described skin nerve branches.
c. *Flexor digitorum longus muscle:* the branches from the tibial nerve containing fibers from the fifth lumbar to second sacral nerves (L5, S1, S2) innervate the muscle.
d. *Posterior tibialis muscle:* the branches from the tibial nerve containing fibers from the fifth lumbar and first sacral nerves (L5, S1) innervate the muscle.
e. The needle is passed posterior to the tibial nerve, artery and vein. If the needle is punctured in a slightly posterior direction, it will be passed into the tibial nerve and an electrical sensation will radiate to the foot.
f. *Flexor hallucis longus muscle:* the branches from the tibial nerve containing fibers from the fifth lumbar to second sacral nerves (L5, S1, S2) innervate the muscle.

Functions
Tonifies the function of the Kidney, regulates menstruation, reduces Heat and induces diuresis.

Clinical indications
Gonorrhea, enterocolitis, orchitis, edema, uterine prolapse, uterine bleeding, constipation, hernia.

51.
(HSUANCHIUNG) XUANZHONG, GB 39, FOOT SHAO YANG GALLBLADDER MERIDIAN

Location
In a seated or lateral recumbent position, the point is located 3 inches above the lateral malleolus of the fibula, between the posterior margin of the fibula and the tendon of the peroneus longus muscle.

Needle and moxibustion method
Perpendicular insertion penetrating to Sanyinjiao [SP 6] 1.0–2.0 inches.
— *Needle sensation:* local soreness and distension radiating distally.
— *Moxibustion dosage:* 3–5 cones; stick 5–20 minutes.

Cross-sectional anatomy of the needle passage
(Fig. 2.18)
a. *Skin:* the branches from the lateral sural cutaneous nerve containing fibers from the fifth lumbar nerve (L5) innervate the skin.
b. *Subcutaneous tissue:* includes the previously described skin nerve branches.
c. *Extensor digitorum longus muscle:* the muscle is located at the anterior lateral leg. The branches from the deep peroneal nerve containing fibers from the fourth lumbar to first sacral nerves (L4, L5, S1) innervate the muscle.
d. *Interosseous membrane:* the branches from the deep peroneal nerve containing fibers from the fourth lumbar to first sacral nerves (L4, L5, S1) innervate the anterior part of the interosseous membrane and the branches from the tibial nerve innervate the posterior part.
e. *Peroneal artery and vein:* located between the interosseous membrane and the extensor digitorum longus muscle. The peroneal artery, together with the peroneal vein, is a branch of the posterior tibial artery.

Functions
Clears and activates the channels and collaterals, strengthens the muscles and tendons and reinforces the bones.

Clinical indications
Paralysis and pain of the lower extremities, neck stiff-

ness, ankle and surrounding soft tissue disease, beriberi, tonsillitis, nephritis, rhinitis.

52.

(TAISHI) TAIXI, KI 3, FOOT SHAO YIN KIDNEY MERIDIAN, STREAM AND SOURCE POINT

Location
In a seated or supine position, the point is located in the midpoint between the posterior border of the medial malleolus and the anterior border of the tendon calcaneus.

Needle and moxibustion method
Perpendicular insertion penetrating to Kunlun [BL 60] 0.5 inch.
— *Needle sensation:* local soreness and distension.
   Perpendicular insertion slightly directed towards the medial malleolus 0.3–0.5 inch (treating plantalgia).
— *Needle sensation:* electrical numbness radiating to the sole of the foot.
— *Moxibustion dosage:* 3–5 cones; stick 5–15 minutes.

Cross-sectional anatomy of the needle passage
(Fig. 2.19)
a. *Skin:* the branches from the saphenous nerve containing fibers from the fourth lumbar nerve (L4) innervate the skin.
b. *Subcutaneous tissue:* includes the previously described skin nerve branches.
c. The needle is passed posterior to the tendons of the flexor digitorum longus and posterior tibialis muscles, and also it is passed anterior to the tendon calcaneus and the tendon of the plantaris muscle. The branches from the tibial nerve containing fibers from the fifth lumbar nerve to second sacral nerves (L5, S1, S2) innervate the muscles.
d. *Flexor hallucis longus muscle:* the branches from the tibial nerve containing fibers from the fifth lumbar to second sacral nerves (L5, S1, S2) innervate the muscle.
e. If the needle is slightly directed anteriorly and laterally, it will be inserted into the tibial nerve, the posterior tibial artery and the posterior tibial vein. An electric numbness radiating to the foot will be felt.

Functions
Nourishes Yin to reduce pathogenic empty Heat, tonifies the Kidney and restores Qi.

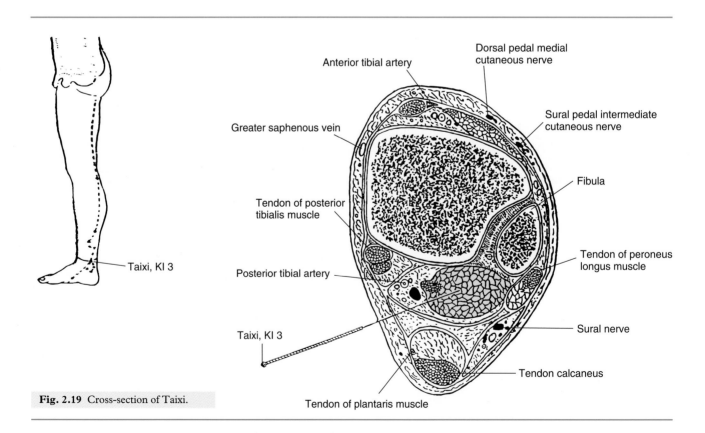

Fig. 2.19 Cross-section of Taixi.

Clinical indications

Nephritis, cystitis, dysmenorrhea, toothache, chronic throat inflammation, dizziness, emphysema, hypochondriasis, lower back pain, paralysis of the lower extremities.

53.

(TACHUNG) DAZHONG, KI 4, FOOT SHAO YIN KIDNEY MERIDIAN, CONNECTING POINT

Location

In a seated or supine position, the point is located posterior and inferior to the medial malleolus in between the Achilles tendon and the calcaneus; or 0.5 inch posterior and inferior to Taixi (KI 3).

Needle and moxibustion method

Perpendicular insertion 0.3–0.5 inch.
— *Needle sensation:* local soreness and distension.
— *Moxibustion dosage:* 3–5 cones; stick 10 minutes.

Cross-sectional anatomy of the needle passage

a. *Skin:* the branches from the saphenous nerve containing fibers from the fourth lumbar nerve (L4) innervate the skin.
b. *Subcutaneous tissue:* includes the previously described skin nerve branches.
c. *Tendon calcaneus:* the needle is passed anterior to the tendon calcaneus and posterior to the calcaneus. The branches from the tibial nerve containing fibers from the fifth lumbar to second sacral nerves (L5, S1, S2) innervate the tendon calcaneus.
d. *Medial calcaneal nerve, artery and vein:* the needle is passed posterior to the medial calcaneal nerve, artery and vein. The tibial nerve gives rise to the medial calcaneal nerve. The posterior tibial artery gives rise to the medial calcaneal artery.

Functions

Strengthens the function of the Kidney, regulates the Blood flow, and tranquilizes the mind and allays excitement.

Clinical indications

Asthma, emphysema, schizophrenia, constipation, lower back pain, dementia, hysteria, vomiting, stomatitis.

54.

(SHUICHUAN) SHUIQUAN, KI 5, FOOT SHAO YIN KIDNEY MERIDIAN, CLEFT POINT

Location

In a seated or supine position, the point is located posterior to the medial malleolus, 1 inch below Taixi [KI 3].

Needle and moxibustion method

Perpendicular insertion 0.3–0.5 inch.
— *Needle sensation:* local soreness and distension.
— *Moxibustion dosage:* 3–5 cones; stick 10 minutes.

Cross-sectional anatomy of the needle passage

a. *Skin:* the branches from the saphenous nerve containing fibers from the fourth lumbar nerve (L4) innervate the skin.
b. *Subcutaneous tissue:* includes the previously described skin nerve branches.
c. *Tendon calcaneus:* the needle is passed anterior to the tendon calcaneus. The branches from the tibial nerve containing fibers from the fifth lumbar to second sacral nerves (L5, S1, S2) innervate the tendon.
d. *Medial calcaneal nerve, artery and vein:* the needle is passed posterior to the medial calcaneal nerve, artery and vein. The tibial nerve gives rise to the medial calcaneal nerve. The posterior tibial artery gives rise to the medial calcaneal artery.

Functions

Regulates the Chong and Ren meridians, and regulates and promotes the functioning of the Lower Jiao (Lower Warmer).

Clinical indications

Dysmenorrhea, myopia, uterine prolapse, endometritis, irregular menstruation, cystitis, gonorrhea.

55.

(SHANGCHIU) SHANGQIU, SP 5, FOOT TAI YANG SPLEEN MERIDIAN, RIVER POINT

Location

In a seated or supine position, draw a straight line at the anterior margin of the medial malleolus of the tibia and another straight line at the inferior margin of the medial malleolus of the tibia, the point is located in the intersection of the two lines; or midway between the medial malleolus of the tibia and the tubercule of the navicular bone.

Needle and moxibustion method
Perpendicular insertion 0.3–0.5 inch, or horizontal insertion penetrating to Jiexi [ST 41] 1.0–1.5 inches.
— *Needle sensation:* local soreness and distension.
— *Moxibustion dosage:* 1–3 cones; stick 5–20 minutes.

Cross-sectional anatomy of the needle passage
(Fig. 2.20)
a. *Skin:* the branches from the saphenous nerve containing fibers from the fourth lumbar nerve (L4) innervate the skin.
b. *Subcutaneous tissue:* includes the previously described skin nerve branches and the greater saphenous vein.
c. *Deltoid ligament:* a triangular shaped ligament, located at the medial ankle joint. It consists of the tibionavicular, anterior tibiotalar, tibiocalcaneal and posterior tibiotalar ligaments. If the needle is inserted into the ligament, a strong resistance will be felt.
d. The needle reaches the medial malleolus of the tibia.

Functions
Regulates the function of the Intestines and Stomach, reduces fever and removes Dampness.

Clinical indications
Gastritis, indigestion, beriberi, edema, ankle and surrounding soft tissue disease, constipation, hemorrhoids, jaundice, vomiting, convulsions, hysteria.

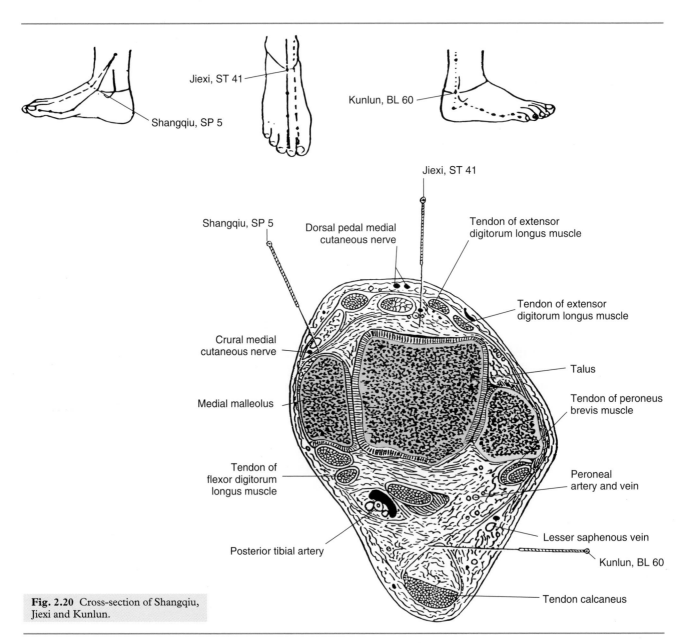

Fig. 2.20 Cross-section of Shangqiu, Jiexi and Kunlun.

56.

(CHUNGFENG) ZHONGFENG, LIV 4, FOOT JUE YIN LIVER MERIDIAN, RIVER POINT

Location
In a seated or supine position, the point is located on the medial side of the foot 1 inch anterior to the medial malleolus of the tibia, and between the tendons of the tibialis anterior and extensor hallucis longus muscles.

Needle and moxibustion method
Perpendicular insertion 0.3–0.5 inch.
— *Needle sensation:* local soreness and distension.
— *Moxibustion dosage:* 3–5 cones; stick 10 minutes.

Cross-sectional anatomy of the needle passage
a. *Skin:* the branches from the saphenous nerve containing fibers from the fourth lumbar nerve (L4) innervate the skin.
b. *Subcutaneous tissue:* includes the previously described skin nerve branches and the medial subcutaneous dorsal pedis vein.
c. *Tendons of the tibialis anterior and extensor hallucis longus muscles:* the needle is passed between the tendons of the tibialis anterior and extensor hallucis longus muscles. The branches from the deep peroneal nerve containing fibers from the fourth and fifth lumbar nerves (L4, L5) innervate both muscles.
d. *Talus:* The needle reaches the talus.

Functions
Removes Heat from the Liver and strengthens the function of the Spleen, reduces fever and removes Dampness.

Clinical indications
Cystitis, gonorrhea, jaundice, hepatitis, liver cirrhosis, nephritis, body palsy, ankle pain, lower back pain.

57.

(CHIEHHSI) JIEXI, ST 41, FOOT YANG MING STOMACH MERIDIAN, RIVER POINT

Location
In a seated or supine position, the point is located at the midpoint of the skin crease of the anterior ankle joint, and between the tendons of the extensor hallucis longus and extensor digitorum longus muscles.

Needle and moxibustion method
Perpendicular insertion to the synovial joint 0.3–0.5 inch, and bilaterally penetrating 1.0–1.5 inches.

— *Needle sensation:* local soreness and distension radiating to the anterior ankle joint.
— *Moxibustion dosage:* 1–3 cones; stick 5–10 minutes.

Cross-sectional anatomy of the needle passage
(Fig. 2.20)
a. *Skin:* the branches from the superficial peroneal nerve containing fibers from the fifth lumbar nerve (L5) innervate the skin. The needle may be inserted through the superficial peroneal nerve.
b. *Subcutaneous tissue:* includes the previously described skin nerve branches and the dorsal venous plexus.
c. *Inferior extensor reticulum:* the thickened dense connective tissue, which reinforces the tendon, is located at the anterior ankle.
d. The needle passes between the tendons of the extensor hallucis longus and extensor digitorum longus muscles. The branches from the deep peroneal nerve containing fibers from the fourth lumbar to first sacral nerves (L4, L5, S1) innervate both muscles.
e. *Deep peroneal nerve and anterior tibial artery and vein:* the deep peroneal nerve, together with the anterior tibial artery and vein to the dorsal foot, is a branch of the common peroneal nerve. The needle is inserted through the deep peroneal nerve and the anterior tibial artery and vein.
f. The point is located over the calcaneus. If the needle is inserted through the ankle joint to the calcaneus, a strong resistance will be felt.

Functions
Regulates the function of the Spleen to remove Dampness, and reduces heat to tranquilize the Mind.

Clinical indications
Ankle and surrounding soft tissue disease, paralysis of the lower extremities, facial edema, headache, dizziness, abdominal distension, constipation.

58.

(CHAOHAI) ZHAOHAI, KI 6, FOOT SHAO YIN KIDNEY MERIDIAN

Location
In a seated or supine position, the point is located in the fossa below the medial malleolus of the tibia, between the medial malleolus and the talus.

Needle and moxibustion method
Perpendicular insertion 0.3–0.5 inch.
— *Needle sensation:* local soreness and distension radiating to the leg or the foot joint.
— *Moxibustion dosage:* 3–5 cones; stick 10 minutes.

Cross-sectional anatomy of the needle passage

a. *Skin:* the branches from the saphenous nerve containing fibers from the fourth lumbar nerve (L4) innervate the skin.

b. *Subcutaneous tissue:* includes the previously described skin nerve branches.

c. *Tibial nerve and posterior tibial artery and vein:* the tibial nerve is a branch of the sciatic nerve. The posterior tibial artery is a branch of the popliteal artery.

d. *Abductor hallucis muscle:* the branches from the tibial nerve containing fibers from the fifth lumbar and first sacral nerves (L5, S1) innervate the muscle.

Functions

Strengthens the function of the Kidney, regulates the menstruation, reduces fever and relieves sore throat.

Clinical indications

Hysteria, convulsions, insomnia, tonsillitis, uterine prolapse, sore throat, cystitis, gonorrhea, irregular menstruation, constipation, rheumatic arthritis.

59.

(KUNLUN) KUNLUN, BL 60, FOOT TAI YANG BLADDER MERIDIAN, RIVER POINT

Location

In a seated or supine position, the point is located in the midpoint between the posterior margin of the lateral malleolus of the fibula and the anterior margin of the tendon calcaneus, level with the high point of the lateral malleolus.

Needle and moxibustion method

Perpendicular insertion penetrating to Taixi [KI 3] or oblique insertion, slightly laterally 0.5 inch, or penetrating to Fuyang [BL 59] 1.0–3.0 inches (treating goiter).

— *Needle sensation:* local numbness and distension radiating to the toes.

— *Moxibustion dosage:* 3–5 cones; stick 15 minutes.

Cross-sectional anatomy of the needle passage

(Fig. 2.20)

a. *Skin:* the branches from the sural nerve containing fibers from the first sacral nerve (S1) innervate the skin.

b. *Subcutaneous tissue:* includes the previously described skin nerve branches and the lesser saphenous vein.

c. The needle is passed anterior to the Achilles tendon, through tissue consisting of adipose tissue and loose connective tissue. The Achilles tendon, attached to the calcaneum, is the tendon of the gastrocnemius muscle and soleus muscle. The branches from the tibial nerve containing fibers from the fifth lumbar to second sacral nerves (L5, S1, S2) innervate these muscles. A strong needle resistance is felt if the needle penetrates into the tendon.

d. If the needle is inserted through to Taixi [KI 3], it can puncture the tibial nerve and the posterior artery and vein.

e. If the needle is inserted slightly in the anterior medial direction, it will reach the calcaneus, with a strong resistance felt.

Functions

Dredges and clears the channel Qi, strengthens the lumbar region and the function of the Kidney.

Clinical indications

Paralysis of the lower extremities, sciatic nerve pain, lower back pain, ankle and surrounding soft tissue disease, headache, dizziness, convulsions, infantile convulsions, epistaxis.

60.

(SHENMAI) SHENMAI, BL 62, FOOT TAI YANG BLADDER MERIDIAN

Location

In a seated position, the point is located in the fossa 0.5 inch inferior to the lateral malleolus of the fibula.

Needle and moxibustion method

Perpendicular insertion 0.3–0.5 inch.

— *Needle sensation:* local soreness and distension.

— *Moxibustion dosage:* 3–7 cones; stick 10 minutes.

Cross-sectional anatomy of the needle passage

a. *Skin:* the branches from the sural nerve containing fibers from the first sacral nerve (S1) innervate the skin.

b. *Subcutaneous tissue:* includes the previously described skin nerve branches.

c. *Lateral plantar artery plexus:* the lateral plantar artery gives rise to the lateral plantar artery plexus.

d. *Abductor digiti minimi muscle:* the needle is inserted at the superior margin of the muscle. The branches from the tibial nerve containing fibers from the first and second sacral nerves (S1, S2) innervate the muscle.

Functions

Promotes the Blood circulation and clears the channels, refreshes the mind and relieves mental stress.

Clinical indications

Headache, dizziness, lower back and leg pain, convulsions, amnesia, cerebrovascular disease, beriberi.

61.

(PUSHEN) PUSHEN, BL 61, FOOT TAI YANG BLADDER MERIDIAN

Location

In a seated position, the point is located 1.5 inches below Kunlun [BL 60] in the fossa of the calcaneum.

Needle and moxibustion method

Perpendicular insertion 0.3–0.5 inch.
— *Needle sensation:* local soreness and distension.
— *Moxibustion dosage:* 3–5 cones; stick 15 minutes.

Cross-sectional anatomy of the needle passage

a. *Skin:* the lateral branches from the sural nerve containing fibers from the first sacral nerve (S1) innervate the skin.
b. *Subcutaneous tissue:* includes the previously described skin nerve branches.
c. *Lateral branch of the peroneal artery and vein:* the lateral branch of the peroneal artery, together with the peroneal vein, is a branch of the peroneal artery.

Functions

Relieves rigidity of the muscles and tendons, activates the collaterals, and removes swelling to alleviate pain.

Clinical indications

Convulsions, schizophrenia, cerebral palsy, infantile convulsions, syncope, lower back pain, foot atrophy, beriberi, local muscle spasm, knee arthritis.

62.

(CHINMEN) JINMEN, BL 63, FOOT TAI YANG BLADDER MERIDIAN, CLEFT POINT

Location

In a seated position, the point is located anterior and inferior to the lateral malleolus 1 inch anterior to Shenmai [BL 62], and at the inferior fossa of the cuboid; or at the midpoint between Shenmai [BL 62] and the posterior margin of the tuberosity of the fifth metatarsal.

Needle and moxibustion method

Perpendicular insertion 0.3–0.5 inch.
— *Needle sensation:* local soreness and distension.
— *Moxibustion dosage:* 3–5 cones; stick 5–20 minutes.

Cross-sectional anatomy of the needle passage

a. *Skin:* the branches from the lateral dorsal pedis nerve containing fibers from the first sacral nerve (S1) innervate the skin.
b. *Subcutaneous tissue:* includes the previously described skin nerve branches.
c. *Tendon of peroneus longus muscle and abductor digiti minimi muscle:* the needle is passed between the tendons of the peroneus longus and abductor digiti minimi muscles. The branches from the superficial peroneal nerve containing fibers from the fifth lumbar and first sacral nerves (L5, S1) innervate the peroneus longus muscle. The branches from the tibial nerve containing fibers from the first and second sacral nerves (S1, S2) innervate the abductor digiti minimi muscle.
d. *Lateral plantar nerve, artery and vein:* the posterior tibial artery gives rise to the lateral plantar artery. The tibial nerve gives rise to the lateral plantar nerve.

Functions

Clears the channels to alleviate pain, and relieves mental stress.

Clinical indications

Convulsions, syncope, infantile convulsions, pelvic pain, dizziness, lateral ankle pain, knee pain and numbness.

63.

(CHIUHSU) QIUXU, GB 40, FOOT SHAO YANG GALLBLADDER MERIDIAN, SOURCE POINT

Location

On the dorsum of the foot, in the fossa anterior and inferior to the lateral malleolus of the fibula, and at the midpoint between Jiexi [ST 41] and the trochlear tubercle of the calcaneus. Located by drawing a vertical line at the anterior margin of the lateral malleolus of the fibula and another horizontal line at the inferior margin of the lateral malleolus, the point is located at the intersection of these two lines.

Needle and moxibustion method

Perpendicular insertion 1.0–1.5 inches.
— *Needle sensation:* local soreness and distension.
— *Moxibustion dosage:* 1–3 cones; stick 5–20 minutes.

Cross-sectional anatomy of the needle passage

(Fig. 2.21)
a. *Skin:* the branches from the lateral dorsal pedis nerve containing fibers from the fifth sacral nerve (S 5) innervate the skin.

b. *Subcutaneous tissue:* includes the previously described skin nerve branches.

c. *Extensor digitorum brevis muscle:* at the dorsal foot. The deep branches from the peroneal nerve containing fibers from the fourth lumbar to first sacral nerves (L4, L5, S1) innervate the muscle.

d. *Lateral tendon of the talus:* the tendon originates from the tubercle of the talus, and inserts into the lateral part of the calcaneus.

e. The needle is inserted posterior to the talus, and anterior to the calcaneus.

Functions
Clears the collaterals, relieves rigidity of the joints, removes heat from the Liver and Gallbladder.

Clinical indications
Pleurisy, cholecystitis, axillary lymph adnexitis, sciatic nerve pain, ankle and surrounding soft tissue disease, beriberi, chillness and fever, myopia, optic neuritis.

64.
(CHUNGYANG) CHONGYANG, ST 42, FOOT YANG MING STOMACH MERIDIAN, SOURCE POINT

Location
In a seated position, the point is located at the highest point of the dorsum of the foot, 1.5 inches below Jiexi [ST 41] in the fossa between the base of the second and third metatarsals and the cuneiform.

Needle and moxibustion method
Perpendicular insertion 0.3–0.5 inch. WARNING: Avoid the dorsal pedis artery.
— *Needle sensation:* local soreness and numbness.
— *Moxibustion dosage:* 3–5 cones; stick 10 minutes.

Cross-sectional anatomy of the needle passage
a. *Skin:* the branches from the superficial peroneal nerve containing fibers from the fifth lumbar nerve (L 5) innervate the skin.

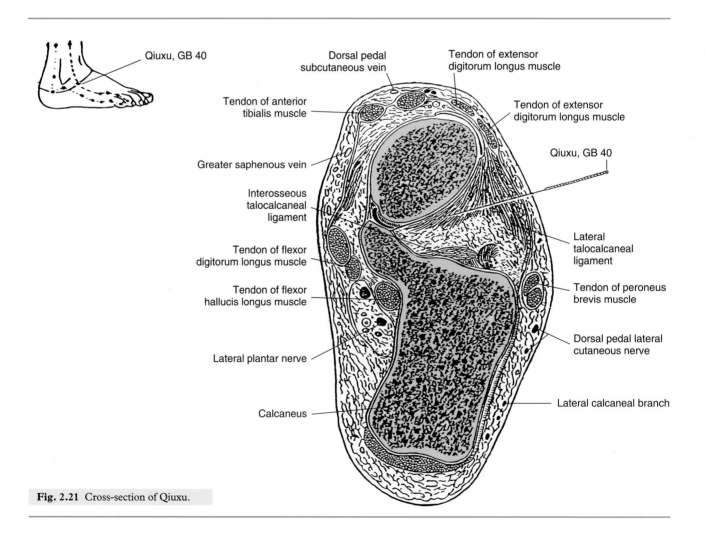

Fig. 2.21 Cross-section of Qiuxu.

b. *Subcutaneous tissue:* includes the previously described skin nerve branches, and the dorsal venous plexus.

c. *Tendon of extensor digitorum longus muscle:* the needle is passed to the medial side of the tendon of the extensor digitorum longus muscle. The branches from the deep peroneal nerve containing fibers from the fifth lumbar and first sacral nerves (L5, S1) innervate the muscle.

d. *Deep peroneal nerve, dorsal pedis artery and vein:* the needle is passed on the lateral side of the deep peroneal nerve, the dorsal pedis artery and the dorsal pedis vein. The common peroneal nerve gives rise to the deep peroneal nerve.

Functions

Regulates the function of the Spleen to remove Dampness, regulates the function of the Stomach, and tranquilizes the Mind.

Clinical indications

Toothache, facial palsy, leg atrophy, facial edema, abdominal distension, dorsal foot pain, psychosis, convulsions, schizophrenia, hysteria, dizziness.

65.

(TSULINCHI) ZULINQI, GB 41, FOOT SHAO YANG GALLBLADDER MERIDIAN, STREAM POINT

Location

In a seated or supine position, the point is located on the dorsum of the foot, in the fossa at the base of the fourth and fifth metatarsals, on the lateral side of the tendon of the fifth extensor digitorum longus muscle.

Needle and moxibustion method

Perpendicular insertion 0.3–0.5 inch.
— *Needle sensation:* local soreness and distension, radiating to the toes.
— *Moxibustion dosage:* 1–3 cones; stick 5–10 minutes.

Cross-sectional anatomy of the needle passage

a. *Skin:* the branches from the superficial peroneal nerve containing fibers from the fifth lumbar nerve (L5) innervate the skin.

b. *Subcutaneous tissue:* includes the previously described skin nerve branches and the dorsal pedis venous plexus.

c. *Fourth dorsal interosseous and third plantar interosseous muscles:* these two muscles are located at the fourth and fifth metatarsals. The deep branches of the lateral plantar nerve containing fibers from the first and second sacral nerves (S1, S2) innervate these two muscles.

d. The needle is inserted between the fourth and fifth metatarsals to the sole of the foot. The needle may be inserted into the oblique head of the adductor hallucis muscle and the lateral plantar nerve, artery and vein.

Functions

Reduces Heat and expels Wind, and improves hearing and acuity of vision.

Clinical indications

Headache, dizziness, pleurisy, pedal pain, fever, paralysis, deafness, tinnitus, dysmenorrhea, mastitis.

66.

(JANKU) RANGU, KI 2, FOOT SHAO YIN KIDNEY MERIDIAN, SPRING POINT

Location

In a seated position, the point is located anterior to the medial malleolus, anterior and inferior to the tuberosity of the navicular bone, approximately 1 inch posterior to Gongsun [SP 4].

Needle and moxibustion method

Perpendicular insertion 0.5–1.0 inch or use a triangular needle to induce bleeding.
— *Needle sensation:* plantar numbness and distension.
— *Moxibustion dosage:* 3–5 cones; stick 10 minutes.

Cross-sectional anatomy of the needle passage

a. *Skin:* the branches from the medial plantar nerve containing fibers from the fourth lumbar nerve (L4) innervate the skin.

b. *Subcutaneous tissue:* includes the previously described skin nerve branches. The subcutaneous tissue consists of a large amount of fibrous connective tissue and a small amount of adipose tissue.

c. *Abductor hallucis muscle:* the muscle is located at the medial side of the foot. The branches from the medial plantar nerve containing fibers from the fifth lumbar and first sacral nerves (L5, S1) innervate the muscle.

d. *Flexor hallucis brevis muscle:* the branches from the medial plantar nerve containing fibers from the fifth lumbar to first sacral nerves (L5, S1) innervate the muscle.

e. *Tendon of flexor digitorum longus muscle:* the branches from the tibial nerve containing fibers from the fifth lumbar to second sacral nerves (L5, S1, S2) innervate the muscle.

Functions

Removes Heat and Dampness, strengthens the function of the Kidney and regulates menstruation.

Clinical indications

Sore throat, myocarditis, tonsillitis, vomiting, diabetes mellitus, cold sweating, cystitis, orchitis, nephritis, nocturnal emission, impotence, irregular menstruation, infertility, tetanus.

67.

(KUNGSUN) GONGSUN, SP 4, FOOT TAI YIN SPLEEN MERIDIAN, CONNECTING POINT

Location

In a seated position, on the medial side of the foot, the point is located in the fossa distal and inferior to the base of the first metatarsal.

Needle and moxibustion method

Perpendicular insertion penetrating to Yongquan [KI 1] 1.0–2.0 inches.
— *Needle sensation:* local soreness and distension, sometimes radiating to the sole of the foot.
— *Moxibustion dosage:* 3–5 cones; stick 5–15 minutes.

Cross-sectional anatomy of the needle passage
(Fig. 2.22)
a. *Skin:* the branches from the saphenous nerve containing fibers from the fourth lumbar nerve (L4) innervate the skin. The saphenous nerve, together with the greater saphenous vein, descends down the medial side of the leg.
b. *Subcutaneous tissue:* consists of a large amount of fibrous connective tissue and a small amount of adipose tissue and includes the previously described skin nerve branches and the greater saphenous vein.
c. *Abductor hallucis muscle:* the muscle is located at the medial side of the foot. The branches from the

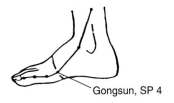

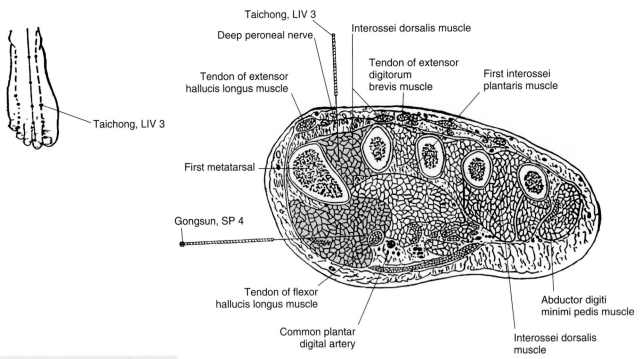

Fig. 2.22 Cross-section of Gongsun and Taichong.

plantar nerve containing fibers from the fifth lumbar and first sacral nerves (L5, S1) innervate the muscle.

d. *Flexor hallucis brevis muscle:* the muscle is located at the lateral side of the abductor hallucis muscle and is attached to the first metatarsal. The branches from the medial plantar nerve containing fibers from the fifth lumbar to second sacral nerves (L5, S1, S2) innervate the muscle.

e. *Tendon of the flexor digitorum longus muscle:* the tendon is located between two heads of the flexor hallucis brevis muscle. The branches from the tibial nerve containing fibers from the fifth lumbar to second sacral nerves (L5, S1, S2) innervate the muscle. If the needle is inserted into the tendon, a strong resistance will be felt.

f. If the needle is inserted inferiorly and laterally to Yongquan [KI 1], it may penetrate the adductor hallucis muscle, the plantar nerve, artery and vein.

Functions
Strengthens the function of the Spleen and Stomach, reduces heat and removes Dampness.

Clinical indications
Stomach pain, gastric ulcer, abdominal pain, diarrhea, bloody stool, indigestion, myocarditis, pleurisies, facial edema, convulsions, hysteria, schizophrenia.

68.

(CHINGKU) JINGGU, BL 64, FOOT TAI YANG BLADDER MERIDIAN, SOURCE POINT

Location
In a seated position, the point is located proximal to the tuberosity of the fifth metatarsal bone on the lateral part of the foot.

Needle and moxibustion method
Perpendicular insertion 0.3–0.5 inch.
— *Needle sensation:* local numbness and distension.
— *Moxibustion dosage:* 3–7 cones; stick 10 minutes.

Cross-sectional anatomy of the needle passage
a. *Skin:* the branches from the lateral dorsal pedis nerve containing fibers from the first sacral nerve (S1) innervate the skin.

b. *Subcutaneous tissue:* includes the previously described skin nerve branches.

c. *Abductor digiti minimi muscle:* the branches from the tibial nerve containing fibers from the first and second sacral nerves (S1, S2) innervate the muscle. The needle is passed through the inferior part of the muscle.

d. *Lateral plantar nerve, artery and vein:* the posterior tibial artery gives rise to the lateral plantar tibial artery. The tibial nerve gives rise to the lateral plantar nerve.

Functions
Clears the channels to alleviate pain, and relieves mental stress.

Clinical indications
Heart disease, meningitis, tachycardia, convulsions, schizophrenia, hypertension, neck stiffness, lower back strain, knee joint arthritis.

69.

(HSIENKU) XIANGU, ST 43, FOOT YANG MING STOMACH MERIDIAN, STREAM POINT

Location
In a seated or supine position, the point is located on the dorsum of the foot in the fossa between the second and third metatarsal bones 2 inches above the toe web.

Needle and moxibustion method
Perpendicular insertion 0.3–0.5 inch or slightly oblique insertion 0.3–0.5 inch.
— *Needle sensation:* local distension.
— *Moxibustion dosage:* 3–7 cones; stick 10 minutes.

Cross-sectional anatomy of the needle passage
a. *Skin:* the branches from the superficial peroneal nerve containing fibers from the fifth lumbar nerve (L5) innervate the skin.

b. *Subcutaneous tissue:* includes the previously described skin nerve branches and the dorsal venous plexus.

c. *Tendon of extensor digitorum muscle:* the needle is passed between the tendons of the extensor digitorum longus muscles of the second and third metatarsals. The branches from the deep peroneal nerve containing fibers from the fourth lumbar to first sacral nerves (L4, L5, S1) innervate the muscles.

d. *Tendon of extensor digitorum brevis muscle:* the branches from the deep peroneal nerve containing fibers from the fourth lumbar to first sacral nerves (L4, L5, S1) innervate the muscle.

e. *Superficial peroneal nerve, second dorsal metatarsal artery and vein:* the superficial nerve is a branch of the common peroneal nerve. The second dorsal metatarsal artery is a branch of the dorsal pedis artery. The second dorsal vein joins the dorsal pedis vein.

f. *Second dorsal interosseous muscle:* the muscle is located at the second and third metatarsals. The branches from the lateral plantar nerve containing fibers from the first and second sacral nerves (S1, S2) innervate the muscle.

Functions
Reduces fever to relieve Exterior syndromes, expels Wind and induces diuresis.

Clinical indications
Facial edema, anasarca, abdominal pain, dorsal foot pain, ascites, hysteria, common cold, bronchitis.

70.

(TAICHUNG) TAICHONG, LIV 3, FOOT JUE YIN LIVER MERIDIAN, STREAM AND SOURCE POINT

Location
In a seated or supine position, the point is located on the dorsum of the foot in the fossa distal to the junction of the first and second metatarsal bones 2 inches above the web of the toe.

Needle and moxibustion method
Perpendicular insertion 0.5–1.0 inch.
— *Needle sensation:* local soreness and distension, or electrical sensation radiating to the sole of the foot, or down the big toe.
— *Moxibustion dosage:* 3–5 cones; stick 5–15 minutes.

Cross-sectional anatomy of the needle passage
(Fig. 2.22)
a. *Skin:* the branches from the deep peroneal nerve containing fibers from the fifth lumbar nerve (L5) innervate the skin.
b. *Subcutaneous tissue:* includes the previously described skin nerve branches and the dorsal venous plexus.
c. The needle is inserted between the tendons of the extensor hallucis longus and extensor digitorum longus muscles. The branches from the deep peroneal nerve containing fibers from the fourth lumbar to first sacral nerves (L4, L5, S1) innervate the muscles.
d. The needle is inserted on the lateral side of the extensor hallucis brevis muscle. The deep branches from the peroneal nerve containing fibers from the fourth lumbar to first sacral nerves (L4, L5, S1) innervate the muscle.
e. *Deep peroneal nerve, first dorsal metatarsal artery and vein:* the deep peroneal nerve is a branch of the common peroneal nerve. The first dorsal metatarsal artery is a branch of the dorsal pedis artery. The first dorsal metatarsal vein joins the dorsal pedis vein.

f. *First dorsal interosseous muscle:* the muscle is located at the first and second metatarsals. The branches from the lateral plantar nerve containing fibers from the first and second sacral nerves (S1, S2) innervate the muscle.
g. If the needle is inserted deeply, it will puncture between the first and second metatarsals and reach the oblique head of the adductor hallucis and flexor hallucis brevis muscles.

Functions
Removes Heat from the Liver, alleviates melancholia, and clears the function of the Liver to dispel Wind.

Clinical indications
Headache, dizziness, hernia, pleurisy, sacral neuritis, pain in the lower extremities, mastitis.

71.

(TIWUHUI) DIWUHUI, GB 42, FOOT SHAO YANG GALLBLADDER MERIDIAN

Location
In a seated or supine position, the point is located 1.5 inches proximal to the toe web, in the fossa between the fourth and fifth metatarsals, on the medial side of the tendon of the extensor digitorum brevis.

Needle and moxibustion method
Perpendicular insertion 0.3–0.5 inch.
— *Needle sensation:* local soreness.
— *Moxibustion dosage:* 3–5 cones; stick 10 minutes.

Cross-sectional anatomy of the needle passage
a. *Skin:* the dorsal pedis branch of the superficial peroneal nerve containing fibers from the fifth lumbar nerve (L5) innervates the skin.
b. *Subcutaneous tissue:* includes the previously described skin nerve branches and the dorsal pedis venous plexus.
c. The needle is passed between the tendons of the fourth and fifth extensor digitorum longus muscles. The branches from the deep peroneal nerve containing fibers from the fourth lumbar to first sacral nerve (L4, L5, S1) innervate the muscle.
d. The needle is inserted on the medial side of the extensor digitorum brevis muscle. The branches from the deep peroneal nerve from the fourth lumbar to first sacral nerves (L4, L5, S1) innervate the muscle.
e. *Fourth dorsal metatarsal artery and vein:* the fourth dorsal metatarsal artery is a branch of the dorsal pedis artery. The fourth dorsal vein joins the dorsal pedis vein.

f. Fourth dorsal interosseous muscle and third plantar interosseous muscle: these two muscles are located at the fourth and fifth metatarsals. The branches from the lateral plantar nerve containing fibers from the first and second sacral nerves (S1, S2) innervate the muscles.

g. The needle is passed between the fourth and fifth metatarsals to the pedal sole.

Functions
Clears and activates the channels and collaterals, and clears away Heat from the Gallbladder.

Clinical indications
Tinnitus, lower back pain, mastitis, rheumatoid arthritis, axillary nerve pain, tuberculosis.

72.
(TAIPAI) TAIBAI, SP 3, FOOT TAI YIN SPLEEN MERIDIAN, STREAM AND SOURCE POINT

Location
In a seated position, the point is located on the medial side of the foot in the fossa proximal and inferior to the head of the first metatarsal bone.

Needle and moxibustion method
Perpendicular insertion 0.3–0.5 inch.
— *Needle sensation:* local soreness and distension.
— *Moxibustion dosage:* 3–5 cones; stick 10 minutes.

Cross-sectional anatomy of the needle passage
a. Skin: the branches from the saphenous nerve and the medial plantar nerve containing fibers from the fourth lumbar nerve (L4) innervate the skin.
b. Subcutaneous tissue: consists of a large amount of fibrous connective tissue and adipose tissue and includes the previously described skin nerve branches.
c. Tendon of abductor hallucis muscle: the tendon is located on the medial side of the foot. The branches from the medial plantar nerve containing fibers from the fifth lumbar and first sacral nerves (L5, S1) innervate the muscle.
d. Flexor hallucis brevis muscle: the muscle is located on the lateral side of the abductor hallucis muscle. The branches from the medial plantar nerve containing fibers from the fifth lumbar to first sacral nerves (L5, S1) innervate the muscle.
e. Tendon of flexor digitorum longus muscle: the branches from the tibial nerve containing fibers from the fifth lumbar to first sacral nerves (L5, S1) innervate the muscle.

f. Medial plantar artery and vein: the posterior tibial artery gives rise to the medial plantar artery.

Functions
Regulates the function of the Stomach and Spleen, reduces fever by eliminating undigested food.

Clinical indications
Fever, abdominal distention, vomiting, epigastric pain, hemorrhoids, constipation, cholera, lower back pain, beriberi.

73.
(HSIAHSI) XIAXI, GB 43, FOOT SHAO YANG GALLBLADDER MERIDIAN, SPRING POINT

Location
In a seated or supine position, the point is located on the dorsum of the foot, in the fossa between the fourth and fifth proximal phalanges at the midpoint of the toe web.

Needle and moxibustion method
Oblique insertion directed upward 0.2–0.5 inch.
— *Needle sensation:* local soreness and distension.
— *Moxibustion dosage:* 3–5 cones; stick 5 minutes.

Cross-sectional anatomy of the needle passage
a. Skin: the branches from the superficial peroneal nerve containing fibers from the fifth lumbar nerve (L5) innervate the skin.
b. Subcutaneous tissue: includes the previously described skin nerve branches and the dorsal venous plexus.
c. Tendons of extensor digitorum longus and brevis muscles: the needle is passed between the tendons of the extensor digitorum longus and extensor digitorum brevis muscles of the fourth and fifth toes. The branches from the deep peroneal nerve containing fibers from the fourth lumbar to first sacral nerves (L4, L5, S1) innervate both muscles.
d. Dorsal metatarsal artery and vein: the fourth dorsal metatarsal artery is a branch of the dorsal pedis artery.
e. The needle is passed between the fourth and fifth phalanges.

Functions
Dispels Wind and reduces fever, and relieves mental anxiety.

Clinical indications
Headache, dizziness, vertigo, deafness, axillary pain, mastitis, fever, common cold, tonsillitis, rheumatic arthritis, schizophrenia.

74.

(YUNGCHUAN) YONGQUAN, KI 1, FOOT SHAO YIN KIDNEY MERIDIAN, WELL POINT

Location

In a supine position with the foot flexed, the point is located on the sole of the foot between the second and third metatarsals in the fossa one third of the distance between the base of the toes and the heel of the foot.

Needle and moxibustion method

Perpendicular insertion 0.5–1.0 inch.
— *Needle sensation:* local pain and distension radiating to the foot joint.
— *Moxibustion dosage:* 1–3 cones; stick 5–10 minutes.

Cross-sectional anatomy of the needle passage
(Fig. 2.23)

a. *Skin:* thickened. The medial and lateral plantar branches of the tibial nerve containing fibers from the first sacral nerve (S1) innervate the skin.

b. *Subcutaneous tissue:* includes the previously described skin nerve branches. Numerous fibrous connective tissues are attached between the skin and the plantar aponeurosis.

c. *Plantar aponeurosis:* a superficial thickened fascia. The branches from the medial and lateral plantar nerves innervate the plantar aponeurosis. If the needle is punctured through the plantar aponeurosis, a strong needle resistance will be felt.

d. The needle is inserted on the lateral side of the second common plantar digitorum nerve, the second plantar metatarsal artery and vein. The point is very close to these structures and the needle may

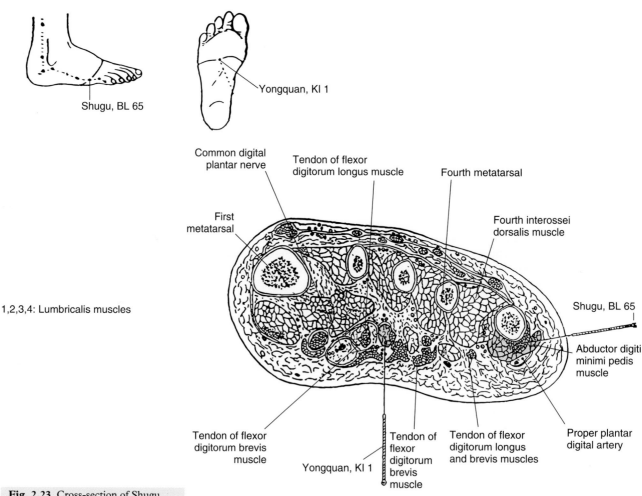

Fig. 2.23 Cross-section of Shugu and Yongquan.

puncture these tissues. The second common plantar digitorum nerve is a branch of the medial plantar nerve.

e. *Second lumbrical muscle:* the lateral plantar branches of the tibial nerve containing fibers from the fifth lumbar to second sacral nerves (L5, S1, S2) innervate the muscle.

f. The needle is passed between the tendons of the flexor digitorum longus and flexor digitorum brevis muscles. The branches from the tibial nerve containing fibers from the fifth lumbar to second sacral nerves (L5, S1, S2) innervate the flexor digitorum longus muscle. The branches from the median nerve containing fibers from the fifth lumbar and first sacral nerves (L5, S1) innervate the flexor digitorum brevis muscle.

Functions
Nourishes Yin to reduce pathogenic Fire, relieves mental stress and revives syncope.

Clinical indications
Headache, shock, heat stroke, hoarseness of the voice, sore throat, cough, acute tonsillitis, tachycardia, jaundice, prolapse of the uterus, spasm of the lower extremities, hernia, edema, impotence.

75.

(SHUKU) SHUGU, BL 65, FOOT TAI YANG BLADDER MERIDIAN, STREAM POINT

Location
In a seated or supine position, the point is located on the lateral side of the foot in the fossa proximal to the head of the fifth metatarsal bone.

Needle and moxibustion method
Perpendicular insertion 0.3–0.5 inch.
— *Needle sensation:* local soreness and distension.
— *Moxibustion dosage:* 1–3 cones; stick 5–10 minutes.

Cross-sectional anatomy of the needle passage
(Fig. 2.23)
a. *Skin:* the lateral dorsal pedis branches of the sural nerve containing fibers from the first sacral nerve (S1) innervate the skin.
b. *Subcutaneous tissue:* includes the previously described skin nerve branches.
c. *Abductor digiti minimi muscle:* the muscle is located at the lateral side of the foot. The branches from the lateral plantar nerve containing fibers from the first and second sacral nerves (S1, S2) innervate the muscle.

d. The needle is passed on the proximal side of the superficial branch of the lateral plantar nerve, a branch from the lateral plantar nerve, and the plantar metatarsal artery, a branch from the plantar arch artery.

e. *Flexor digiti minimi brevis muscle:* the branches from the lateral plantar nerve containing fibers from the first and second sacral nerves (S1, S2) innervate the muscle.

Functions
Clears the channels to promote Blood circulation, and removes Heat and expels Wind.

Clinical indications
Headache, dizziness, deafness, lower back pain, gastrocnemius muscle pain, neck stiffness, hemorrhoids, cerebrovascular disease, convulsions, schizophrenia.

76.

(ZUTUNGKU) ZUTONGGU, BL 66, FOOT TAI YANG BLADDER MERIDIAN, SPRING POINT

Location
In a seated position, the point is located in the lateral skin crease of the fifth toe, in the fossa distal and slightly inferior to the metatarsophalangeal joint.

Needle and moxibustion method
Perpendicular insertion 0.2–0.3 inch.
— *Needle sensation:* local pain and distension.
— *Moxibustion dosage:* 3–7 cones; stick 10 minutes.

Cross-sectional anatomy of the needle passage
a. *Skin:* the branches from the lateral dorsal pedis nerve containing fibers from the first sacral nerve (S1) innervate the skin.
b. *Subcutaneous tissue:* includes the previously described skin nerve branches.
c. *Proper digital plantar nerve, plantar metatarsal artery and vein:* the lateral plantar artery gives rise to the plantar metatarsal artery. The lateral plantar nerve gives rise to the proper digital plantar nerve.

Functions
Dredges and clears the channel Qi, and improves the acuity of vision.

Clinical indications
Neck stiffness, headache, epistaxis, chronic gastritis, convulsions, schizophrenia.

77.

(NEITING) NEITING, ST 44, FOOT YANG MING STOMACH MERIDIAN, SPRING POINT

Location
In a seated or supine position, the point is located on the dorsum of the foot, in the fossa between the second and third proximal phalanges and proximal to the margin of the toe web.

Needle and moxibustion method
Upwards oblique insertion 0.2–0.5 inch.
— *Needle sensation:* local soreness and distension.
— *Moxibustion dosage:* 3–5 cones; stick 5–10 minutes.

Cross-sectional anatomy of the needle passage
a. *Skin:* the branches from the superficial peroneal nerve containing fibers from the fifth lumbar nerve (L5) innervate the skin.
b. *Subcutaneous tissue:* includes the previously described skin nerve branches and the dorsal venous plexus.
c. The needle is passed between the tendons of the extensor digitorum longus muscle and the extensor digitorum brevis muscle of the second and third toes. The branches from the deep peroneal nerve containing fibers from the fourth lumbar to first sacral nerves (L4, L5, S1) innervate these muscles.
d. *Second dorsal metatarsal artery and vein:* the dorsal metatarsal artery is a branch of the dorsal pedis artery.
e. The needle is passed between the second and third phalanges.

Functions
Descends the Lung and stomach Qi, and regulates the function of the Stomach to remove Dampness.

Clinical indications
Headache, toothache, trigeminal neuralgia, tonsillitis, epistaxis, vocal cord spasm, stomach spasm, diaphragm muscle spasm.

78.

(HSINCHIEN) XINGJIAN, LIV 2, FOOT JUE YIN LIVER MERIDIAN, SPRING POINT

Location
In a seated or supine position, the point is located on the dorsum of the foot, in the fossa between the first and second proximal phalanges, and proximal to the margin of the toe web.

Needle and moxibustion method
Upwards oblique insertion 0.3–0.5 inch.
— *Needle sensation:* local soreness and distension.
— *Moxibustion dosage:* 3–5 cones; stick 10 minutes.

Cross-sectional anatomy of the needle passage
a. *Skin:* the deep peroneal branches from the anterior tibial nerve containing fibers from the fifth lumbar nerve (L5) innervate the skin.
b. *Subcutaneous tissue:* includes the previously described skin nerve branches and the dorsal venous plexus.
c. *Tendons of extensor digitorum longus and brevis, and extensor hallucis longus muscles:* the needle is passed between the tendons of the extensor digitorum longus and brevis muscles of the first and second toes, and the extensor hallucis longus muscle. The branches from the deep peroneal nerve containing fibers from the fourth lumbar to first sacral nerves (L4, L5, S1) innervate these muscles.
d. *Dorsal metatarsal artery and vein:* the first dorsal metatarsal artery is a branch of the dorsal pedis artery.

Functions
Regulates menstruation, reinforces the Chong meridian, clears away Heat from the Liver and improves acuity of vision.

Clinical indications
Penile pain, constipation, infantile convulsion, diabetes mellitus, tachycardia, peritonitis, insomnia, hypertension, glaucoma, conjunctivitis.

79.

(TATU) DADU, SP 2, FOOT TAI YIN SPLEEN MERIDIAN, SPRING POINT

Location
In a seated position, the point is located on the medial side of the big toe in the fossa distal and inferior to the first metatarsophalangeal joint.

Needle and moxibustion method
Perpendicular insertion 0.1–0.3 inch.
— *Needle sensation:* local pain.
— *Moxibustion dosage:* 1–3 cones; stick 15 minutes.

Cross-sectional anatomy of the needle passage
a. *Skin:* the branches from the medial plantar nerve from the fourth lumbar nerve (L4) innervate the skin.
b. *Subcutaneous tissue:* includes the previously described skin nerve branches.

c. *Tendon of abductor hallucis muscle:* the branches from the medial plantar nerve containing fibers from the fifth lumbar and first sacral nerves (L5, S1) innervate the muscle.

d. *Medial plantar artery and vein:* the posterior tibial artery gives rise to the medial plantar artery.

Functions

Regulates the function of the Spleen and Middle Jiao (Middle Warmer), restores depleted Yang and rescues the patient from collapse.

Clinical indications

Abdominal distension, stomach pain, constipation, fever, vomiting, lower back pain, pericarditis, infantile convulsion, cerebrovascular disease.

80.

(CHIHYIN) ZHIYIN, BL 67, FOOT TAI YANG BLADDER MERIDIAN, WELL POINT

Location

In a seated or supine position, the point is located on the lateral side of the little toe, about 0.1 inch lateral and proximal to the nail root; or draw a line across the nail base and another line down the lateral nail: the point is located at the intersection of the two lines.

Needle and moxibustion method

Oblique insertion 0.1–0.2 inch or use a triangular needle to induce bleeding.
— *Needle sensation:* local pain.
— *Moxibustion dosage:* 3–5 cones; stick 10–30 minutes.

Cross-sectional anatomy of the needle passage

a. *Skin:* the lateral plantar branches of the sural nerve containing fibers from the first sacral nerve (S1) innervate the skin.

b. *Subcutaneous tissue:* consists of a large amount of dense connective tissue and a small amount of adipose tissue and includes the lateral plantar nerve, dorsal digital artery and vein.

c. *Nail root:* if the needle is inserted into the nail bed, a strong needle resistance will be felt.

Functions

Removes Heat, regulates the flow of Qi, and reverses the position of a fetus.

Clinical indications

Common cold, headache, dizziness, premature ejaculation, eczema, nasal obstruction.

81.

(YINPAI) YINBAI, SP 1, FOOT TAI YIN SPLEEN MERIDIAN, WELL POINT

Location

In a seated or supine position, the point is located on the medial side of the big toe, about 0.1 inch medial and proximal to the nail root; or draw a line across the nail base and another line alongside the medial nail: the point is located at the intersection of these two lines.

Needle and moxibustion method

Oblique proximal insertion 0.1–0.2 inch or use a triangular needle to induce bleeding.
— *Needle sensation:* local pain.
— *Moxibustion dosage:* 3–7 cones; stick 5–20 minutes.

Cross-sectional anatomy of the needle passage

a. *Skin:* the medial plantar branches of the superficial peroneal nerve containing fibers from the first sacral nerve (S1) innervate the skin.

b. *Subcutaneous tissue:* consists of a large amount of dense connective tissue and a small amount of adipose tissue and includes the medial plantar nerve, dorsal digital artery and vein.

c. *Nail root:* if the needle is inserted to the nail base, a strong needle resistance will be felt.

Functions

Regulates the function of the Spleen to restore depleted Yang, and nourishes the Blood circulation to restore consciousness. Use moxa to stop bleeding.

Clinical indications

Coma, peritonitis, acute gastroenteritis, dysmenorrhea, epistaxis, schizophrenia, gastrointestinal bleeding.

82.

(LITUI) LIDUI, ST 45, FOOT YANG MING, STOMACH MERIDIAN, WELL POINT

Location

In a seated or supine position, the point is located at the lateral side of the second toe, about 0.1 inch lateral and proximal to the nail root; or draw a line across the nail base and another line alongside the lateral nail: the point is located at the intersection of the two lines.

Needle and moxibustion method

Oblique insertion 0.1–0.2 inch.
— *Needle sensation:* local aching.
— *Moxibustion dosage:* 3 cones.

Cross-sectional anatomy of the needle passage

a. *Skin:* the medial plantar branches of the superficial peroneal nerve containing fibers from the first sacral nerve (S1) innervate the skin.

b. *Subcutaneous tissue:* consists of a large amount of dense connective tissue and a small amount of adipose tissue and includes the medial plantar nerve branch, dorsal digital artery and vein.

c. *Nail root:* if the needle is punctured into the nail base, a strong needle resistance will be felt.

Functions

Clears the channels to revive syncope, reduces fever and regulates the flow of Qi.

Clinical indications

Facial edema, facial palsy, toothache, epistaxis, enteritis, abdominal distension, fever, convulsions, hysteria, tonsillitis, anemia, hepatitis.

83.

(TATUN) DADUN, LIV 1, FOOT JUE YIN LIVER MERIDIAN, WELL POINT

Location

In a seated or supine position, the point is located at the lateral side of the big toe, about 0.1 inch lateral and proximal to the nail root; or draw a line across the nail base and another line alongside the lateral nail: the point is located in the intersection of the two lines.

Needle and moxibustion method

Oblique proximal insertion 0.1–0.2 inch.
— *Needle sensation:* local soreness and distension.
— *Moxibustion dosage:* 3–7 cones; stick 7 minutes.

Cross-sectional anatomy of the needle passage

a. *Skin:* the medial plantar branches of the superficial peroneal nerve containing fibers from the first sacral nerve (S 1) innervate the skin.

b. *Subcutaneous tissue:* consists of a large amount of dense connective tissue and a small amount of adipose tissue and includes the medial plantar nerve, dorsal digital artery and vein.

c. *Nail root:* if the needle is inserted to the nail base, a strong needle resistance will be felt.

Functions

Removes Heat from the Liver, regulates the flow of Qi, and restores depleted Yang to rescue the patient from collapse.

Clinical indications

Hernia, gonorrhea, orchitis, spermatic cord pain, uterine prolapse, convulsions, syncope, myopia.

84.

(TSUCHIAOYIN) ZUQIAOYIN, GB 44, FOOT SHAO YANG GALLBLADDER MERIDIAN

Location

In a seated or supine position, the point is located at the lateral side of the fourth toe, about 0.1 inch lateral and proximal to the nail root; or draw a line across the nail base and another line alongside the lateral nail, the point is located at the intersection of the two lines.

Needle and moxibustion method

Oblique proximal insertion 0.1–0.2 inch.
— *Needle sensation:* local pain.
— *Moxibustion dosage:* 2–3 cones; stick 5 minutes.

Cross-sectional anatomy of the needle passage

a. *Skin:* the branches from the superficial peroneal nerve containing fibers from the fifth lumbar nerve (L5) innervate the skin.

b. *Subcutaneous tissue:* consists of a large amount of dense connective tissue and a small amount of adipose tissue and includes the lateral plantar nerve, dorsal digital artery and vein.

c. *Nail root:* if the needle is inserted to the nail base, a strong needle resistance will be felt.

Functions

Clears and activates the channels and collaterals, and clears away Heat from the Liver to refresh the Mind.

Clinical indications

Headache, vertigo, eye pain, deafness, glaucoma, anemia, nightmares, pleuritis.

Cross-sectional anatomy of the head

The head is attached to the neck. The border line of the head and the neck is the inferior margin of the mandible, the angle of the mandible, the mastoid process, the superior nuchal line and the external occipital protuberance.

For superficial measurement during acupuncture treatment, the distance from the anterior frontal hairline to the posterior hairline is 12 inches, the distance between the left and right frontal hair angles is 9 inches, and the distance between the left and right mastoid processes posterior to the auricle is 9 inches.

1.

(PAIHUI) BAIHUI, GV 20, GOVERNING VESSEL

Location

In a seated position, draw the mid-sagittal line of the head and another line connecting the apexes of the two ears. The point is located at the intersection of the two lines. Or assuming that the distance between anterior and posterior hairlines is 12 inches, Baihui is found 5 inches posterior to the anterior hairline on the midline of the body.

Needle and moxibustion method

Anterior, posterior, right and left horizontal insertion 0.5–1.0 inch.
— *Needle sensation:* soreness, distension, and heaviness.
— *Moxibustion dosage:* 3–9 cones; stick 5–10 minutes.

Cross-sectional anatomy of the needle passage

a. *Skin:* the branches from the supraorbital, the greater occipital and the auriculotemporal nerves innervate the skin. The supraorbital nerve is a branch of the ophthalmic division of the trigeminal nerve (CN V). The greater occipital nerve contains fibers from the second cervical nerve (C2), and the auriculotemporal nerve is a branch of the mandibular division of the trigeminal nerve (CN V).

b. *Subcutaneous tissue:* includes the previously described skin nerve branches, the occipital artery and vein, and the superficial temporal artery and vein. The subcutaneous tissue consists of much vertical connective tissue, which connect the skin and the galea aponeurotica and separate the adipose tissue into many small septa. The occipital and superficial temporal arteries are branches of the external carotid artery. The occipital vein, together with the occipital artery, joins the external jugular vein. The superficial temporal artery is a terminal branch of the external carotid artery. The superficial temporal vein, together with the temporal artery, joins the retromandibular vein.

c. *Galea aponeurotica:* a strong dense connective tissue which is connected anteriorly to the frontal muscle and posteriorly to the occipital muscles of the cranial vault, and is tightly connected with the subcutaneous tissue and the skin.

d. *Loose connective tissue beneath the aponeurosis:* a thin loose connective tissue between the epicranium and the scalp. The loose connective tissue is connected anteriorly to the eyelids and posteriorly to the occipital hairline. If the blood is drained into this structure, it may cause a large hematoma.

e. *Periosteum and bone of the skull:* the pericranium is thin and dense, fused firmly to the bone of the skull. Deep needling can reach the parietal bone.

Warning

The subcutaneous tissue contains a large amount of fibrous connective tissue and blood vessels. When the needle passes through these structures, a moderate needle resistance will be felt. To avoid bleeding, no vigorous lifting and thrusting of the needle is permitted. If there are signs of bleeding, use a cotton compress to stop it.

Functions

Refreshes the brain to restore the Mind, and nourishes the Yang to alleviate collapse.

Clinical indications

Headache, dizziness, prolapse of the anus, prolapse of

the uterus, convulsions, cerebrovascular disease, hysteria, schizophrenia, insomnia, syncope.

2.

(HOUTING) HOUDING, GV 19, GOVERNING VESSEL

Location
In a seated position with the head slightly bent forward, the point is located on the mid-sagittal line of the head 1.5 inches inferior to Baihui [GV 20], and 3 inches superior to Naohu [GV 17].

Needle and moxibustion method
Horizontal insertion 0.3–0.5 inch.
— *Needle sensation:* local distension and soreness.
— *Moxibustion dosage:* 3–5 cones; stick 10 minutes.

Cross-sectional anatomy of the needle passage
a. *Skin:* the branches from the greater occipital nerve containing fibers from the second and third cervical nerves (C2, C3) innervate the skin.
b. *Subcutaneous tissue:* includes the previously described skin nerve branches, and the occipital artery and vein. The external carotid artery gives rise to the occipital artery. The occipital vein, together with the occipital artery, joins the external jugular vein.
c. *Galea aponeurotica:* a strong dense connective tissue which is connected anteriorly to the frontal muscle and posteriorly to the occipital muscle, and is tightly connected to the subcutaneous tissue and the skin.
d. *Loose connective tissue beneath the aponeurosis:* a thin loose connective tissue between the epicranium and the scalp. The loose connective tissue is connected anteriorly to the eyelids and posteriorly to the occipital hairline. If the blood drains into these structures, it may cause a large hematoma.
e. *Periosteum and bone of the skull:* the pericranium is thin and dense, fused firmly to the skull. Deep needling reaches the parietal bone.

Functions
Relieves mental stress, tranquilizes the Mind, regulates menstruation, and arrests pain.

Clinical indications
Epilepsy, convulsions, hysteria, schizophrenia, common cold, dizziness, headache, insomnia, neck stiffness.

3.

(CHIENTING) QIANDING, GV 21, GOVERNING VESSEL

Location
In a seated position, the point is located on the mid-sagittal line of the head 1.5 inches anterior to Baihui [GV 20].

Needle and moxibustion method
Horizontal insertion 0.3–0.5 inch.
— *Needle sensation:* local distension and soreness.
— *Moxibustion dosage:* 3–5 cones; stick 10 minutes.

Cross-sectional anatomy of the needle passage
a. *Skin:* the branches from the supraorbital and greater occipital nerves innervate the skin. The supraorbital nerve is a branch of the ophthalmic division of the trigeminal nerve (CN V), and the greater occipital nerve is a branch of the second and third cervical nerves (C2, C3).
b. *Subcutaneous tissue:* includes the previously described skin nerve branches and the superficial temporal artery and vein. The external carotid artery gives rise to the superficial temporal artery.
c. *Galea aponeurotica:* a strong dense connective tissue which is connected anteriorly to the frontal muscle and posteriorly to the occipital muscles.
d. *Loose connective tissue beneath the aponeurosis:* a thin loose connective tissue between the epicranium and the scalp. The loose connective tissue is connected anteriorly to the eyelids, and posteriorly to the occipital hairline. If the blood drains into these structures, it may cause a large hematoma.
e. *Periosteum and bone of the skull:* the pericranium is thin and dense, fused firmly to the skull. Deep needling reaches the parietal bone.

Functions
Strengthens the brain and tranquilizes the Mind, reduces fever and dispels Wind.

Clinical indications
Headache, cerebrovascular disease, hypertension, neurosis, epistaxis, nasal obstruction, facial edema, epilepsy.

4.

(TUNGTIEN) TONGTIAN, BL 7, FOOT TAI YANG BLADDER MERIDIAN

Location
In a seated position, the point is located 1.5 inches lateral to the Governing Vessel, 1.5 inches posterior to

Chengguang [BL 6], and 4 inches posterior to the front hairline.

Needle and moxibustion method

Horizontal insertion 0.3–0.5 inch.
— *Needle sensation:* local distension and soreness.
— *Moxibustion dosage:* 3 cones; stick 10 minutes.

Cross-sectional anatomy of the needle passage

a. *Skin:* the branches from the greater occipital nerve containing fibers from the second and third cervical nerves (C2, C3) innervate the skin.
b. *Subcutaneous tissue:* includes the previously described skin nerve branches, the superficial temporal artery and vein, and the occipital artery and vein. The external carotid artery gives rise to the superficial temporal and occipital arteries.
c. *Galea aponeurotica:* a strong dense connective tissue which is connected anteriorly to the frontal muscle and posteriorly to the occipital muscle.
d. *Loose connective tissue beneath the aponeurosis:* a thin loose connective tissue between epicranium and scalp. The loose connective tissue is connected anteriorly to the eyelids and posteriorly to the occipital hairline. If the blood drains into these structures, it may cause a large hematoma.
e. *Periosteum and bone of the skull:* the pericranium is thin and dense, and fused firmly to the skull. Deep needling can reach the parietal bone.

Functions

Expels Wind, reduces fever, activates the channels and collaterals and induces resuscitation.

Clinical indications

Dizziness, headache, hemiplegia, cervical stiffness, nasal obstruction, nasal discharge, epistaxis, nasal polyps.

5.

(CHENGKUANG) CHENGGUANG, BL 6, FOOT TAI YANG BLADDER MERIDIAN

Location

In a seated position, the point is located 1.5 inches lateral to the Governing Vessel (midline of the head), and 1.5 inches posterior to Wuchu [BL 5].

Needle and moxibustion method

Horizontal insertion 0.3–0.5 inch.
— *Needle sensation:* local distension and soreness.
— *Moxibustion dosage:* 3 cones; stick 10 minutes.

Cross-sectional anatomy of the needle passage

a. *Skin:* the lateral branches of the frontal and greater occipital nerves containing fibers from the second and third cervical nerves (C2, C3) innervate the skin.
b. *Subcutaneous tissue:* includes the previously described skin nerve branches, the supraorbital artery, the superficial temporal artery and vein, and the occipital artery and vein. The superficial temporal and occipital arteries are the terminal branches of the external carotid artery. The supraorbital artery is a branch of the ophthalmic artery.
c. *Galea aponeurotica:* a strong dense connective tissue which is connected anteriorly to the frontal muscle and posteriorly to the occipital muscle.
d. *Loose connective tissue beneath the aponeurosis:* a thin loose connective tissue between epicranium and scalp. The loose connective tissue is connected anteriorly to the eyelids and posteriorly to the occipital hairline.
e. *Periosteum and bone of the skull:* the pericranium is thin and dense, fused firmly to the skull.

Functions

Reduces fever and expels Wind, and clears the collaterals to improve visual acuity.

Clinical indications

Headache, dizziness, nasal obstruction, nasal discharge, glaucoma, myopia, nausea.

6.

(LOCHUEH) LUOQUE, BL 8, FOOT TAI YANG BLADDER MERIDIAN

Location

1.5 inches posterior to Tongtian [BL 7], and 1.5 inches lateral to the Governing Vessel (midline of the head).

Needle and moxibustion method

Horizontal insertion 0.3–0.5 inch.
— *Needle sensation:* distension and pain.
— *Moxibustion dosage:* 3 cones; stick 10 minutes.

Cross-sectional anatomy of the needle passage

a. *Skin:* the branches from the greater occipital nerve containing fibers from the second and third cervical nerves (C2, C3) innervate the skin.
b. *Subcutaneous tissue:* includes the previously described skin nerve branches, and the occipital artery and vein. The external carotid artery gives rise to the occipital artery.
c. *Occipital muscle:* the points are located at the insertion of the occipital muscle. The posterior auricular

branches of the facial nerve (CN VII) innervate the muscle.
d. Loose connective tissue of the aponeurosis.
e. Periosteum of the parietal bone.

Functions
Relieves convulsions, resolves Phlegm, improves visual acuity and induces resuscitation.

Clinical indications
Dizziness, vertigo, glaucoma, myopia, nasal obstruction, convulsions.

7.
(MEICHUNG) MEICHONG, BL 3, FOOT TAI YANG BLADDER MERIDIAN

Location
In a seated position, the point is located 0.5 inches within the anterior hairline and above the medial border of the eyebrow, or at the midpoint between Shenting [GV 24] and Qu Chai [BL 4].

Needle and moxibustion method
Horizontal insertion 0.3–0.5 inch.
— *Needle sensation:* local distension and soreness.
— *Moxibustion dosage:* 3 cones; stick 10 minutes.

Cross-sectional anatomy of the needle passage
a. *Skin:* branches from the frontal nerve containing fibers from the ophthalmic division of the trigeminal nerve (CN V) innervate the skin.
b. *Subcutaneous tissue:* includes the previously described skin nerve branches, and the supraorbital artery and vein. The supraorbital artery is a branch of the ophthalmic artery.
c. *Frontal muscle:* the branches containing fibers from the temporal branch of the facial nerve (C 7) innervate the frontal muscle.

Functions
Reduces fever and expels Wind, and relieves mental depression.

Clinical indications
Convulsions, headache, dizziness, trigeminal neuralgia, conjunctivitis, nasal obstruction.

8.
(SHENTING) SHENTING, GV 24, GOVERNING VESSEL

Location
In a seated or supine position, the point is located on the mid-sagittal line of the head 1 inch posterior to the front hairline, or 4 inches anterior to Baihui [GV 20].

Needle and moxibustion method
Horizontal insertion 0.3–0.5 inch or use a triangular needle to induce bleeding.
— *Needle sensation:* local distension and soreness.
— *Moxibustion dosage:* 3–5 cones; stick 10 minutes.

Cross-sectional anatomy of the needle passage
a. *Skin:* the branches from the supraorbital nerve containing fibers from the ophthalmic division of the trigeminal nerve (CN V) innervate the skin.
b. *Subcutaneous tissue:* includes the previously described skin nerve branches, and the supraorbital artery and vein. The ophthalmic artery gives rise to the supraorbital artery.
c. *Frontal muscle:* the branches containing fibers from the temporal branch of the facial nerve (CN VII) innervate the muscle. The needle is passed between the two frontal muscles.
d. *Loose connective tissue of the aponeurosis.*
e. *Periosteum of the frontal bone.*

Functions
Reduces fever and stops convulsions, and arrests vomiting.

Clinical indications
Vomiting, tachycardia, pterygium, rhinitis, epilepsy, trismus, convulsions, hysteria, schizophrenia, neurosis.

9.
(CHUCHA) QUCHA, BL 4, FOOT TAI YANG BLADDER MERIDIAN

Location
In a seated or supine position, the point is located at the medial third of the distance between Shenting [GV 24] and Touwei [ST 8], 0.5 inch inside the anterior hair line.

Needle and moxibustion method
Horizontal insertion 0.3–0.4 inch.
— *Needle sensation:* local distension and soreness.
— *Moxibustion dosage:* 3–5 cones; stick 10 minutes.

Cross-sectional anatomy of the needle passage

a. *Skin:* the lateral branches from the frontal nerve containing fibers from the ophthalmic division of the trigeminal nerve (CN V) innervate the skin.

b. *Subcutaneous tissue:* includes the previously described skin nerve branches, and the supraorbital artery and vein. The supraorbital artery is a branch of the ophthalmic artery.

c. *Frontal muscle:* the branches containing fibers from the temporal branch of the facial nerve (CN VII) innervate the muscle.

Functions

Reduces fever and expels Wind, and clears the head to improve visual acuity.

Clinical indications

Nasal obstruction, epistaxis, asthma, frontal headache, blindness, optic neuritis, dizziness, common cold.

10.

(WUCHU) WUCHU, BL 5, FOOT TAI YANG BLADDER MERIDIAN

Location

In a seated position, the point is located 1.5 inches lateral to Shangxing [GV 23], 0.5 inch posterior to Qucha [BL 4], and 1 inch posterior to the front hairline.

Needle and moxibustion method

Horizontal insertion 0.3 inches.
— *Needle sensation:* local distension and heaviness.
— *Moxibustion dosage:* 3 cones; stick 10 minutes.

Cross-sectional anatomy of the needle passage

a. *Skin:* the lateral branches of the frontal nerve containing fibers from the ophthalmic division of the trigeminal nerve (CN V) innervate the skin.

b. *Subcutaneous tissue:* includes the previously described skin nerve branches, and the supraorbital artery and vein. The supraorbital artery is a branch of the ophthalmic artery.

c. *Frontal muscle:* the branches containing fibers from the temporal branch of the facial nerve (CN VII) innervate the frontal muscle.

Functions

Reduces fever, expels Wind, and clears the channels and collaterals to improve acuity of vision.

Clinical indications

Headache, convulsions, back rigidity, epistaxis, blindness, glaucoma, conjunctivitis.

11.

(TOULINCHI) TOULINQI, GB 15, FOOT SHAO YANG GALLBLADDER MERIDIAN

Location

In a seated or supine position, the point is located 0.5 inch inside the frontal hairline, directly above Yangbai [GB 14] and at the mid-point between Touwei [ST 8] and Shenting [GV 24].

Needle and moxibustion method

Horizontal superior insertion 0.3–0.5 inch.
— *Needle sensation:* local distension and soreness.
— *Moxibustion dosage:* 3 cones; stick 5 minutes.

Cross-sectional anatomy of the needle passage

a. *Skin:* the medial and lateral branches of the frontal nerve containing fibers from the ophthalmic division of the trigeminal nerve (CN V) innervate the skin.

b. *Subcutaneous tissue:* includes the previously described skin nerve branches and the frontal artery and vein. The ophthalmic artery gives rise to the frontal artery.

c. *Frontal muscle:* the branches containing fibers from the temporal branch of the facial nerve (CN VII) innervate the muscle.

Functions

Removes Heat from the Liver and Gallbladder, and tranquilizes the Mind to ease mental anxiety.

Clinical indications

Dizziness, eye pain, nasal obstruction, convulsions, deafness, coma.

12.

(SHANGHSING) SHANGXING, GV 23, GOVERNING VESSEL

Location

In a seated or supine position, the point is located on the mid-sagittal line of the head 1 inch posterior to the anterior hairline.

Needle and moxibustion method

Horizontal insertion 0.5–0.8 inch or use a triangular needle to induce bleeding.
— *Needle sensation:* local distension and soreness.
— *Moxibustion dosage:* moxibustion contraindicated.

Cross-sectional anatomy of the needle passage

a. *Skin:* the branches from the supratrochlear and supraorbital nerves containing fibers from the ophthalmic division of the trigeminal nerve (CN V) innervate the skin.

b. *Subcutaneous tissue:* includes the previously described skin nerve branches, and the supratrochlear artery and vein. The subcutaneous tissue contains much vertical dense connective tissue, which connects the skin and epicranium, separating the adipose tissue into many small septa. The supratrochlear artery is a terminal branch of the ophthalmic artery.

c. *Galea aponeurotica:* a strong dense connective tissue which is connected anteriorly to the frontal muscle and posteriorly to the occipital muscle.

Functions

Arrests convulsions, tranquilizes the Mind, and clears and activates the channels and collaterals.

Clinical indications

Headache, dizziness, sinusitis, epistaxis, conjunctivitis, convulsions, hysteria, schizophrenia, hypertension, arteriosclerosis, cerebrovascular disease.

13.

(TOUWEI) TOUWEI, ST 8, FOOT YANG MING STOMACH MERIDIAN

Location

In a seated position, the point is located at the coronal suture 4.5 inches lateral to the midline of the head, and 0.5 inch posterior to the corner of the anterior hairline.

Needle and moxibustion method

Posterior horizontal insertion 0.5–1.0 inch.
— *Needle sensation:* local soreness, or a sensation radiating to the surrounding area.
— *Moxibustion dosage:* moxibustion contraindicated.

Cross-sectional anatomy of the needle passage
(Fig. 3.1)

a. *Skin:* the branches containing fibers from the zygomaticotemporal and auriculotemporal nerves innervate the skin. The zygomaticotemporal nerve is a branch from the maxillary division of the trigeminal nerve (CN V). The auriculotemporal nerve is a branch from the mandibular division of the trigeminal nerve (CN V).

b. *Subcutaneous tissue:* includes the previously described skin nerve branches, the temporal branch of the facial nerve, and the superficial temporal artery and vein. The superficial temporal artery is a terminal branch of the external carotid artery.

c. *Galea aponeurotica of superior margin of temporal muscle:* the temporal muscle, located at the temporal

bone, is a flat fan-shaped muscle. The temporal branches containing fibers from the mandibular division of the trigeminal nerve (CN V) innervate the temporal muscle. The epicranium is a strong dense connective tissue connected anteriorly to the frontal muscle and posteriorly to the occipital bone.

d. *Loose connective tissue beneath the aponeurosis.*

e. *Periosteum of the parietal bone.*

Functions

Expels Wind and purges pathogenic Fire, alleviates pain and improves visual acuity.

Clinical indications

Headache, migraine, schizophrenia, facial palsy, optic neuritis, conjunctivitis.

14.

(MUCHUANG) MUCHUANG, GB 16, FOOT SHAO YANG GALLBLADDER MERIDIAN

Location

In a seated position, the point is located 1.5 inches posterior to Toulinqi [GB 15].

Needle and moxibustion method

Posterior horizontal insertion 0.3–0.4 inch.
— *Needle sensation:* local distension and soreness.
— *Moxibustion dosage:* 3–5 cones; stick 10 minutes.

Cross-sectional anatomy of the needle passage

a. *Skin:* the branches from the medial and lateral frontal nerves containing fibers from the ophthalmic division of the trigeminal nerve (CN V) innervate the skin.

b. *Subcutaneous tissue:* includes the previously described skin nerve branches, and the superficial temporal artery and vein. The external carotid artery gives rise to the superficial temporal artery.

c. *Galea aponeurotica:* a strong dense connective tissue which is connected anteriorly to the frontal muscle and posteriorly to the occipital muscle.

d. *Loose connective tissue beneath the aponeurosis.*

e. *Periosteum of the parietal bone.*

Functions

Clears and activates the channels and collaterals, and improves visual acuity and hearing.

Clinical indications

Headache, dizziness, myopia, nasal obstruction, facial edema, toothache, cerebrovascular disease, hearing loss.

15.

(CHENGYING) ZHENGYING, GB 17, FOOT SHAO YANG GALLBLADDER MERIDIAN

Location
In a seated position, the point is located 1.5 inches posterior to Muchuang [GB 16].

Needle and moxibustion method
Horizontal insertion 0.3–0.5 inch.
— *Needle sensation:* local distension and soreness.
— *Moxibustion dosage:* 3–5 cones; stick 10 minutes.

Cross-sectional anatomy of the needle passage
a. *Skin:* the branches containing fibers from the frontal and greater occipital nerves innervate the skin. The frontal nerve is a branch from the ophthalmic division of the trigeminal nerve (CN V), and the greater occipital nerve is a branch from the second and third cervical nerves (C2, C3).
b. *Subcutaneous tissue:* includes the previously described skin nerve branches, the superficial temporal artery and vein, and the occipital artery. The external carotid artery gives rise to the superficial temporal and the occipital arteries.
c. *Galea aponeurotica:* a strong dense connective tissue which is connected anteriorly to the frontal muscle and posteriorly to the occipital muscle.
d. *Loose connective tissue of the aponeurosis.*
e. *Periosteum of the parietal bone.*

Functions
Clears and activates the channels and collaterals, and arrests vomiting.

Clinical indications
Headache, dizziness, nausea, vomiting, toothache.

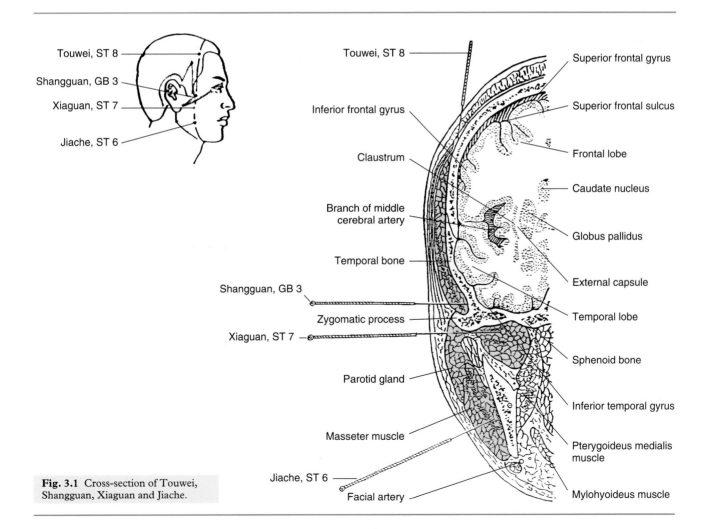

Fig. 3.1 Cross-section of Touwei, Shangguan, Xiaguan and Jiache.

16.

(CHENGLING) CHENGLING, GB 18, FOOT SHAO YANG GALLBLADDER MERIDIAN

Location

In a seated position, the point is located 1.5 inches posterior to Zhengying [GB 17].

Needle and moxibustion method

Horizontal insertion 0.3–0.5 inch.
— *Needle sensation:* local distension and soreness.
— *Moxibustion dosage:* 3–5 cones; stick 10 minutes.

Cross-sectional anatomy of the needle passage

a. *Skin:* the branches containing fibers from the greater occipital nerve from the ophthalmic division of the trigeminal nerve (CN V) innervate the skin.
b. *Subcutaneous tissue:* includes the previously described skin nerve branches, and the occipital artery and vein. The external carotid artery gives rise to the occipital artery.
c. *Galea aponeurotica:* a strong dense connective tissue which is connected anteriorly to the frontal muscle and posteriorly to the occipital muscle.
d. *Loose connective tissue beneath the aponeurosis.*
e. *Epicranium of the parietal bone.*

Functions

Refreshes the head and Mind, and activates the collaterals to dispel Wind.

Clinical indications

Headache, nasal obstruction, nasal discharge, epistaxis, dizziness, asthma, eye pain, fever and chills.

17.

(PENSHEN) BENSHEN, GB 13, FOOT SHAO YANG GALLBLADDER MERIDIAN

Location

In a seated position, the point is located 0.5 inch posterior to the anterior hairline 3 inches lateral to Shenting [GV 24], or two thirds of the distance from Shenting [GV 24] to Touwei [ST 8].

Needle and moxibustion method

Horizontal insertion 0.3–0.5 inch.
— *Needle sensation:* local distension or soreness.
— *Moxibustion dosage:* 3–5 cones; stick 10 minutes.

Cross-sectional anatomy of the needle passage

a. *Skin:* the lateral branches of the frontal nerve containing fibers from the ophthalmic division of the

trigeminal nerve (CN V) innervate the skin.
b. *Subcutaneous tissue:* includes the previously described skin nerve branches, the superficial temporal artery and vein, and the frontal artery and vein. The external carotid artery gives rise to the superficial temporal and frontal arteries.
c. *Frontal muscle:* the branches containing fibers from the temporal branch of the facial nerve (CN VII) innervate the muscle.

Functions

Stops dizziness, alleviates headache, and tranquilizes the Mind to ease mental anxiety.

Clinical indications

Headache, dizziness, vomiting, convulsions, facial palsy, neck stiffness, insomnia, paralysis of the lower extremities.

18.

(HANYAN) HANYAN, GB 4, FOOT SHAO YANG GALLBLADDER MERIDIAN

Location

At the anterior temporal region, the point is located one quarter of the distance between Touwei [ST 8] and Qubin [GB 7]; or 1 inch inferior and posterior to Touwei [ST 8] and 0.5 inch inside the temporal hairline.

Needle and moxibustion method

Horizontal insertion 0.3–0.5 inch.
— *Needle sensation:* local distension and soreness.
— *Moxibustion dosage:* 3 cones; stick 10 minutes.

Cross-sectional anatomy of the needle passage

a. *Skin:* the temporal branches of the auriculotemporal nerve containing fibers from the mandibular division of the trigeminal nerve (CN V) innervate the skin.
b. *Subcutaneous tissue:* includes the previously described skin nerve branches, and the superficial temporal artery and vein. The external carotid artery gives rise to the superficial temporal artery.
c. *Temporal muscle:* the branches containing fibers from the temporal branch of the facial nerve (CN VII) innervate the muscle.

Functions

Dispels Wind, activates the collaterals, alleviates pain, and improves visual acuity.

Clinical indications

Migraine, tinnitus, dizziness, toothache, rhinitis, convulsions, trigeminal neuralgia, rheumatoid arthritis, facial palsy.

19.

(NAOHU) NAOHU, GV 17, GOVERNING VESSEL

Location

In a seated position with the head bent forward, or in a prone position, the point is located on the mid-sagittal line of the head, 1.5 inches superior to Fengfu [GV 16], and superior to the external occipital protuberance.

Needle and moxibustion method

Horizontal insertion 0.3–0.5 inch. Some texts say it is contraindicated for acupuncture.
— *Needle sensation:* soreness and distension.
— *Moxibustion dosage:* stick 5 minutes.

Cross-sectional anatomy of the needle passage

a. *Skin:* the branches from the greater occipital nerve containing fibers from the second and third cervical nerves (C2, C3) innervate the skin.
b. *Subcutaneous tissue:* includes the previously described skin nerve branches, the occipital artery and vein, and the emissary vessel. The external carotid artery gives rise to the occipital artery.
c. *Occipital muscle:* the needle is passed between the two occipital muscles. The branches containing fibers from the posterior auricular branch of the facial nerve (CN VII) innervate the muscle.
d. *Loose connective tissue of the aponeurosis.*
e. The needle is inserted superior to the external occipital protuberance.

Functions

Reduces fever, improves visual acuity, arrests spasms and tranquilizes the Mind.

Clinical indications

Epilepsy, hysteria, infantile convulsion, hypertension, optic neuritis, conjunctivitis, neck stiffness, jaundice, dizziness.

20.

(CHIANGCHIEN) QIANGJIAN, GV 18, GOVERNING VESSEL

Location

In a seated position with the head slightly bent forward or in a prone position, the point is located on the mid-saggital line at the occipital region, 1.5 inches superior to Naohu [GV 17]; or at the midpoint between Fengfu [GV 16] and Baihui [GV 20].

Needle and moxibustion method

Anterior or posterior horizontal insertion 0.3–0.5 inch.
— *Needle sensation:* aching and distension.
— *Moxibustion dosage:* 3–5 cones; stick 10 minutes.

Cross-sectional anatomy of the needle passage

a. *Skin:* branches from the greater occipital nerve containing fibers from the second and third cervical nerves (C2, C3) innervate the skin.
b. *Subcutaneous tissue:* includes the previously described skin nerve branches, and the occipital artery and vein. The external carotid artery gives rise to the occipital artery.
c. *Galea aponeurotica:* a strong dense connective tissue which is connected anteriorly to the frontal muscle and posteriorly to the occipital muscle.
d. *Loose connective tissue of the aponeurosis.*
e. *Periosteum of the occipital and temporal bones.*

Functions

Clears Heat from the Heart to tranquilize the Mind, and relieves rigidity of muscles and tendons in the neck to alleviate pain.

Clinical indications

Headache, epilepsy, hysteria, dizziness, vomiting, neck stiffness, insomnia.

21.

(TIENCHUNG) TIANCHONG, GB 9, FOOT SHAO YANG GALLBLADDER MERIDIAN

Location

In a seated position, the point is located superior to the ear, 0.5 inch posterior to Shuaigu [GB 8]; or at the intersection between a vertical line running through the mastoid process of the temporal bone and a horizontal line from Shuaigu [GB 8].

Needle and moxibustion method

Anterior or posterior horizontal insertion 0.3–0.5 inch.
— *Needle sensation:* soreness and distension.
— *Moxibustion dosage:* 3 cones; stick 10 minutes.

Cross-sectional anatomy of the needle passage

a. *Skin:* branches from the greater occipital nerve containing fibers from the second and third cervical nerves (C2, C3) innervate the skin.
b. *Subcutaneous tissue:* includes the previously described skin nerve branches, and the posterior auricular artery and vein. The external carotid artery gives rise to the posterior auricular artery.

c. *Superior auricular muscle:* a thin fan-shaped muscle. The branches containing fibers from the temporal branch of the facial nerve (CN VII) innervate the muscle.

d. *Temporal muscle:* branches containing fibers from the temporal branch of the facial nerve (CN VII) innervate the muscle.

e. *Galea aponeurotica:* a strong dense connective tissue which is connected anteriorly to the frontal muscle and posteriorly to the occipital muscle.

Functions

Relieves mental stress, and promotes Blood circulation to remove Blood Stasis.

Clinical indications

Headache, convulsions, migraine, hysteria, gingival cyst.

22.

(SHUAIKU) SHUAIGU, GB 8, FOOT SHAO YANG GALLBLADDER MERIDIAN

Location

In a seated position, the point is located 1.5 inches superior to the apex of the ear, at the midpoint between the tip of the ear and the tubercule of the parietal bone.

Needle and moxibustion method

Horizontal insertion 0.3–0.5 inch.
— *Needle sensation:* local aching and distension.
— *Moxibustion dosage:* 3–5 cones; stick 10 minutes.

Cross-sectional anatomy of the needle passage

a. *Skin:* the temporal nerve containing fibers from the auriculotemporal nerve of the mandibular division of the trigeminal nerve (CN V), and the greater occipital nerve containing fibers from the second and third cervical nerves (C2, C3) innervate the skin.

b. *Subcutaneous tissue:* includes the previously described skin nerve branches and the superficial temporal artery and vein. The external carotid artery gives rise to the superficial temporal artery.

c. *Superior auricular muscle:* a thin fan-shaped muscle. Branches containing fibers from the temporal branch of the facial nerve (CN VII) innervate the muscle.

d. *Temporal muscle:* branches containing fibers from the temporal branch of the facial nerve (CN VII) innervate the muscle.

e. *Galea aponeurotica:* a strong dense connective tissue which is connected anteriorly to the frontal muscle and posteriorly to the occipital muscle.

Functions

Reduces Heat and dispels Wind, and clears and activates the channels and collaterals.

Clinical indications

Cough, expectoration, vomiting, migraine, infantile convulsion, eye diseases, facial palsy, bronchitis.

23.

(CHIAOSUN) JIAOSUN, TB 20, HAND SHAO YANG TRIPLE BURNER MERIDIAN

Location

In a seated position, the point is located in the superior posterior auricular sulcus and superior to the tip of the ear.

Needle and moxibustion method

Horizontal insertion 0.3–0.5 inch.
— *Needle sensation:* local distension and soreness radiating to the auricular region.
— *Moxibustion dosage:* 3 cones; stick 5–10 minutes.

Cross-sectional anatomy of the needle passage

a. *Skin:* the branches from the auriculotemporal nerve containing fibers from the mandibular division of the trigeminal nerve innervate the skin.

b. *Subcutaneous tissue:* includes the previously described skin nerve branches and the anterior auricular branch of the superficial temporal artery and vein. The external carotid artery gives rise to the superficial temporal artery.

c. *Superior auricular muscle:* a thin fan-shaped muscle. The branches containing fibers from the temporal branch of the facial nerve (CN VII) innervate the muscle.

d. *Superior auricular concha.*

Functions

Improves visual acuity and hearing, and clears Wind and Heat.

Clinical indications

Pterygium, optic neuritis, migraine, gingivitis, toothache, mumps, tinnitus, deafness, neck stiffness.

24.

(LUHSI) LUXI, TB 19, HAND SHAO YANG TRIPLE BURNER MERIDIAN

Location
In a seated position, the point is located posterior to the ear and superior to the mastoid process of the temporal bone, at the superior third of the distance between Jiaosun [TB 20] and Yifeng [TB 17] when a curved line is drawn between these two points; or 1 inch superior to Chimai [TB 18].

Needle and moxibustion method
Upwards or anterior oblique insertion 0.3–0.5 inch or use a triangular needle to induce bleeding.
— *Needle sensation:* soreness and distension.
— *Moxibustion dosage:* 1–3 cones; stick 5–10 minutes.

Cross-sectional anatomy of the needle passage
a. *Skin:* the branches from the greater occipital nerve containing fibers from the second and third cervical nerves (C2, C3), and the lesser occipital nerve containing fibers from the second cervical nerve (C2) innervate the skin.
b. *Subcutaneous tissue:* includes the previously described skin nerve branches, and the posterior auricular artery and vein. The external carotid artery gives rise to the posterior auricular artery.
c. *Posterior auricular muscle:* branches containing fibers from the posterior auricular branch of the facial nerve (CN VII) innervate the muscle.
d. *Posterior auricular concha.*

Functions
Improves hearing, reduces fever and dispels Wind and settles the Mind.

Clinical indications
Ear pain, tinnitus, deafness, otitis media, bronchial asthma, infantile vomiting, convulsions, common cold, migraine.

25.

(FUPAI) FUBAI, GB 10, FOOT SHAO YANG GALLBLADDER MERIDIAN

Location
The point is located posterior to the ear, at the posterior superior part of the mastoid process of the temporal bone, 1 inch posterior and inferior to Tianchong [GB 9]; or 1 inch posterior to the superior margin of the auricle; or at the midpoint of the slightly curved line between Tianchong [GB 9] and Touqiaoyin [GB 11].

Needle and moxibustion method
Downward horizontal insertion under the skin 0.3–0.5 inch.
— *Needle sensation:* local soreness and distension.
— *Moxibustion dosage:* 3 cones; stick 10 minutes.

Cross-sectional anatomy of the needle passage
a. *Skin:* the branches from the greater occipital nerve containing fibers from the second and third cervical nerves (C2, C3) innervate the skin.
b. *Subcutaneous tissue:* includes the previously described skin nerve branches, and the posterior auricular artery and vein. The external carotid artery gives rise to the posterior auricular artery.
c. *Posterior auricular muscle:* branches containing fibers from the posterior auricular branch of the facial nerve (CN VII) innervate the muscle.
d. *Temporal muscle:* the branches containing fibers from the temporal branch of the facial nerve (CN VII) innervate the muscle.

Functions
Dispels Wind, and regulates the flow of Qi to alleviate pain.

Clinical indications
Headache, migraine, conjunctivitis, optic neuritis, tinnitus, deafness, shoulder pain, bronchitis, paralysis of the lower extremities.

26.

(NAOKUNG) NAOKONG, GB 19, FOOT SHAO YANG GALLBLADDER MERIDIAN

Location
In a seated position with the head bent slightly forward or in a prone position, the point is located lateral to the occipital protuberance 1.5 inches superior to Fenchi [GB 20], and 2 inches lateral to Naohu [GV 17].

Needle and moxibustion method
Horizontal insertion 0.3–0.4 inch.
— *Needle sensation:* local distension.
— *Moxibustion dosage:* 3–5 cones; stick 10 minutes.

Cross-sectional anatomy of the needle passage
a. *Skin:* the branches from the greater occipital nerve containing fibers from the second and third cervical nerves (C2, C3) innervate the skin.
b. *Subcutaneous tissue:* includes the previously described skin nerve branches, and the occipital artery and vein. The external carotid artery gives rise to the occipital artery.

c. *Occipital muscle:* the branches containing fibers from the posterior auricular branch of the facial nerve (CN VII) innervate the muscle.

Functions
Regulates Qi and Blood, and improves visual and auditory acuity.

Clinical indications
Headache, dizziness, convulsions, hysteria, schizophrenia, asthma, common cold, tachycardia, tinnitus, cervical stiffness, optic neuritis, glaucoma.

27.
(YUCHEN) YUZHEN, BL 9, FOOT TAI YANG BLADDER MERIDIAN

Location
In a seated position with the head slightly bent forward or in a prone position, the point is located 1.5 inches posterior to Luoque [BL 8], 1.3 inches lateral to Naohu [GV 17], and 1.3 inches lateral to the superior nuchal line of the external occipital protuberance, between Naohu [GV 17] and Naokong [GB 19].

Needle and moxibustion method
Downward horizontal insertion 0.3–0.5 inch.
— *Needle sensation:* local heaviness and distension.
— *Moxibustion dosage:* 3–5 cones; stick 15 minutes.

Cross-sectional anatomy of the needle passage
a. *Skin:* the branches from the greater occipital nerve containing fibers from the second and third cervical nerves (C2, C3) innervate the skin.
b. *Subcutaneous tissue:* includes the previously described skin nerve branches and the occipital artery and vein. The external carotid artery gives rise to the occipital artery.
c. *Occipital muscle:* the branches containing fibers from the posterior auricular branch of the facial nerve (CN VII) innervate the muscle.

Functions
Improves visual acuity, and clears and activates the channels and collaterals.

Clinical indications
Headache, eye pain, myopia, glaucoma, optic neuritis, nasal obstruction, dizziness.

28.
(CHIMAI) CHIMAI, TB 18, HAND SHAO YANG TRIPLE BURNER MERIDIAN

Location
In a seated position, the point is located posterior to the ear and inferior to the mastoid process of the temporal bone at the inferior one third of the curved posterior auricular line drawn between Yifeng [TB 17] and Jiaosun [TB 20].

Needle and moxibustion method
Inferior anterior oblique insertion towards the mastoid process of the temporal bone 0.3–0.5 inch or use a triangular needle to induce bleeding.
— *Needle sensation:* soreness and distension.
— *Moxibustion dosage:* 3 cones; stick 5–10 minutes.

Cross-sectional anatomy of the needle passage
a. *Skin:* the posterior auricular branch of the greater auricular nerve arising from the cutaneous branch of the cervical plexus innervates the skin.
b. *Subcutaneous tissue:* includes the previously described skin nerve branches and the posterior auricular branch of the occipital artery and vein.
c. *Posterior auricular muscle:* branches containing fibers from the posterior auricular branch of the facial nerve (CN VII) innervate the muscle.
d. *Posterior auricular concha.*

Functions
Clears and activates the channels and collaterals, and improves hearing.

Clinical indications
Headache, dizziness, deafness, infantile convulsions, dysentery, vomiting, blindness, optic neuritis.

29.
(TOUCHIAOYIN) TOUQIAOYIN, GB 11, FOOT SHAO YANG GALLBLADDER MERIDIAN

Location
In a seated position, the point is located behind the ear in the posterior superior fossa of the mastoid process of the temporal bone, at the midpoint between Fubai [GB 10] and Wangu [GB 12]; or 1 inch inferior to Fubai [GB 10].

Needle and moxibustion method
Oblique insertion 0.3–0.5 inch.
— *Needle sensation:* local soreness and distension.
— *Moxibustion dosage:* 3–5 cones; stick 10 minutes.

Cross-sectional anatomy of the needle passage

a. *Skin:* the branches of the greater occipital nerve containing fibers from the second and third cervical nerves (C2, C3) and the lesser occipital containing fibers from the second cervical nerve (C2) innervate the skin.

b. *Subcutaneous tissue:* includes the previously described skin nerve branches and the posterior auricular artery and vein. The external carotid artery gives rise to the posterior auricular artery.

c. *Posterior auricular muscle:* the branches containing fibers from the posterior auricular branch of the facial nerve (CN VII) innervate the muscle.

Functions

Regulates the flow of Qi to lift melancholia, and improves visual acuity.

Clinical indications

Nuchal headache, ear pain, deafness, tinnitus, cough, convulsions, chest pain.

30.

(WANKU) WANGU, GB 12, FOOT SHAO YANG GALLBLADDER MERIDIAN

Location

In a seated position posterior to the ear and 0.7 inch inferior to Touqiaoyin [GB 11], the point is located in the posterior inferior fossa of the mastoid process of the temporal bone.

Needle and moxibustion method

Downward oblique insertion 0.3–0.5 inch.
— *Needle sensation:* local numbness and distension.
— *Moxibustion dosage:* 3–7 cones; stick 10 minutes.

Cross-sectional anatomy of the needle passage

a. *Skin:* the branches from the lesser occipital nerve containing fibers from the second cervical nerve (C2) innervate the skin.

b. *Subcutaneous tissue:* includes the previously described skin nerve branches and the posterior auricular artery and vein. The external carotid artery gives rise to the posterior auricular artery.

c. *Sternocleidomastoid muscle:* the needle is passed into the superior part of the sternocleidomastoid muscle. The branches containing fibers from the spinal accessory nerve (CN XI) and the branches of the second and third cervical nerves (C2, C3) innervate the muscle.

Functions

Dispels Wind and reduces fever, and dredges and activates the channels and collaterals.

Clinical indications

Headache, nuchal pain, toothache, gingival cyst, facial hemiplegia, insomnia, paralysis of the lower extremities, convulsions.

31.

(HSINHUI) XINHUI, GV 22, GOVERNING VESSEL

Location

On the mid-sagittal line of the head, 3 inches anterior to Baihui [GV 20], and 1 inch posterior to Shangxing [GV 23].

Needle and moxibustion method

Horizontal insertion under the skin 0.3–0.5 inch.
— *Needle sensation:* local numbness and distension.
— *Moxibustion dosage:* 3–5 cones; stick 10 minutes.

Cross-sectional anatomy of the needle passage

a. *Skin:* the branches from the supraorbital nerve containing fibers from the ophthalmic division of the trigeminal nerve (CN V) innervate the skin.

b. *Subcutaneous tissue:* includes the previously described skin nerve branches, the superficial temporal artery and vein, and the supraorbital artery and vein pass. The supraorbital artery is a branch of the ophthalmic artery.

c. *Galea aponeurotica:* a strong dense connective tissue which is connected anteriorly to the frontal muscle and posteriorly to the occipital muscle.

d. *Loose connective tissue beneath the aponeurosis.*

e. *Periosteum of the parietal bone.*

Functions

Reduces fever and dispels Wind, and stops convulsions.

Clinical indications

Infantile convulsions, headache, dizziness, hypertension, facial edema, epistaxis, nasal obstruction, insomnia.

32.

(CHIACHE) JIACHE, ST 6, FOOT YANG MING STOMACH MERIDIAN

Location

In a seated or lateral recumbent position, the point is located 1 inch superior to the anterior angle of the mandible, at the highest point of the masseter muscle while clenching the teeth tightly.

Needle and moxibustion method
Perpendicular insertion 0.3–0.5 inch.
— *Needle sensation:* local soreness and distension.

Oblique insertion penetrating to Dicang [ST 4] 2.0–3.0 inches (for treating facial palsy).
— *Needle sensation:* local soreness and distension, and radiating to the surrounding region.

Insertion towards the maxillary or mandibular teeth (treating toothache).
— *Moxibustion dosage:* 3 cones; stick 5–10 minutes.

Cross-sectional anatomy of the needle passage
(Fig. 3.1)
a. *Skin:* the branches from the greater auricular nerve containing fibers from the second and third cervical nerves (C2, C3) innervate the skin.
b. *Subcutaneous tissue:* includes the previously described skin nerve branches, and the mandibular division of the trigeminal nerve.
c. *Masseter muscle:* this has superficial and deep layers. The branches from the buccal nerve containing fibers from the mandibular division of the trigeminal nerve innervate the muscle.
d. With perpendicular insertion, the deepest layer of the needle reaches the mandible. With oblique insertion penetrating to Dicang [ST 4], the needle is passed through the risorius, depressor oris, orbicularis oris and zygomaticus major muscles. The branches containing fibers from the facial nerve (CN VII) innervate the muscles.

Functions
Opens the jaw and clears the collaterals, expels Wind and regulates the flow of Qi.

Clinical indications
Facial palsy, facial muscle spasm, trismus, toothache, mumps, hysteria.

33.

(YINTANG) YINTANG, EX-HN 3, EXTRA MERIDIAN OF HEAD AND NECK

Location
In a supine position, the point is located at the midpoint between the two eyebrows.

Needle and moxibustion method
Oblique downward insertion, and directed to the nasal tip; or left and right penetrating to Zanzhu [BL 2] and Jingming [BL 1] 0.5–1.0 inch.

— *Needle sensation:* local soreness and distension, or radiating to the nasal tip.

Use a triangular needle to induce bleeding.
— *Moxibustion dosage:* 3–5 cones.

Cross-sectional anatomy of the needle passage
a. *Skin:* the branches from the supratrochlear nerve containing fibers from the ophthalmic division of the trigeminal nerve innervate the skin.
b. *Subcutaneous tissue:* includes the previously described skin nerve branches, and the supratrochlear artery and vein. The supratrochlear artery, together with the supratrochlear vein, is a terminal branch of the ophthalmic artery.
c. *Procerus muscle:* the procerus muscle is part of the frontal muscle. The temporal branches containing fibers from the facial nerve (CN VII) innervate the muscle.
d. Deep needling reaches the nasal bone.

Warning
Do not use lateral inferior deep insertion or lifting and thrusting, as this may damage the eyeballs.

Functions
Clears Wind, calms the Mind, opens the Nose.

Clinical indications
Frontal headache, dizziness, insomnia, nasal disease, hypertension, hypotension, infantile convulsions.

34.

(YANGPAI) YANGBAI, GB 14, FOOT SHAO YANG GALLBLADDER MERIDIAN

Location
In a supine position, the point is located 1 inch above the midpoint of the eyebrow directly above the pupil when looking straight ahead.

Needle and moxibustion method
Horizontal downward insertion penetrating to Yuyao [EX-HN 4], or left and right to Sizkukong [TB 23] and Zanzhu [BL 2] respectively, 0.2–0.3 inch.
— *Needle sensation:* distension at the frontal region, or radiating to the top of the skull.
— *Moxibustion dosage:* usually no direct moxibustion; stick 3–5 minutes.

Cross-sectional anatomy of the needle passage
a. *Skin:* the lateral branches of the supraorbital nerve containing fibers from the ophthalmic division of the trigeminal nerve (CN V) innervate the skin.
b. *Subcutaneous tissue:* includes the previously described skin nerve branches, and the supraorbital artery and vein. The supraorbital artery is a branch of the ophthalmic artery.

c. *Occipitofrontal muscle:* the branches containing fibers from the temporal branch of the facial nerve (CN VII) innervate the muscle.

d. The deep layer of the needle reaches the periosteum of the frontal bone.

Functions

Dispels Wind and activates the collaterals, reduces fever, and improves visual acuity.

Clinical indications

Supraorbital nerve palsy, facial palsy, eye diseases, myopia, ptosis, conjunctivitis, night blindness.

35.

(TSANCHU) ZANZHU, BL 2, FOOT TAI YANG BLADDER MERIDIAN

Location

In a supine position, the point is located at the medial end of the eyebrow, in the supraorbital fissure.

Needle and moxibustion method

Inferior oblique insertion penetrating to Jingming [BL 1] 0.3–0.5 inch (treats eye diseases).
— *Needle sensation:* local or periorbital distension and soreness.

Horizontal insertion penetrating to Yuyao [Ex-HN 4] 1.0–1.5 inches (treats facial palsy and headache).
— *Needle sensation:* local and periorbital distension and soreness.

Inferior laterally oblique insertion to the supraorbital foramen 0.5 inch (treats supraorbital nerve pain).
— *Needle sensation:* electrical sensation radiating to the neck.
No moxibustion.

Cross-sectional anatomy of the needle passage

a. *Skin:* the branches from the frontal nerve containing fibers from the ophthalmic division of the trigeminal nerve (CN V) innervate the skin.

b. *Subcutaneous tissue:* includes the previously described skin nerve branches, and the supraorbital artery and vein. The supraorbital artery is a branch of the ophthalmic artery.

c. *Orbicularis oculi muscle:* the zygomatic and temporal branches containing fibers from the facial nerve (CN VII) innervate the muscle.

d. *Corrugator supercilii muscle:* located at the deep layer of the orbital orbicularis oculi and frontal muscles. The temporal branches from the facial nerve (CN VII) innervate the muscle.

e. The deep layer of the needle reaches the periosteum of the frontal bone.

Functions

Reduces fever and expels Wind, and clears channels to improve visual acuity.

Clinical indications

Headache, myopia, acute conjunctivitis, facial palsy, nystagmus, glaucoma, night blindness, excessive tearing.

36.

(YUYAO) YUYAO, EX-HN 4, EXTRA POINT OF THE HEAD AND NECK

Location

In a seated position, with the two eyes looking straight ahead, the point is located in the middle of the eyebrow, directly above the pupil.

Needle and moxibustion method

Horizontal insertion laterally under the skin penetrating to Zanzhu [BL 2] or Sizhukong [TB 23] 0.5–1.0 inch (treats supraorbital nerve pain).
— *Needle sensation:* local distension which can radiate to the eyeball.

Oblique inferior insertion at 30° 0.3–0.5 inch.
— *Needle sensation:* electrical sensation radiating to the surrounding region.
No moxibustion.

Cross-sectional anatomy of the needle passage

a. *Skin:* the lateral branches from the supraorbital nerve containing fibers from the ophthalmic division of the trigeminal nerve (CN V) innervate the skin.

b. *Subcutaneous tissue:* includes the previously described skin nerve branches, the supraorbital artery and vein, and the temporal and zygomatic branches of the facial nerve. The ophthalmic artery gives rise to the supraorbital artery which runs together with the supraorbital nerve to the frontal region. The temporal branches from the facial nerve (CN VII), passing the upper parotid gland to the temporal area, innervate the upper part of the orbital orbicularis oculi and occipitotemporal muscles. The zygomatic branches from the facial nerve (CN VII), passing the upper parotid gland and the zygomatic bone, innervate the lower part of the orbital orbicularis oculi, zygomaticus major, and levator labii superioris muscles.

c. *Orbicularis oculi muscle:* a flat muscle, encircling the eyes. The temporal and zygomatic branches from the facial nerve (CN VII) innervate the muscle.

d. *Occipitofrontal muscle:* a flat muscle at the frontal bone. The temporal branches from the facial nerve (CN VII) innervate the muscle.

e. Deep needling reaches the superciliary arch of the frontal bone.

Clinical indications
Myopia, supraorbital nerve pain, acute conjunctivitis, orbital muscle palsy, facial palsy.

37.
(SZUCHUKUNG) SIZHUKONG, TB 23, HAND SHAO YANG TRIPLE BURNER MERIDIAN

Location
In a seated position, the point is located in the lateral fossa of the eyebrow.

Needle and moxibustion method
Horizontal posterior insertion along with the skin, or penetrating to Yuyao [EX-HN 4] 0.5–1.0 inch.
— *Needle sensation:* local distension.
No moxibustion.

Cross-sectional anatomy of the needle passage
a. Skin: the branches from the supraorbital nerve containing fibers from the ophthalmic division of the trigeminal nerve (CN V), and the branches from the zygomatic nerve containing fibers from the maxillary division of the trigeminal nerve (CN V) innervate the skin.
b. Subcutaneous tissue: includes the previously described skin nerve branches, the superficial temporal artery and vein. The external carotid artery gives rise to the superficial temporal artery, and the superficial vein joins the retromandibular vein.
c. Orbicularis oculi muscle: a flat muscle encircling the eyes. The temporal and zygomatic branches from the facial nerve (CN VII) innervate the muscle.

Functions
Reduces fever and dispels Wind, and activates the collaterals to improve visual acuity.

Clinical indications
Headache, eye diseases, conjunctivitis, optic neuritis, facial palsy, convulsion, schizophrenia.

38.
(CHIUHOU) QIUHUO, EX-HN 7, EXTRA MERIDIAN OF HEAD AND NECK

Location
In a seated or supine position, with the eyes looking straight ahead, the point is located at the lateral quarter of the infraorbital margin.

Needle and moxibustion method
Perpendicular insertion. Ask the patient to look up. The practitioner then uses the index finger to fix the eyeballs, and performs a slow perpendicular and slightly medial insertion towards the optic nerve 0.5–1.0 inch. WARNING: No twirling, lifting and thrusting of the needle.
— *Needle sensation:* soreness and distension radiating to the whole eyeball.
No moxibustion.

Cross-sectional anatomy of the needle passage
(Fig. 3.2)
a. Skin: the branches from the infraorbital nerve containing fibers from the maxillary division of the trigeminal nerve (CN V) innervate the skin.
b. Subcutaneous tissue: includes the previously described skin nerve branches, and the infraorbital artery and vein. The internal maxillary artery gives rise to the infraorbital artery. The infraorbital vein joins the pterygoid plexus and facial vein.
c. Orbicularis oculi muscle: a flat muscle encircling the eye. The temporal and zygomatic branches from the facial nerve (CN VII) innervate the muscle.
d. Fatty tissue of orbit: the supporting tissue of the eyeballs and the extrinsic muscle of the eye and bony orbit. When the needle is punctured through the fatty tissue, little resistance will be felt.
e. Inferior oblique muscle and inferior orbit: the inferior oblique muscle is the extrinsic muscle of the eye. The inferior branches from the oculomotor nerve (CN III) innervate the muscle.

Warning
1. The point bleeds very easily. If the patient complains of a swelling and protruding sensation of the eyeball, withdraw the needle immediately and press the point for 2–3 minutes to prevent further bleeding. With moderate bleeding, there will be local ecchymosis. Use a cold compress to stop bleeding and then a hot compress to increase the blood circulation. Usually these complications will be resolved within 10 days, and without any sequelae.
2. Use a fine needle and do not perform deep twirling, lifting or thrusting of the needle, as it is very easy to penetrate into the intracranial cavity and damage the surrounding structures and to cause bleeding while inserting the point.

Clinical indications
Glaucoma, myopia, cataract, optic neuritis, atrophy of the optic nerve.

39.

(TUNGTZULIAO) TONGZILIAO, GB 1, FOOT SHAO YANG GALLBLADDER MERIDIAN

Location
In a seated or supine position, the point is located 0.5 inch lateral to the lateral ocular angle.

Needle and moxibustion method
Horizontal posterior insertion from the anterior to posterior direction penetrating to Taiyang [EX-HN 5] 0.3–0.5 inch.
— *Needle sensation:* local distension, sometimes radiating to the acoustic meatus.
  Use a triangular needle to induce bleeding.
— *Moxibustion dosage:* 3–5 cones; stick 10 minutes.

Cross-sectional anatomy of the needle passage
a. *Skin:* the zygomatic and zygomaticotemporal branches from the zygomatic nerve containing fibers from the maxillary division of the trigeminal nerve (CN V) innervate the skin.
b. *Subcutaneous tissue:* includes the previously described skin nerve branches.
c. *Orbicularis oculi muscle:* a flat muscle encircling the eyes. The temporal and zygomatic branches from the facial nerve (CN VII) innervate the muscle.
d. *Temporal fascia:* a strong thickened fascia which covers the temporal muscle. There are superficial and deep layers of the fascia; the insertion of the superficial layer is the superficial surface of the zygomatic process of the temporal bone and the insertion of the deep layer is the deep surface between them filled with adipose tissue.
e. *Temporal muscle:* a fan-shaped flat muscle. The deep temporal nerve from the branches of the mandibular division of the trigeminal nerve (CN V) innervates the muscle.

Functions
Reduces fever and dispels Wind, alleviates pain and improves visual acuity.

Clinical indications
Headache, conjunctivitis, night blindness, optic nerve atrophy, glaucoma, myopia, optic neuritis, facial palsy, trigeminal neuralgia.

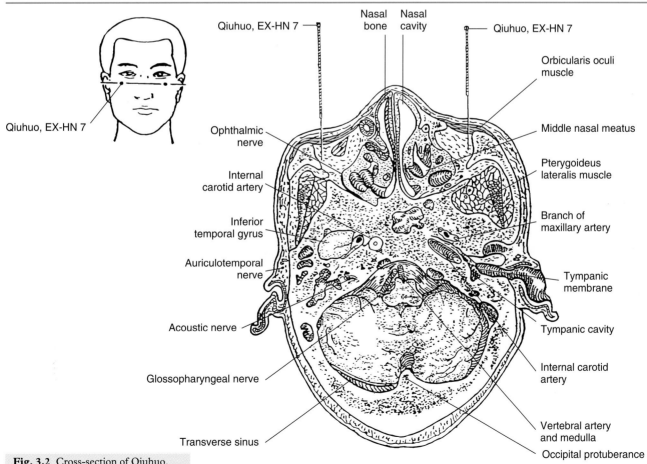

Fig. 3.2 Cross-section of Qiuhuo.

40.

(CHUANLIAO) QUANLIAO, SI 18, HAND TAI YANG SMALL INTESTINE MERIDIAN

Location
In a seated position, the point is located directly below the external ocular angle at the inferior margin of the zygomatic bone, and at the same height as Yingxiang [LI 20].

Needle and moxibustion method
Perpendicular insertion 0.3–0.5 inch.
— *Needle sensation:* local distension.
No direct moxibustion.

Cross-sectional anatomy of the needle passage
a. *Skin:* the infraorbital nerve from the terminal branch of the maxillary division of the trigeminal nerve (CN V) innervates the skin.
b. *Subcutaneous tissue:* includes the previously described skin nerve branches, the transverse facial artery and vein. The superficial temporal artery gives rise to the transverse facial artery, and the transverse facial vein joins the retromandibular vein.
c. *Zygomaticus major muscle:* the zygomatic branches containing fibers from the facial nerve (CN VII) innervate the muscle.
d. *Masseter muscle:* the branches from the masseter nerve containing fibers from the mandibular division of the trigeminal nerve (CN V) innervate the muscle.
e. *Temporal muscle:* a fan-shaped flat muscle. The branches from the deep temporal nerve containing fibers from the mandibular division of the trigeminal nerve (CN V) innervate the muscle.

Functions
Reduces fever and expels Wind, and activates the channels to remove Blood Stasis.

Clinical indications
Facial palsy, facial nerve spasm, trigeminal neuralgia, maxillary toothache, gingivitis, mumps.

41.

(CHULIAO) JULIAO, ST 3, FOOT YANG MING STOMACH MERIDIAN

Location
In a seated or supine position, the point is located at the intersection of a vertical line drawn from the pupils and a horizontal line from the lower border of the ala nasi, and about 0.8 inch lateral to the nostril.

Needle and moxibustion method
Perpendicular insertion 0.3–0.5 inch.
— *Needle sensation:* local distension and soreness.
— *Moxibustion dosage:* 3–5 cones; stick 15 minutes.

Cross-sectional anatomy of the needle passage
a. *Skin:* the branches from the infraorbital nerve containing fibers from the maxillary division of the trigeminal nerve (CN V) innervate the skin.
b. *Subcutaneous tissue:* includes the previously described skin nerve branches, the facial artery and vein, and the infraorbital artery and vein. The external carotid artery gives rise to the facial artery, and the infraorbital artery is a branch of the facial artery.
c. *Quadratus labii superioris muscle:* the buccal branches from the facial nerve (CN VII) innervate the muscle.
d. *Levator anguli oris muscle:* the buccal branches from the facial nerve (CN VII) innervate the muscle.

Functions
Reduces fever, removes Blood Stasis, improves visual acuity, and removes nebula.

Clinical indications
Glaucoma, conjunctiva congestion, lacrimation, myopia, epistaxis, toothache, facial hemiplegia.

42.

(YINGHSIANG) YINGXIANG, LI 20, HAND YANG MING LARGE INTESTINE MERIDIAN

Location
In a supine position, the point is located on the superior part of the nasolabial groove 0.5 inches lateral to the midpoint of the lateral border of the ala nasi, or 1 inch superior and lateral to Kouheliao [LI 19].

Needle and moxibustion method
Penetrating to Bitong [Ex-HN 14] 0.5–0.8 inch (treating nasal diseases).

Penetrating to Sibai [ST 2] 0.5–1.0 inch (treating ascariasis disease of the gallbladder).
— *Needle sensation:* local soreness, distension and lacrimation, and sometimes radiating to the nose.

Cross-sectional anatomy of the needle passage
(Fig. 3.3)
a. *Skin:* the branches from the infraorbital nerve containing fibers from the maxillary division of the trigeminal nerve (CN V) innervate the skin.
b. *Subcutaneous tissue:* includes the previously described skin nerve branches and the facial artery and vein. The external carotid artery gives rise to the facial artery. The facial vein, together with the facial artery,

comes from the submental vein, and then enters the external jugular vein.

c. *Levator labii superioris muscle:* the buccal branches from the facial nerve (CN VII) innervate the muscle. The muscle originates from the infraorbital margin and infraorbital foramen of the maxillary bone, and inserts at the skin of the upper lip, nasal alae, and nasolabial groove.

d. Deep needling reaches the maxillary bone. If the needle is inserted to Bitong [EX-HN 14], it may be passed through the levator labii superioris alaeque nasi muscle. If the needle is inserted to Sibai [ST 2], it may reach the infraorbital foramen which contains

the infraorbital nerve, artery, and vein. Don't insert to Sibai [ST 2] too deep, as this may damage the infraorbital nerve, artery, and vein.

Functions
Reduces fever, expels Wind, clears the channels and induces resuscitation.

Clinical indications
Sinusitis, parasinusitis, epistaxis, nasal polyps, conjunctivitis, facial palsy, ascariasis disease of the gallbladder, constipation.

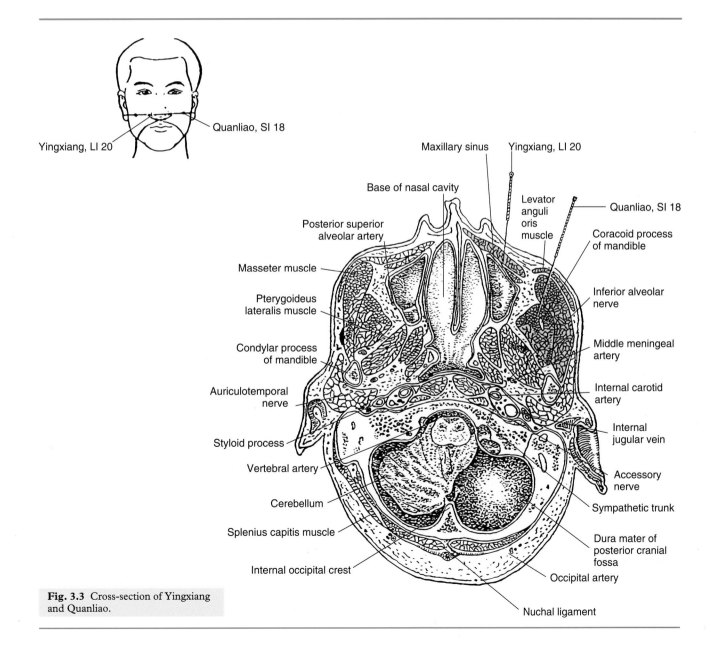

Fig. 3.3 Cross-section of Yingxiang and Quanliao.

43.

(SHANGYINGHSIANG) SHANGYINGXIANG (BITONG), EX-HN 8, EXTRA POINT OF THE HEAD AND NECK

Location

In the inferior fossa of the nasal bone, at the superior end of the nasolabial groove at the intersection of the nose and the face.

Needle and moxibustion method

Superior medial oblique insertion 0.3–0.5 inch.
— *Needle sensation:* lacrimation and local distension, sometimes radiating to the nose. Usually no moxibustion.

Cross-sectional anatomy of the needle passage

a. *Skin:* the branches from the infraorbital nerve containing fibers from the maxillary division of the trigeminal nerve (CN V) and the infratrochlear nerve containing fibers from the ophthalmic division of the trigeminal nerve (CN V) innervate the skin.
b. *Subcutaneous tissue:* includes the previously described skin nerve branches and the angular artery. The angular artery is a terminal branch of the facial artery.
c. *Levator labii superioris alaeque nasi muscle:* the buccal branches from the facial nerve (CN VII) innervate the muscle. The muscle originates from the maxillary bone, and inserts at the skin of the upper lip, ala nasi, and nasolabial groove.

Clinical indications

Sinusitis, nasal polyps.

44.

(SULIAO) SULIAO, GV 25, GOVERNING VESSEL

Location

In a seated or supine position, the point is located at the tip of the nose.

Needle and moxibustion method

Superior oblique insertion 0.3–0.5 inch.
— *Needle sensation:* soreness and numbness, radiating to the nasal meatus and the nasal root.
   Use a triangular needle to induce bleeding.
No moxibustion.

Cross-sectional anatomy of the needle passage

a. *Skin:* the branches from the anterior ethmoid nerve containing fibers from the ophthalmic division of the trigeminal nerve (CN V) innervate the skin.
b. *Subcutaneous tissue:* contains a small amount of adipose tissue, closely connecting the subcutaneous tissue and the skin and includes the previously described skin nerve branches, the dorsal nasal artery and vein. The facial artery gives rise to the dorsal nasal artery, together with the dorsal nasal vein.
c. *Nasal cartilage:* a hyaline cartilage.

Functions

Reduces fever, restores depleted Yang and rescues the patient from collapse.

Clinical indications

Shock, hypotension, infantile convulsion, bradycardia, epistaxis, sinusitis, nasal polyp, rosacea.

45.

(HOLIAO) HELIAO, LI 19, HAND YANG MING LARGE INTESTINE MERIDIAN

Location

Above the upper lip at the intersection of lines drawn vertically from the lateral margin of the nostril and horizontally from Shuigou [GV 26].

Needle and moxibustion method

Horizontal medial insertion 0.3–0.5 inch.
— *Needle sensation:* local soreness.
No moxibustion.

Cross-sectional anatomy of the needle passage

(Fig. 3.4)
a. *Skin:* the branches from the infraorbital nerve containing fibers from the maxillary division of the trigeminal nerve (CN V) innervate the skin.
b. *Subcutaneous tissue:* includes the previously described skin nerve branches and the superior labial artery. The superior labial artery is a branch of the facial artery.
c. *Orbicularis oris muscle:* an oval-shaped flat muscle encircling the mouth. The buccal and mandibular branches containing fibers from the facial nerve (CN VII) innervate the muscle.

Functions

Reduces fever, expels Wind, clears the channels and induces resuscitation.

Clinical indications

Sinusitis, epistaxis, facial palsy.

46.

(YIFENG) YIFENG, TB 17, HAND SHAO YANG TRIPLE BURNER MERIDIAN

Location

Posterior to the ear lobe, in the fossa which appears when opening the mouth, at the midpoint between the mastoid process of the temporal bone and the mandibular bone.

Needle and moxibustion method

Oblique insertion from lateral posterior to medial inferior direction 0.5–1.5 inches (treating deafness).
— *Needle sensation:* local soreness and numbness, and sometimes radiating to the pharynx.

Perpendicular insertion 0.5–1.0 inch (treating facial paralysis and mumps).
— *Needle sensation:* ear soreness and distension, or sometimes radiating to the anterior tongue.
— *Moxibustion dosage:* 3–5 cones; stick 5–10 minutes.

Cross-sectional anatomy of the needle passage
(Fig. 3.4)

a. *Skin:* the branches from the greater auricular nerve containing fibers from the second and third cervical nerves (C2, C3) innervate the skin.

b. *Subcutaneous tissue:* includes the previously described skin nerve branches.

c. *Parotid gland:* the largest pair of the salivary glands, and deltoid-shaped. The parotid glands are located at the anterior inferior surface of the external auditory meatus, the posterior surface of masseter muscle, and the posterior border of mandible. The parotid glands are encapsulated by the masseteric fascia. The external carotid artery, the posterior mandibular vein, the facial nerve, and the auriculotemporal nerve innervate the parotid gland.

d. *Sternocleidomastoid muscle:* the branches from the spinal accessory nerve (CN XI), and the anterior branches containing fibers from the second and third cervical nerves (C2, C3) innervate the muscle.

e. *Splenius capitis muscle:* at the deep layer of the sternocleidomastoid muscle. The posterior branches

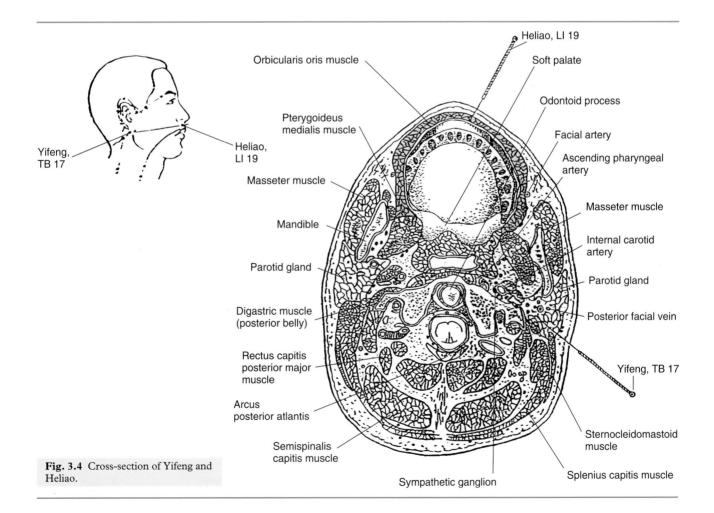

Fig. 3.4 Cross-section of Yifeng and Heliao.

containing fibers from the second and third cervical nerves (C2, C3) innervate the muscle.

f. *Longus capitis muscle:* one of the sacrospinalis muscles. The posterior branches containing fibers from the first to eighth cervical nerves (C1–C8) innervate the muscle.

g. *Digastric muscle, posterior belly:* the digastric muscle consists of the anterior and posterior belly which is connected by the intermediate tendon. The branches containing fibers from the facial nerve (CN VII) innervate the posterior belly of the digastric muscle. The branches containing fibers from the trigeminal nerve (CN V) innervate the anterior belly of the muscle.

Functions
Dispels Wind and clears the collaterals, and improves hearing.

Clinical indications
Dizziness, deafness, otitis media, mumps, toothache, eye pain, facial palsy, mandibular joint arthritis.

47.

(SHUIGOU) SHUIGOU, GV 26, GOVERNING VESSEL

Location
In a seated or supine position, the point is located below the nose in the superior one third of the nasolabial groove.

Needle and moxibustion method
Oblique upward insertion 0.5–1.0 inch.
— *Needle sensation:* local pain. Twirling the needle sometimes causes soreness and distension.

Triple penetration method: the needle is inserted first towards the nasal septal, then withdrawn up to the skin level, and then is inserted towards both alae nasi (treating salivation).
— *Needle sensation:* local soreness and distension.

Use the nail to press the point.
— *Moxibustion dosage:* 3–5 cones; stick 10 minutes. Usually no moxibustion is permitted.

Cross-sectional anatomy of the needle passage
a. *Skin:* the branches from the infraorbital nerve containing fibers from the maxillary division of the trigeminal nerve (CN V) innervate the skin.
b. *Subcutaneous tissue:* includes the previously described skin nerve branches, and the superior labial artery and vein. The facial artery gives rise to the superior

labial artery. The superior labial vein is a branch of the facial vein.
c. *Orbicularis oris muscle:* the oval-shaped flat muscle encircling the mouth. The buccal and mandibular branches from the facial nerve (CN VII) innervate the muscle.

Functions
Reduces fever, revives the spirit, regulates the flow of Qi and promotes Blood circulation.

Clinical indications
Shock, coma, heat stroke, convulsions, hysteria, acute lumbar sprain, sea sickness, car sickness.

48.

(TITSANG) DICANG, ST 4, FOOT YANG MING STOMACH MERIDIAN

Location
In a lateral recumbent position, the point is located 0.4 inch lateral to the oral angle.

Needle and moxibustion method
Penetrating through to Jiache [ST 6] 1.5–2.0 inches (treating facial paralysis).

Penetrating through Yingxiang [LI 20] 1.0–2.0 inches (treating trigeminal neuralgia).
— *Needle sensation:* local or half facial soreness and distension.
— *Moxibustion dosage:* 3–5 cones; stick 10 minutes. Usually moxibustion is contraindicated.

Cross-sectional anatomy of the needle passage
a. *Skin:* the branches from the buccal nerve containing fibers from the mandibular division of the trigeminal nerve (CN V), and the branches from the infraorbital nerve containing fibers from the maxillary division of the trigeminal nerve (CN V) innervate the skin.
b. *Subcutaneous tissue:* includes the previously described skin nerve branches, and the facial artery and vein. The external carotid artery gives rise to the facial artery.
c. *Orbicularis oris muscle:* the oval-shaped flat muscle encircling the mouth. The buccal and mandibular branches containing fibers from the facial nerve (CN VII) innervate the muscle.
d. *Buccinator muscle:* at the deepest layer of the face, a rectangular flat muscle. The buccal branches containing fibers from the facial nerve (CN VII) innervate the muscle.

Functions

Expels Wind and activates the collaterals, to relieve facial pain.

Clinical indications

Facial palsy, facial muscle spasm, salivation, trigeminal neuralgia, infantile convulsions.

49.

(CHENGCHIANG) CHENGJIANG, CV 24, CONCEPTION VESSEL

Location

In a supine position, the point is located on the anterior midline in the fossa of the mentolabial sulcus.

Needle and moxibustion method

Upward oblique insertion 0.3–0.5 inch.
— *Needle sensation:* local soreness and distension.
— *Moxibustion dosage:* 3–5 cones; stick 5–10 minutes.

Cross-sectional anatomy of the needle passage

a. *Skin:* the mentalis nerve from the terminal branch of the inferior alveolar nerve containing fibers from the mandibular division of the trigeminal nerve (CN V) innervates the skin. The mentalis nerve supplies the mandibular teeth, the mandibular gingiva, the skin and mucosa of the mental and lower lip.
b. *Subcutaneous tissue:* includes the previously described skin nerve branches, the mentalis artery and vein, and the submentalis artery and vein. The mentalis artery, together with the mentalis vein, is a terminal branch of the inferior alveolar artery. The facial artery gives rise to the submentalis artery, supplying the lower lip, mental muscles and skin. The submentalis vein is a branch of the facial vein.
c. *Orbicularis oris muscle:* the oval-shaped flat muscle encircling the mouth. The buccal and mandibular branches containing fibers from the facial nerve (CN VII) innervate the muscle.
d. *Depressor labii muscle:* a deltoid-shaped flat muscle. The mandibular branches containing fibers from the facial nerve (CN V) innervate the muscle.
e. *Mentalis muscle:* at the deep layer of the depressor labii muscle, a pyramid-shaped muscle. The mandibular branches containing fibers from the facial nerve (CN VII) innervate the muscle.
f. Deep insertion of the needle reaches the mandibular bone.

Functions

Reduces fever and dispels Wind, and tranquilizes the Mind.

Clinical indications

Facial palsy, cerebrovascular disease, toothache, mouth ulcer, excessive salivation.

50.

(CHIACHENGCHIANG) JIACHENGJIANG, EX-HN-18, EXTRA POINT OF THE HEAD AND NECK

Location

In a supine position, the point is located 1 inch lateral to Chengjiang [CV 24], directly inferior to Dicang [ST 4].

Needle and moxibustion method

Perpendicular insertion 0.2–0.5 inch.
— *Needle sensation:* local soreness and distension.
    Oblique insertion in an inferior medial oblique direction 0.3–0.5 inch (treating trigeminal neuralgia).
— *Needle sensation:* electrical sensation radiating to the lower lip.

Cross-sectional anatomy of the needle passage

a. *Skin:* the mentalis nerve from the terminal branch of the inferior alveolar nerve containing fibers from the mandibular division of the trigeminal nerve (CN V) innervates the skin.
b. *Subcutaneous tissue:* includes the previously described skin nerve branches, the mentalis artery and vein, and the submentalis artery and vein. The mentalis artery, together with the mentalis vein, is a terminal branch of the inferior alveolar artery. The facial artery gives rise to the submentalis artery. The submentalis vein is a branch of the facial vein.
c. *Orbicularis oris muscle:* the oval-shaped flat muscle encircling the mouth. The buccal and mandibular branches containing fibers from the facial nerve (CN VII) innervate the muscle.
d. *Depressor labii muscle:* a deltoid-shaped flat muscle which originates from the lateral nose and inserts to the mental tubercle. The mandibular branches from the facial nerve (CN VII) innervate the muscle.
e. Deep insertion of the needle reaches the lateral side of the mental foramen.

Clinical indications

Trigeminal neuralgia, facial palsy, facial muscle spasm.

51.

(TAYING) DAYING, ST 5, FOOT YANG MING STOMACH MERIDIAN

Location

In a seated position, the point is located 1.3 inches anterior to the mandibular angle; or on clenching the teeth, the point is located in the groove at the anterior margin of the masseter muscle, in the fossa of the mandibular bone.

Needle and moxibustion method

Oblique insertion 0.3–0.5 inch (WARNING: avoid vessel) or penetrating to Jiache [ST 6] or Chengjiang [CV 24] 0.3–1.0 inch.
— *Needle sensation:* facial distension and numbness.
— *Moxibustion dosage:* 3–5 cones; stick 15 minutes.

Cross-sectional anatomy of the needle passage

a. *Skin:* the branches from the mentalis nerve containing fibers from the mandibular division of the trigeminal nerve (CN V), and the branches from the facial nerve (CN VII) innervate the skin.
b. *Subcutaneous tissue:* includes the previously described skin nerve branches.
c. *Masseter muscle:* the needle is inserted at the anterior margin of the masseter muscle. The branches containing fibers from the masseter nerve from the mandibular division of the trigeminal nerve (CN V) innervate the muscle.
d. *Facial artery and vein:* the needle is passed posterior to the facial artery and vein. The external carotid artery gives rise to the facial artery and vein.

Functions

Regulates the channels and collaterals, and promotes the flow of Qi and Blood.

Clinical indications

Toothache, facial edema, fever, facial palsy, trismus, wry mouth, stiff tongue.

52.

(TUITUAN) DUIDUAN, GV 27, GOVERNING VESSEL

Location

In a seated or supine position, the point is located in the middle of the upper lip at the junction of the mucosa of the upper lip and the skin of the philtrum.

Needle and moxibustion method

Upwards oblique insertion 0.2–0.3 inch.
— *Needle sensation:* local soreness and distension.
— *Moxibustion dosage:* 1–3 cones; stick 3–5 minutes.

Cross-sectional anatomy of the needle passage

a. *Skin:* the buccal branches containing fibers from the facial nerve (CN VII) and the branches from the infraorbital nerve containing fibers from the trigeminal nerve (CN V) innervate the skin.
b. *Subcutaneous tissue:* includes the previously described skin nerve branches, and the superior labial artery and vein. The facial artery gives rise to the superior labial artery, together with the superior labial vein.
c. *Orbicularis oris muscle:* an oval-shaped muscle encircling the mouth. The buccal branches containing fibers from the facial nerve (CN VII) innervate the muscle.

Functions

Reduces fever and dispels Wind, and refreshes the Mind.

Clinical indications

Nasal obstruction, nasal polyps, epistaxis, toothache, diabetes mellitus, pterygium, jaundice, convulsions, hysteria, schizophrenia.

53.

(YINCHIAO) YINJIAO, GV 28, GOVERNING VESSEL

Location

In a seated position with the upper lip raised, the point is located in the junction between the frenulum of the upper lip and the gingiva.

Needle and moxibustion method

Upwards oblique insertion 0.1–0.2 inch or use a triangular needle to induce bleeding.
— *Needle sensation:* local soreness and distension.
Moxibustion contraindicated.

Cross-sectional anatomy of the needle passage

a. *Skin:* the superior alveolar branches containing fibers from the maxillary division of the trigeminal nerve (CN V) innervate the skin.
b. *Subcutaneous tissue:* includes the previously described skin nerve branches, and the superior labial artery and vein. The facial artery gives rise to the superior labial artery and vein.
c. *Orbicularis oris muscle:* an oval-shaped muscle encircling the mouth. The buccal branches containing

fibers from the facial nerve (CN VII) innervate the muscle.

d. Deep needling reaches the frenulum of the upper lip.

Functions
Promotes the Blood circulation to clear the collaterals, and removes Heat from fever.

Clinical indications
Pterygium, nasal polyp, nasal obstruction, gingival cyst, jaundice, psychosis.

54.

(TAIYANG) TAIYANG, EX-HN 5, EXTRA MERIDIAN OF HEAD AND NECK

Location
In a seated or lateral recumbent position, drawing a vertical line from the lateral eyebrow, and another horizontal line from the lateral ocular angle, the point is located in the depression 1 inch posterior to the intersection.

Needle and moxibustion method
Perpendicular insertion 0.5–1.0 inch.
— *Needle sensation:* local soreness and distension.

Horizontal insertion, along the skin posteriorly penetrating 1.0–2.0 inches (treating migraine).
— *Needle sensation:* soreness and distension radiating to the temporal region.

Horizontal insertion, downwards under the skin penetrating to Jiache [ST 6] 3 inches (treating facial palsy).

Use a triangular needle to induce bleeding (treating acute conjunctivitis or headache).
No moxibustion.

Cross-sectional anatomy of the needle passage
a. *Skin:* the branches from the zygomatic nerve containing fibers from the maxillary division of the trigeminal nerve (CN V) innervate the skin.
b. *Subcutaneous tissue:* includes the previously described skin nerve branches, and the superficial temporal artery and vein. The superficial temporal artery is a terminal branch of the external carotid artery. The superficial temporal vein, together with the superficial temporal artery, joins the retromandibular vein.
c. *Orbicularis oculi muscle:* the oval-shaped flat muscle encircling the eye. The temporal and zygomatic branches containing fibers from the facial nerve (CN VII) innervate the muscle.
d. *Temporal fascia:* a strong thick fascia, which covers the temporal muscle.

e. *Temporal muscle:* covered with the strong temporal fascia and adipose tissue. The branches from the deep temporal nerve containing fibers from the mandibular division of the trigeminal nerve innervate the muscle.

Clinical indications
Migraine, trigeminal neuralgia, facial palsy, facial muscle spasm, vertigo, dizziness, conjunctiva congestion, optic neuritis, optic nerve atrophy.

55.

(HSIAKUAN) XIAGUAN, ST 7, FOOT YANG MING STOMACH MERIDIAN

Location
The point is located at the inferior margin of the zygomatic process of the temporal bone and the anterior part of the condyloid process of the mandible. Open the mouth to locate the point.

Needle and moxibustion method
Inferior perpendicular insertion 1.5 inches (treating trigeminal neuralgia).
— *Needle sensation:* local soreness and distension, or radiating to the mandibular alveolar.

Anterior posterior oblique insertion 0.8–1.0 inch (treating mandibular joint inflammation).
— *Needle sensation:* soreness and distension radiating to the whole temporomandibular joint.

Horizontal insertion along the external mandible to the maxillary teeth (oral angle) and the mandibular teeth (Jiache [ST 6]) 1.5–2.0 inches (treating toothache).
— *Needle sensation:* soreness and distension radiating to the maxillary and mandibular teeth.

Posteriorly oblique insertion 1.5 inches (treating auricular disease).
— *Needle sensation:* soreness and distension radiating to the auricular region.

Inferior oblique insertion 1.5–2.0 inches (treating masseter muscle spasm).
— *Needle sensation:* local soreness and distension.
— *Moxibustion dosage:* 3–5 cones; stick 5–10 minutes.

Cross-sectional anatomy of the needle passage
(Figs 3.1 & 3.5)
a. *Skin:* the branches from the auriculotemporal nerve containing fibers from the mandibular division of the trigeminal nerve (CN V) innervate the skin.
b. *Subcutaneous tissue:* includes the previously described skin nerve branches, the temporal branch of the facial nerve, and the transverse facial artery and vein.

The temporal branches containing fibers from the facial nerve (CN VII) innervate the orbicularis oculi, temporal, and levator labii superioris muscles. The transverse artery is a branch of the superficial temporal artery. The transverse facial vein joins the posterior submandibular vein.

c. *Parotid gland:* the largest salivary gland. The facial ganglion, the auriculotemporal nerve, the superficial temporal artery and vein, and the maxillary artery and vein pass through the parotid gland.

d. *Masseter muscle:* a rectangular flat muscle. The branches from the masseter nerve containing fibers from the mandibular division of the trigeminal nerve (CN V) innervate the muscle.

e. *Posterior temporal muscle and mandibular notch:* the branches from the deep temporal nerve containing fibers from the mandibular division of the trigeminal nerve (CN V) innervate the temporal muscle. The mandibular notch is between the carotid process and the condyle of the mandible. The needle is passed posterior to the temporal muscle through the mandibular notch.

f. *Maxillary artery and vein:* the external carotid artery gives rise to the maxillary artery, and the maxillary vein joins the retromandibular vein.

g. *Lateral pterygoid muscle:* beneath the infratemporal fossa, a deltoid-shaped muscle. The branches from the lateral pterygoid nerve containing fibers from the mandibular division of the trigeminal nerve (CN V) innervate the muscle.

h. The deepest layer of the needle reaches the mandibular alveolar nerve, the lingual nerve, and the middle meningeal artery. The mandibular alveolar and lingual nerves are the branches of the mandibular division of the trigeminal nerve (CN V). If the needle punctures these structures, soreness and distension of the surrounding region or electrical sensation radiating to the mandibular alveolar will be felt. The middle meningeal artery is a branch of the maxillary artery. To avoid puncturing the needle into

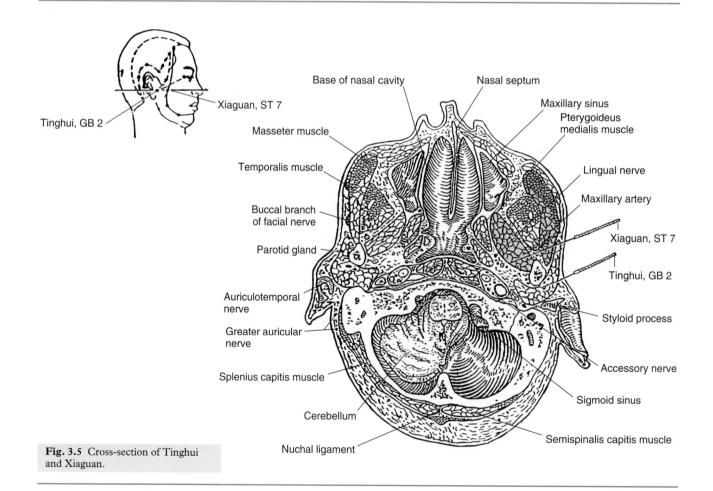

Fig. 3.5 Cross-section of Tinghui and Xiaguan.

the middle meningeal artery, which may cause massive bleeding, don't insert the needle too deeply.

Functions
Expels Wind and activates the collaterals, and regulates the flow of Qi to alleviate pain.

Clinical indications
Facial palsy, facial muscle spasm, trigeminal neuralgia, toothache, otitis media, inflammation of the mandibular joint.

56.

(SHANGKUAN) SHANGGUAN, GB 3, FOOT SHAO YANG GALLBLADDER MERIDIAN

Location
The point is located anterior to the ear superior to Xiaguan [ST 7], in the fossa of the superior margin of the zygomatic process of the temporal bone.

Needle and moxibustion method
Perpendicular insertion 0.3–0.5 inch (WARNING: no deep insertion.)
— *Needle sensation:* local distension and soreness.
— *Moxibustion dosage:* 3 cones; stick 5 minutes.

Cross-sectional anatomy of the needle passage
(Fig. 3.1)
a. *Skin:* the zygomaticofacial branches containing fibers from the maxillary division of the trigeminal nerve (CN V) and the zygomatic branches from the facial nerve (CN VII) innervate the skin.
b. *Subcutaneous tissue:* includes the previously described skin nerve branches, and the superficial temporal artery and vein. The external carotid artery gives rise to the superficial temporal artery.
c. *Temporal muscle:* the temporal branches containing fibers from the facial nerve (CN VII) innervate the muscle.
d. *Maxillary artery and vein:* the external carotid artery gives rise to the maxillary artery, and the maxillary vein joins the retromandibular vein.
e. The needle reaches the superior margin of the zygomatic process of the temporal bone.

Functions
Improves hearing and visual acuity, and dispels Wind.

Clinical indications
Tinnitus, deafness, toothache, migraine, dizziness, convulsions, facial paralysis, optic neuritis, glaucoma.

57.

(TINGHUI) TINGHUI, GB 2, FOOT SHAO YANG GALLBLADDER MERIDIAN

Location
In a seated or lateral recumbent position, the point is located in the anterior fossa of the intertragic notch at the posterior margin of the condyle of the mandible while opening the mouth. The point is directly below Tinggong [SI 19].

Needle and moxibustion method
Opening the mouth, use a slightly obliquely posterior perpendicular insertion 1.0–1.5 inches.
— *Needle sensation:* local soreness and distension.
— *Moxibustion dosage:* 3–5 cones; stick 10 minutes.

Cross-sectional anatomy of the needle passage
(Fig. 3.5)
a. *Skin:* the branches from the auriculotemporal nerve containing fibers from the mandibular division of the trigeminal nerve (CN V) and the greater auricular nerve containing fibers from the second and third cervical nerves (C2, C3) innervate the skin.
b. *Subcutaneous tissue:* includes the previously described skin nerve branches, and the superficial temporal artery and vein. The superficial temporal artery is a terminal branch of the external carotid artery and supplies nutrients to the parotid glands, the skin and muscle of the frontal and temporal region. The superficial temporal vein joins the posterior mandibular vein.
c. *Parotid fascia:* encircling the parotid gland, this is the superficial layer of the deep carotid fascia which is divided into the superficial and deep layers at the posterior margin of the parotid gland.
d. *Parotid gland:* the largest salivary gland. The facial plexus, the auriculotemporal nerve, the superficial temporal artery and vein, and the maxillary artery and vein.

Functions
Removes Heat from the Liver and Gallbladder, and improves hearing.

Clinical indications
Deafness, tinnitus, otitis media, auditory hallucinations, toothache, mumps, facial palsy.

58.

(ERHMEN) ERMEN, TB 21, HAND SHAO YANG TRIPLE BURNER MERIDIAN

Location
In a seated or lateral recumbent position, with the mouth open, the point is located anterior to the supra-tragic notch, or in the fossa at the posterior margin of the condyle of the mandible.

Needle and moxibustion method
Slightly posterior oblique insertion 0.5–1.0 inch or inferior penetration to Tinggong [SI 19], and Tinghui [GB 2] 1.0–1.5 inches.
— *Needle sensation:* local soreness and distension, or radiating to the side of the face.
— *Moxibustion dosage:* 3–5 cones.

Cross-sectional anatomy of the needle passage
(Fig. 3.6)
a. *Skin:* the branches from the auriculotemporal nerve containing fibers from the mandibular division of the trigeminal nerve (CN V) innervate the skin.
b. *Subcutaneous tissue:* includes the previously described skin nerve branches, and the superficial temporal artery and vein. The superficial temporal artery is a terminal branch of the external carotid artery. The superficial temporal vein joins the posterior mandibular vein.
c. *Superior part of parotid gland:* the largest salivary gland. The facial plexus, the auriculotemporal nerve, the superficial temporal artery, and the maxillary artery and vein pass.

Functions
Promotes and regulates the functional activities of the Qi of the ear and improves hearing.

Clinical indications
Tinnitus, deafness, otitis media, toothache, inflammation of mandibular joint.

59.

(CHUPIN) QUPIN, GB 7, FOOT SHAO YANG GALLBLADDER MERIDIAN

Location
In a seated or lateral recumbent position, draw a horizontal line from Jiaosun [TB 20] and a vertical

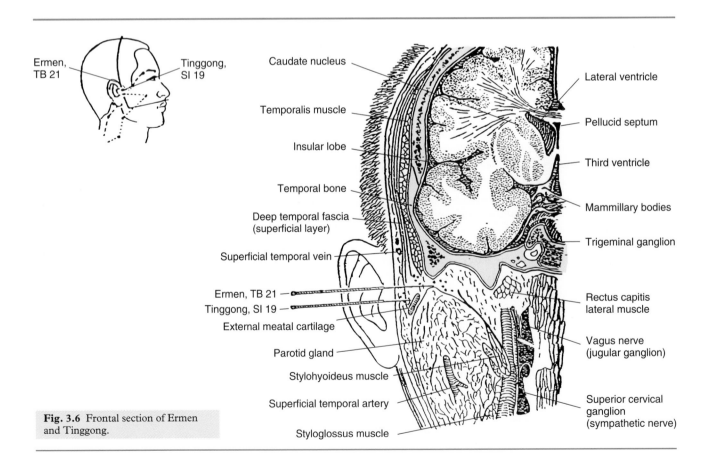

Fig. 3.6 Frontal section of Ermen and Tinggong.

line from the anterior helix of the ear, the point is located at the intersection of the two lines (approximately one finger width anterior to Jiaohsun [TB 20]).

Needle and moxibustion method

Horizontal insertion 0.3–0.5 inch.
— *Needle sensation:* local aching and distension.
— *Moxibustion dosage:* 3–5 cones; stick 3–5 minutes.

Cross-sectional anatomy of the needle passage

a. *Skin:* the temporal branches from the auriculotemporal nerve containing fibers from the mandibular division of the trigeminal nerve (CN V) innervate the skin.
b. *Subcutaneous tissue:* includes the previously described skin nerve branches, and the superficial temporal artery and vein. The external carotid artery gives rise to the superficial temporal artery. The superficial temporal vein joins the posterior mandibular vein.
c. *Temporal muscle:* the temporal branches containing fibers from the facial nerve (CN VII) innervate the muscle.

Functions

Refreshes the head and dispels Wind, and activates the collaterals.

Clinical indications

Migraine, toothache, vomiting, infantile convulsions, eye diseases, optic neuritis, conjunctivitis.

60.

(HSUANLU) XUANLU, GB 5, FOOT SHAO YANG BLADDER MERIDIAN

Location

In a seated position, the point is located at the midpoint of the line between Touwei [ST 8] and Qubin [GB 7] in the anterior frontal region.

Needle and moxibustion method

Posterior horizontal insertion 0.2–0.3 inch.
— *Needle sensation:* local soreness and distension.
— *Moxibustion dosage:* 3–5 cones; stick 3 minutes.

Cross-sectional anatomy of the needle passage

a. *Skin:* the temporal branches of the auriculotemporal nerve containing fibers from the mandibular division of the trigeminal nerve (CN V) innervate the skin.
b. *Subcutaneous tissue:* includes the previously described skin nerve branches, and the superficial temporal artery and vein. The external carotid artery gives rise

to the superficial temporal artery. The superficial temporal vein joins the posterior mandibular vein.
c. *Temporal muscle:* the temporal branches containing fibers from the facial nerve (CN VII) innervate the muscle.

Functions

Dispels Wind and activates the collaterals, alleviates pain and reduces swelling.

Clinical indications

Eye pain, toothache, migraine, rhinitis, common cold, trigeminal neuralgia.

61.

(HSUANLI) XUANLI, GB 6, FOOT SHAO YANG GALLBLADDER MERIDIAN

Location

In a seated position, the point is located in the hairline of the temporal region three quarters of the distance from Touwei [ST 8] to Qubin [GB 7]; or at the midpoint between Xuanlu [GB 5] and Qubin [GB 7].

Needle and moxibustion method

Posterior horizontal insertion 0.3–0.5 inch.
— *Needle sensation:* local distension and soreness.
— *Moxibustion dosage:* 3–5 cones; stick 3 minutes.

Cross-sectional anatomy of the needle passage

a. *Skin:* the temporal branches of the auriculotemporal nerve containing fibers from the mandibular division of the trigeminal nerve (CN V) innervate the skin.
b. *Subcutaneous tissue:* includes the previously described skin nerve branches, and the superficial temporal artery and vein. The external carotid artery gives rise to the superficial temporal artery. The superficial temporal vein joins the posterior mandibular vein.
c. *Temporal muscle:* the temporal branches containing fibers from the facial nerve (CN VII) innervate the muscle.

Functions

Reduces fever and dispels Wind, and dredges and activates the channels and collaterals.

Clinical indications

Migraine, common cold, vomiting, intermittent fever, convulsions, trigeminal neuralgia, tinnitus, rhinitis.

62.

(ERHHOLIAO) ERHELIAO, TB 22, HAND SHAO YANG TRIPLE BURNER MERIDIAN

Location
In a seated or lateral recumbent position, the point is located level with the root of the ear anterior and superior to Ermen [TB 21] at the posterior margin of the superficial temporal artery; or at the midpoint between Qubin [GB 7] and Shangguan [GB 3].

Needle and moxibustion method
Oblique insertion 0.1–0.3 inch (WARNING: avoid the superficial temporal artery.)
— *Needle sensation:* local soreness and distension.
— *Moxibustion dosage:* 1–2 cones; stick 5–10 minutes.

Cross-sectional anatomy of the needle passage
a. *Skin:* the branches from the auriculotemporal nerve containing fibers from the mandibular division of the trigeminal nerve (CN V) and the temporoparietal branches from the facial nerve (CN VII) innervate the skin.
b. *Subcutaneous tissue:* includes the previously described skin nerve branches, and the superficial temporal artery and vein. The superficial temporal artery is a branch of the external carotid artery. The superficial temporal vein joins the posterior mandibular vein.
c. *Temporal muscle:* the temporal branches containing fibers from the facial nerve (CN VII) innervate the muscle.
d. The needle reaches the zygomatic process of the temporal bone.

Functions
Improves hearing, reduces fever and dispels Wind.

Clinical indications
Headache, tinnitus, nasal discharge, trismus, migraine.

63.

(TINGKUNG) TINGGONG, SI 19, HAND TAI YANG SMALL INTESTINE MERIDIAN

Location
In a seated or lateral recumbent position, with the mouth slightly open, the point is located in between the tragus and the mandibular joint, or at the midpoint between Ermen [TB 21] and Tinghui [GB 2].

Needle and moxibustion method
Slightly inferior perpendicular insertion 0.5–1.0 inch.
— *Needle sensation:* local soreness and distension, or radiating to the ipsilateral face, or spreading into the inner part of the ear.
— *Moxibustion dosage:* 3–5 cones; stick 10 minutes.

Cross-sectional anatomy of the needle passage
(Fig. 3.6)
a. *Skin:* the branches from the auriculotemporal nerve containing fibers from the mandibular division of the trigeminal nerve (CN V) innervate the skin.
b. *Subcutaneous tissue:* includes the previously described skin nerve branches, and the superficial temporal artery and vein. The superficial temporal artery is a terminal branch of the external carotid artery. The superficial temporal vein joins the posterior mandibular vein.
c. *Cartilage of external auditory meatus:* the external one third of the auditory meatus is cartilage and the inner two thirds are bone. The needle is inserted into the cartilaginous auditory meatus.

Functions
Reduces fever and activates the collaterals, alleviates tinnitus and improves hearing.

Clinical indications
Tinnitus, deafness, otitis media, otitis externa, facial palsy, schizophrenia, convulsions.

4

Cross-sectional anatomy of the neck

The border of the neck and the head has been described in Section 3. The border line of the neck and the trunk is the superior margin of the manubrium of the sternum anteriorly, the clavicle and acromion laterally, and the line of the acromion to the spinous process of the seventh cervical vertebra posteriorly.

1.

(LIENCHUAN) LIANQUAN, CV 23, CONCEPTION VESSEL

Location
In a supine position, on the anterior midline of the neck, the point is located in the fossa superior to the thyroid cartilage between the hyoid and mandibular bones.

Needle and moxibustion method
Perpendicular insertion towards the tongue root 0.5–0.8 inch.
— *Needle sensation:* local distension, or radiating to the tongue.
— *Moxibustion dosage:* 3–5 cones; stick 10 minutes.

Cross-sectional anatomy of the needle passage
a. *Skin:* the ascending branches of the transverse cervical nerve containing fibers from the second and third cervical nerves (C2, C3) innervate the skin.
b. *Subcutaneous tissue:* includes the previously described skin nerve branches, and the anterior jugular vein. The subcutaneous tissue consists of the platysma muscle and the submental lymph node. The anterior jugular vein joins the subclavicular vein. The platysma muscle is a thin wide muscle, firmly attached to the skin. The cervical branches of the facial nerve (CN VII) innervate the platysma muscle.
c. *Digastric muscle:* the muscle contains the anterior and posterior bellies united by an intermediate round tendon. The posterior belly is innervated by the branches containing fibers from the facial nerve (CN VII), and the anterior belly by the mylohyoid nerve containing fibers from the inferior alveolar branches

of the trigeminal nerve (CN V). The needle is passed between the anterior and posterior bellies.
d. *Mylohyoid muscle:* a flat triangular-shaped muscle, at the medial part of the mandible, and between the mandibular and hyoid bones. The muscle is supplied by the inferior alveolar branches from the mandibular division of the trigeminal nerve (CN V).
e. *Geniohyoideus muscle:* a small rectangular-shaped muscle, at the superior part of the hyoid muscle and the inferior part of the tongue. The hypoglossal nerve from the first cervical nerve (C1) innervates the muscle.

Functions
Regulates the throat, reduces fever and regulates the flow of Qi.

Clinical indications
Tongue numbness, tongue muscle atrophy, cough, tonsillitis, pharyngitis, paralysis of the vocal cords, bronchitis, bronchial asthma, deafness.

2.

(FUTU) FUTU, LI 18, HAND YANG MING LARGE INTESTINE MERIDIAN

Location
In a seated or supine position, the point is located on the lateral side of the neck in between the sternal and clavicular heads of the sternocleidomastoid muscle, and 3 inches lateral to the apex of the Adam's apple.

Needle and moxibustion method
Perpendicular insertion towards the cervical spine 0.5–1.0 inch.
— *Needle sensation:* swelling and tightness of the throat, or electrical sensation radiating to the hand.
— *Moxibustion dosage:* 1–3 cones; stick 5–10 minutes.

Cross-sectional anatomy of the needle passage
(Fig. 4.1)

a. *Skin:* the transverse nerve from the cutaneous branches of the second and third cervical nerves (C2, C3) innervate the skin.

b. *Subcutaneous tissue:* includes the transverse nerve, the platysma muscle, and the cervical branch of the facial nerve. The platysma muscle is a thin wide muscle firmly attached to the skin. The cervical branches containing fibers from the facial nerve (CN VII) innervate the platysma muscle.

c. *Sternocleidomastoid muscle:* covered with the superficial layer of the cervical fascia. Two heads of the muscle originate from the anterior sternum and the medial part of the clavicle, and the insertion of the muscle is the mastoid process of the temporal bone. The needle is passed between the junction of the sternal and clavicular heads of the muscle. The branches containing fibers from the spinal accessory nerve (CN XI) and the anterior rami of the second and third cervical nerves (C2, C3) innervate the muscle.

d. The needle is inserted at the anterior margin of the carotid sheath. The carotid sheath consists of the common carotid artery, the internal jugular vein, and the vagus nerve. To avoid damage to the vessel and nerve, don't insert the needle deeply.

Functions
Regulates the flow of Qi and Blood circulation, and removes Heat from the throat and chest.

Clinical indications
Asthma, sputum, hoarseness of voice, sore throat, difficulty in swallowing, acupuncture anesthesia in thyroid operations, neurosis, hysteria, schizophrenia.

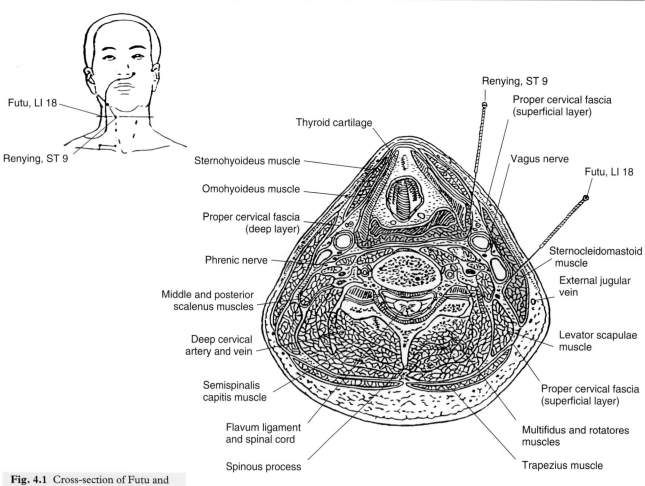

Futu, LI 18

Renying, ST 9

Renying, ST 9
Proper cervical fascia (superficial layer)
Thyroid cartilage
Sternohyoideus muscle
Omohyoideus muscle
Proper cervical fascia (deep layer)
Phrenic nerve
Middle and posterior scalenus muscles
Deep cervical artery and vein
Semispinalis capitis muscle
Flavum ligament and spinal cord
Spinous process
Vagus nerve
Futu, LI 18
Sternocleidomastoid muscle
External jugular vein
Levator scapulae muscle
Proper cervical fascia (superficial layer)
Multifidus and rotatores muscles
Trapezius muscle

Fig. 4.1 Cross-section of Futu and Renying.

3.

(YIMING) YIMING (ANMIAN), EX-HN 14, EXTRA POINT OF THE HEAD AND NECK

Location

In a lateral seated position with the head slightly bent forward, the point is located posterior to the ear at the same height as the ear lobe at the midpoint between Fengchi [GB 20] and Yifeng [TB 17].

Needle and moxibustion method

Perpendicular insertion 0.5–1.0 inch.
— *Needle sensation:* ipsilateral soreness, distension and electrical sensation.

Cross-sectional anatomy of the needle passage

(Fig. 4.2)

a. Skin: the branches from the greater auricular nerve containing fibers from the second and third cervical nerves (C2, C3) and the lesser auricular nerve arising from the second cervical nerve (C2) innervate the skin.

b. Subcutaneous tissue: includes the previously described skin nerve branches, and the posterior auricular artery and vein. The external carotid artery gives rise to the posterior auricular artery, together with the posterior auricular vein. The posterior auricular vein joins the external jugular vein.

c. Sternocleidomastoid muscle: two heads of the muscle originate from the anterior sternum and medial part of the clavicle, and the insertion of the muscle is the mastoid process of the temporal bone. The branches containing fibers from the spinal accessory nerve (CN XI) and the anterior rami of the second and third cervical nerves (C2, C3) innervate the muscle.

d. Splenius capitis muscle: at the deep layer of the sternocleidomastoid muscle, an irregular deltoid-shaped muscle. The lateral branches of the dorsal primary divisions of the middle and lower clavicle nerves innervate the muscle.

e. Longus capitis muscle: the middle part of the sacrospinalis muscle. The branches containing fibers from the first, second and third cervical nerves (C1, C2, C3) innervate the muscle.

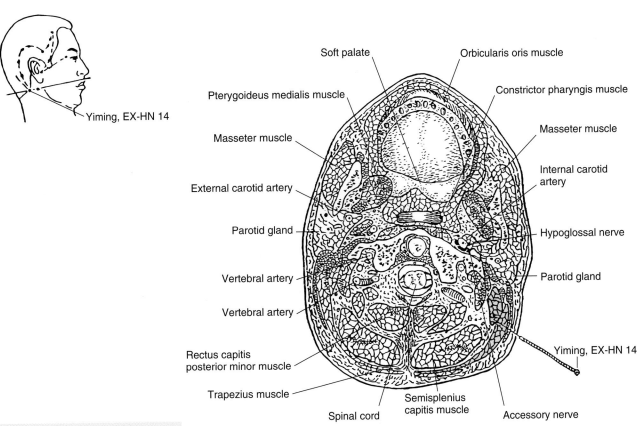

Fig. 4.2 Cross-section of Yiming.

Warning

The deep layer of the point is composed of the carotid artery and vein, and the cervical artery. To avoid damage to these structures, don't insert the needle too deeply.

Clinical indications

Myopia, cataract, night blindness, optic nerve atrophy, tinnitus, dizziness, insomnia.

4.

(TIENYU) TIANYOU, TB 16, HAND SHAO YANG TRIPLE BURNER MERIDIAN

Location

In a seated or lateral recumbent position, the point is located in the posterior inferior part of the mastoid process of the temporal bone at the posterior margin of the sternocleidomastoid muscle; or drawing a horizontal line from the inferior mandibular angle, and another vertical line from the posterior margin of the mastoid process of the temporal bone, the point is located at the intersection of the two lines.

Needle and moxibustion method

Perpendicular insertion 0.5–1.0 inch.
— *Needle sensation:* local soreness and distension radiating to the head.
— *Moxibustion dosage:* 3 cones; stick 3–5 minutes.

Cross-sectional anatomy of the needle passage
(Fig. 4.3)

a. *Skin:* the branches from the greater occipital nerve containing fibers from the second and third cervical nerves (C2, C3) and the lesser occipital nerve arising from the second cervical nerve (C2) innervate the skin.

b. *Subcutaneous tissue:* includes the previously described skin nerve branches.

c. *Sternocleidomastoid and trapezius muscles:* the needle is passed between these two muscles. The branches containing fibers from the spinal accessory nerve (CN XI) and the anterior rami of the second and third cervical nerves (C2, C3) innervate the sternocleido-mastoid muscle. The trapezius muscle runs from the neck down the back of the body, and is a broadened deltoid-shaped muscle. The branches from the spinal accessory nerve (CN XI) and the ventral primary division of the third and fourth cervical nerves (C3, C4) innervate the trapezius muscle.

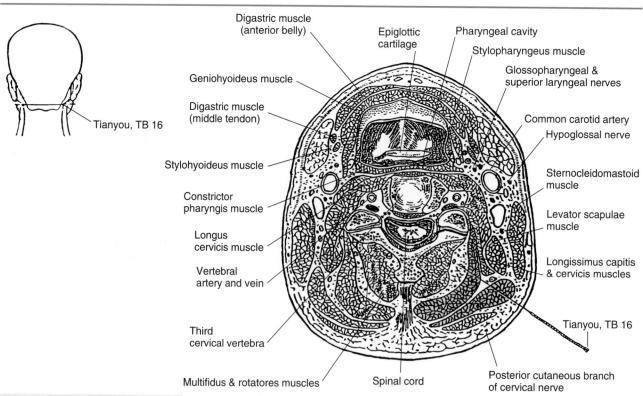

Tianyou, TB 16

Digastric muscle (anterior belly)
Epiglottic cartilage
Pharyngeal cavity
Stylopharyngeus muscle
Glossopharyngeal & superior laryngeal nerves
Geniohyoideus muscle
Digastric muscle (middle tendon)
Common carotid artery
Hypoglossal nerve
Stylohyoideus muscle
Sternocleidomastoid muscle
Constrictor pharyngis muscle
Levator scapulae muscle
Longus cervicis muscle
Longissimus capitis & cervicis muscles
Vertebral artery and vein
Tianyou, TB 16
Third cervical vertebra
Multifidus & rotatores muscles
Spinal cord
Posterior cutaneous branch of cervical nerve

Fig. 4.3 Cross-section of Tianyou.

d. *Splenius capitis and cervicis muscles:* the branches containing fibers from the dorsal divisions of the second to fifth cervical nerves (C2–C5) innervate both muscles.

e. *Deep cervical artery and vein:* the deep cervical artery is a branch of the costocervical trunk. The deep cervical vein joins the brachiocephalic vein.

f. *Semispinalis capitis and cervicis muscles:* the muscles are located at the deep layer of the splenius capitis and cervicis muscles, and the semispinalis cervicis muscle is located at the deepest layer of the muscle groups. The branches containing fibers from the dorsal division of the second to fourth cervical nerves (C2–C4) innervate these two muscles.

Functions
Refreshes the mind, improves hearing, and promotes Blood circulation to remove Blood Stasis.

Clinical indications
Deafness, tinnitus, sore throat, neck stiffness.

5.
(TIENJUNG) TIANRONG, SI 17, HAND TAI YANG SMALL INTESTINE MERIDIAN

Location
In a seated or lateral recumbent position, the point is located on the lateral superior part of the neck in the fossa at the posterior angle of the mandible, at the anterior margin of the sternocleidomastoid muscle.

Needle and moxibustion method
Perpendicular insertion 0.5–1.0 inch.
— *Needle sensation:* local soreness and distension, and radiating to the tongue root or the throat.
— *Moxibustion dosage:* 3 cones; stick 3–5 minutes.

Cross-sectional anatomy of the needle passage
(Fig. 4.4)
a. *Skin:* the branches from the greater auricular nerve containing fibers from the second and third cervical nerves (C2, C3) innervate the skin.
b. *Subcutaneous tissue:* includes the previously described skin nerve branches, and the external jugular vein.

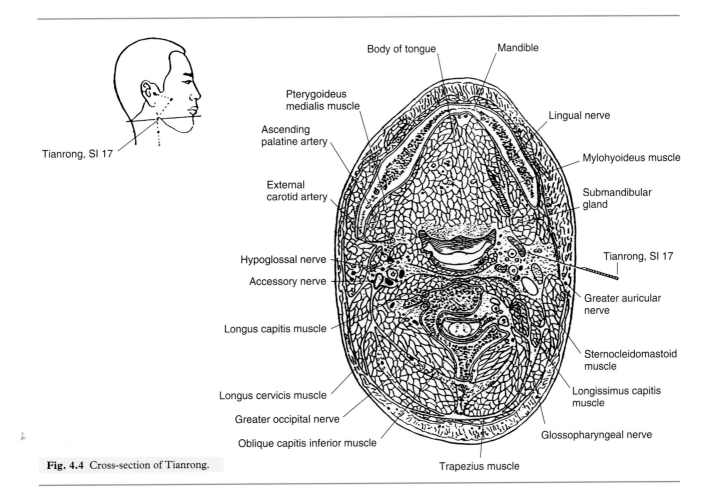

Fig. 4.4 Cross-section of Tianrong.

The external jugular vein, the largest superficial vein, obliquely ascends the external surface of the sternocleidomastoid muscle and joins the subclavian vein.

c. *Digastric and stylohyoid muscles:* the posterior belly of the digastric muscle is innervated by the branches containing fibers from the facial nerve (CN VII), and the anterior belly by branches containing fibers from the trigeminal nerve (CN V). The stylohyoid muscular branches containing fibers from the facial nerve (CN VII) innervate the stylohyoid muscle.

d. The deepest level of the needle can reach the anterior part of the external carotid artery. Deep insertion is contraindicated.

Functions

Reduces fever and alleviates swelling, and improves Blood circulation to activate the collaterals.

Clinical indications

Tonsillitis, sore throat, cervical cyst, asthma, otitis media, deafness, tinnitus, mumps, neck stiffness.

6.

(TIENCHU) TIANZHU, BL 10, FOOT TAI YANG BLADDER MERIDIAN

Location

In a seated position with the head bent forward, or in a prone position, the point is located 1.3 inches lateral to Yamen [GV 15], at the lateral margin of the trapezius muscle.

Needle and moxibustion method

Perpendicular insertion 0.5–1.0 inch.
— *Needle sensation:* local distension and soreness, and radiating to the head and neck.
— *Moxibustion dosage:* 5–10 cones; stick 3–5 minutes.

Cross-sectional anatomy of the needle passage

a. *Skin:* the branches from the third occipital nerve containing fibers from the third cervical nerve (C3) innervate the skin.

b. *Subcutaneous tissue:* includes the previously described skin nerve branches, and the subcutaneous vein.

c. *Trapezius muscle:* a broadened deltoid-shaped muscle. The branches of the spinal accessory nerve containing fibers from the vertebral primary division of the third and fourth cervical nerves (C3, C4) innervate the muscle.

d. *Splenius capitis muscle:* at the deep layer of the sternocleidomastoid muscle and an irregular flat deltoid-shaped muscle. The branches containing fibers from the dorsal division from the second to fifth cervical nerves (C2–C5) innervate the muscle.

e. *Semispinalis capitis muscle:* this small muscle is located at the deep layer of the splenius capitis muscle. The branches containing fibers from the dorsal division from the second to fourth cervical nerves (C2–C4) innervate the muscle.

Warning

1. If the needle is inserted more than 1 inch, it may reach the greater occipital nerve and the rectus capitis posterior major muscle. The greater occipital nerve is one of the branches of the dorsal rami of the second cervical nerve (C2). The branches from the dorsal rami of the suboccipital nerve containing fibers from the first cervical nerve (C1) innervate the rectus capitis posterior major muscle.

2. Don't puncture the needle deeply in the medial superior direction, as it may penetrate into the medulla oblongata.

Functions

Reduces fever, expels Wind, and clears and activates the channels and collaterals.

Clinical indications

Headache, neck stiffness, sore throat, hysteria, convulsions, infantile convulsions, schizophrenia, hypochondriasis, common cold, insomnia.

7.

(TIENCHUANG) TIANCHUANG, SI 16, HAND TAI YANG SMALL INTESTINE MERIDIAN

Location

In a seated position, the point is located on the lateral aspect of the neck on the posterior margin of the sternocleidomastoid muscle, and 0.5 inch posterior to Futu [LI 18].

Needle and moxibustion method

Perpendicular insertion 0.3–0.7 inch.
— *Needle sensation:* electrical sensation radiating to the thumb.
— *Moxibustion dosage:* 3–5 cones; stick 10 minutes.

Cross-sectional anatomy of the needle passage

a. *Skin:* the branches from the greater auricular nerve containing fibers from the second and third cervical nerves (C2, C3), and the cervical cutaneous nerves containing fibers from the third cervical nerve (C3) innervate the skin.

b. *Subcutaneous tissue:* includes the previously described skin nerve branches, and the ascending cervical artery.

c. *Sternocleidomastoid muscle:* the needle is inserted at

the posterior margin of the sternocleidomastoid muscle. The branches containing fibers from the spinal accessory nerve and the anterior rami of the second and third cervical nerves (C2, C3) innervate the muscle.

d. *Trapezius muscle:* a broadened deltoid-shaped muscle. The needle is inserted at the anterior margin of the muscle. The branches from the spinal accessory nerve containing fibers from the vertebral primary division of the third and fourth cervical nerves (C3, C4) innervate the muscle.

e. *Splenius capitis muscle:* the deep layer muscle of the sternocleidomastoid muscle, an irregular flat deltoid-shaped muscle. The branches from the dorsal divisions containing fibers from the second to fifth cervical nerves (C2–C5) innervate the muscle.

Functions

Reduces fever and relieves sore throat, improves hearing and induces resuscitation.

Clinical indications

Sore throat, common cold, deafness, tinnitus, cervical stiffness, aphasia of cerebrovascular disease, schizophrenia, hypertension.

8.

(TIENTING) TIANDING, LI 17, HAND YANG MING LARGE INTESTINE MERIDIAN

Location

In a seated position, the point is located above the midpoint of the supraclavicular fossa 0.5 inch posterior to the posterior margin of the sternocleidomastoid muscle, at the midpoint between Futu [LI 18] and Quepen [ST 12], or 1 inch below Futu [LI 18].

Needle and moxibustion method

Perpendicular insertion 0.3–0.5 inch.
— *Needle sensation:* distension and soreness radiating to the throat or the upper extremities.
— *Moxibustion dosage:* 3–7 cones; stick 15 minutes.

Cross-sectional anatomy of the needle passage

a. *Skin:* the branches from the supraclavicular nerve containing fibers from the third and fourth cervical nerves (C3, C4) and the cervical cutaneous nerve containing fibers from the third cervical nerve (C3) innervate the skin.

b. *Subcutaneous tissue:* includes the previously described skin nerve branches, the platysma muscle, and the external jugular vein. The external jugular vein joins the subclavicular vein. The branches containing fibers from the cervical branch of the facial nerve (CN VII) innervate the platysma muscle.

c. *Sternocleidomastoid muscle:* the needle is inserted at the posterior margin of the sternocleidomastoid muscle. The branches containing fibers from the spinal accessory nerve (CN XI) and the anterior rami of the second and third cervical nerves (C2, C3) innervate the muscle.

d. *Middle scalene muscle:* the needle is inserted at the origin of the middle scalene muscle. The branches containing fibers from the fifth to eighth cervical nerves (C5–C8) innervate the muscle.

e. *Phrenic nerve:* the phrenic nerve is located at the posterior lateral part of the internal jugular vein. The phrenic nerve originates from the third, fourth and fifth cervical nerves (C3, C4, C5).

Functions

Promotes the flow of Qi to remove Blood Stasis, and relieves sore throat.

Clinical indications

Hoarseness, sore throat, tonsillitis, numbness of the upper extremities.

Cross-sectional anatomy of the trunk

The border line of the trunk and the neck, upper extremities and the lower extremities has been described in Sections 1, 2 and 4.

For surface measurement during acupuncture treatment, the distance from the superior margin of the sternum (jugular notch) to the junction of the body and the xiphoid process of the sternum is 9 inches, the distance between the two nipples is 8 inches, from the umbilicus to the junction of the body and the xiphoid process of the sternum is 8 inches, from the umbilicus to the superior margin of the pubic symphysis is 5 inches, from the middle of the axilla to the eleventh rib is 12 inches, from the eleventh rib to the greater trochanter of the femur is 9 inches, from the posterior middle line to the vertebral margin of the scapula is 3 inches, and from the spinous process of the first thoracic vertebra to the inferior margin of the median sacral crest is 9 inches.

1.

(CHUNGFU) ZHONGFU, LU 1, HAND TAI YIN LUNG MERIDIAN, FRONT-MU POINT OF THE LUNG

Location
In a supine or seated position, the point is located on the lateral superior part of the chest in the first intercostal space, 6 inches lateral to the midline of the sternum.

Needle and moxibustion method
Lateral superior oblique insertion 0.5–1.0 inch.
— *Needle sensation:* distension and soreness radiating to the chest and the upper extremities.
— *Moxibustion dosage:* 3–5 cones; stick 5–10 minutes.

Cross-sectional anatomy of the needle passage
(Fig. 5.1)
a. *Skin:* the branches from the supraclavicular nerve containing fibers from the fourth cervical nerve (C4) innervate the skin.
b. *Subcutaneous tissue:* includes the previously described skin nerve branches.

c. *Anterior margin of deltoid muscle:* the needle is inserted at the superior part of the anterior margin of the deltoid muscle. The branches from the axillary nerve containing fibers from the anterior branches of the fifth and sixth cervical nerves (C5, C6) innervate the muscle.
d. The needle is inserted medial to the cephalic vein, which joins the axillary vein.
f. *Pectoralis major muscle:* a flat fan-shaped muscle. The medial and lateral pectoral nerves containing fibers from the brachial plexus of the fifth cervical to the first thoracic nerves (C5–T1) innervate the muscle. The needle is inserted lateral to the pectoral nerve.
g. *Pectoralis minor muscle:* at the deeper layer of the pectoralis major muscle. The branches from the medial pectoral nerve from the brachial plexus of the fifth cervical to the first thoracic nerves (C5–T1) innervate the muscle.
h. *Coracobrachialis and biceps brachii muscles:* the coracobrachialis muscle is located at the medial side of the short head of the biceps brachii muscle. The branches from the musculocutaneous nerve containing fibers from the fifth to seventh cervical nerves (C5–C7) and fifth to sixth cervical nerves (C5, C6) innervate the coracobrachialis and biceps brachii muscles, respectively.

Functions
Clears and disperses the Upper Jiao (Upper Warmer), and promotes Lung Qi.

Clinical indications
Bronchitis, pneumonia, asthma, tuberculosis, tonsillitis.

2.

(HSUANCHI) XUANJI, CV 21, CONCEPTION VESSEL

Location
In a seated or supine position, the point is located on the anterior midline of the chest in the middle of the manubrium of the sternum; or in the fossa 1 inch below Tiantu [CV 22].

Needle and moxibustion method
Horizontal downward insertion 0.3–0.5 inch.
— *Needle sensation:* local distension and soreness.
— *Moxibustion method:* 3–5 cones; stick 5–15 minutes.

Cross-sectional anatomy of the needle passage
(Fig. 5.2)
a. *Skin:* the branches from the supraclavicular nerve containing fibers from the third and fourth cervical nerves (C3, C4) innervate the skin.

b. *Subcutaneous tissue:* includes the previously described skin nerve branches, and the anterior perforating branches of the internal thoracic artery and vein. The internal thoracic artery is a branch of the subclavicular artery. The internal thoracic vein drains into the brachiocephalic vein.

c. *Pectoralis major muscle:* a flat fan-shaped muscle. The medial and lateral pectoral nerves containing fibers from the brachial plexus of the fifth cervical to first thoracic nerves (C5–T1) innervate the muscle.

d. Deep needling reaches the manubrium of the sternum.

Functions
Regulates the flow of Qi to relieve cough and asthma.

Clinical indications
Bronchial asthma, chronic bronchitis, esophageal spasm, tonsillitis, emphysema, pleuritis, stomach spasm.

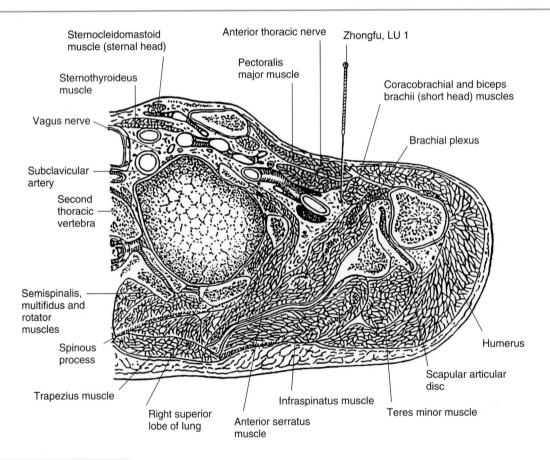

Fig. 5.1 Cross-section of Zhongfu.

3.
(HUAKAI) HUAGAI, CV 20, CONCEPTION VESSEL

Location

In a supine position, the point is located on the anterior midline of the chest, level with the first intercostal space.

Needle and moxibustion method

Horizontal insertion 0.3–0.5 inch.

— *Needle sensation:* local distension.

— *Moxibustion dosage:* 3–5 cones; stick 10 minutes.

Cross-sectional anatomy of the needle passage

a. Skin: the anterior cutaneous branches containing fibers from the anterior division of the first intercostal nerve innervate the skin.

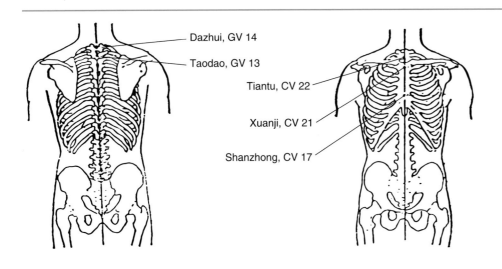

Dazhui, GV 14
Taodao, GV 13
Tiantu, CV 22
Xuanji, CV 21
Shanzhong, CV 17

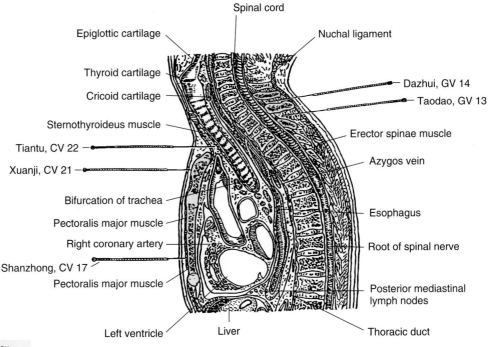

Spinal cord
Epiglottic cartilage
Nuchal ligament
Thyroid cartilage
Cricoid cartilage
Dazhui, GV 14
Taodao, GV 13
Sternothyroideus muscle
Erector spinae muscle
Tiantu, CV 22
Xuanji, CV 21
Azygos vein
Bifurcation of trachea
Pectoralis major muscle
Esophagus
Right coronary artery
Root of spinal nerve
Shanzhong, CV 17
Pectoralis major muscle
Posterior mediastinal lymph nodes
Left ventricle
Liver
Thoracic duct

Fig. 5.2 Sagittal section of Tiantu, Xuanji, Shanzhong, Dazhui and Taodao.

b. *Subcutaneous tissue:* includes the previously described skin nerve branches, and the anterior perforating branch of the internal thoracic artery and vein. The internal thoracic artery is a branch of the subclavicular artery. The internal thoracic vein drains into the brachiocephalic vein.

c. *Pectoralis major muscle:* the medial and lateral pectoral nerves containing fibers from the brachial plexus of the fifth cervical to first thoracic nerves (C5–T1) innervate the muscle.

d. The needle reaches the manubrium of the sternum.

Warning

Don't insert the needle deeply, as it may puncture through a child's thymus or an adult's thoracic cavity into the trachea.

Functions

Soothes chest oppression, alleviates diaphragm pain, and clears Heat from the Lung to relieve cough.

Clinical indications

Cough, sensation of fullness in the chest, asthma, bronchitis, emphysema, tonsillitis.

4.

(SHANCHUNG) SHANZHONG, CV 17, CONCEPTION VESSEL

Location

In a supine position, the point is located on the anterior midline of the chest at the midpoint between the two nipples in men. In women the point can be located at the level of the fourth intercostal space.

Needle and moxibustion method

Downward horizontal insertion or directing the needle bilaterally to the nipples 0.3–0.5 inch.
— *Needle sensation:* local distension, soreness or heaviness of the chest.
— *Moxibustion dosage:* 5–9 cones; stick 5–15 minutes.

Cross-sectional anatomy of the needle passage
(Fig. 5.2)

a. *Skin:* the medial cutaneous branches containing fibers from the anterior cutaneous divisions from the fourth intercostal nerve innervate the skin.

b. *Subcutaneous tissue:* includes the previously described skin nerve branches, and the perforating branch of the internal thoracic artery and vein. The internal thoracic artery is a branch of the subclavicular artery. The internal thoracic vein drains into the brachiocephalic vein.

c. *Pectoralis major muscle:* a flat fan-shaped muscle. The

medial and lateral pectoral nerves containing fibers from the brachial plexus of the fifth cervical to first thoracic nerves (C5–T1) innervate the muscle. The needle can be inserted bilaterally to the pectoralis major muscles.

d. Deep needling reaches the body of the sternum.

Functions

Soothes chest oppression and alleviates diaphragm pain, and relieves cough and asthma.

Clinical indications

Bronchial asthma, bronchitis, chest pain, mastitis, pleurisy, coma, angina pectoris, pericarditis, pneumonia, lung abscess, pleuritis.

5.

(TAOTAO) TAODAO, GV 13, GOVERNING VESSEL

Location

In a prone position, the point is located on the midline of the back, in the fossa between the spinous processes of the first and second thoracic vertebrae.

Needle and moxibustion method

Slightly superior oblique insertion 0.5–1.0 inch.
— *Needle sensation:* local distension and soreness, and radiating inferiorly or bilaterally to the shoulder.
— *Moxibustion dosage:* 3–7 cones; stick 5–15 minutes.

Cross-sectional anatomy of the needle passage
(Fig. 5.2)

a. *Skin:* the medial branches containing fibers from the dorsal rami of the first thoracic nerve (T1) innervate the skin.

b. *Subcutaneous tissue:* includes the previously described skin nerve branches.

c. *Tendon of trapezius muscle:* the branches containing fibers from the spinal accessory nerve (CN XI) and the ventral primary division of the third and fourth cervical nerves (C3, C4) innervate the muscle.

d. *Supraspinal ligament:* the medial branches from the dorsal rami of the eighth cervical nerve (C8) innervate the ligament.

e. *Interspinal ligament:* between the spinous process of the first and second thoracic vertebrae. The medial branches containing fibers from the dorsal rami of the first thoracic nerve (T1) innervate the ligament.

f. *Ligamentum flavum:* between the first and second thoracic vertebral arches. If the needle is inserted deeply, it will puncture through the ligamentum flavum into the spinal canal.

Warning

Don't insert the needle deeply, as it may puncture the spinal cord. When the needle penetrates through the ligamentum flavum, resistance may suddenly cease. Stop inserting the needle. If the needle punctures the spinal cord, a strong electrical sensation will be felt and panic may ensue. Extract the needle immediately. No lifting, thrusting and twirling of the needle are permitted.

Functions

Nourishes Yin to restore Yang, arrests malarial disease and reduces fever.

Clinical indications

Fever, heat stroke, schizophrenia, convulsions, bronchitis, asthma, tuberculosis, pneumothorax, hepatitis, eczema, hemiparalysis, shoulder pain.

6.

(TZUKUNG) ZIGONG, CV 19, CONCEPTION VESSEL

Location

In a supine position, the point is located on the anterior midline of the chest and at the same height as the second intercostal space.

Needle and moxibustion method

Horizontal insertion 0.3–0.5 inch.
— *Needle sensation:* local numbness and distension.
— *Moxibustion dosage:* 3–5 cones; stick 10 minutes.

Cross-sectional anatomy of the needle passage

a. *Skin:* the anterior cutaneous branches containing fibers from the anterior rami of the second intercostal nerve innervate the skin.
b. *Subcutaneous tissue:* includes the previously described skin nerve branches, and the anterior perforating branch of the internal thoracic artery and vein. The internal thoracic artery is a branch of the subclavicular artery. The internal thoracic vein drains into the brachiocephalic vein.
c. *Pectoralis major muscle:* the medial and lateral pectoral nerves containing fibers from the brachial plexus of the fifth cervical to first thoracic nerves (C5–T1) innervate the muscle.
d. The needle reaches the body of the sternum.

Warning

Don't insert the needle deeply, as it may puncture through the thoracic cavity into the pericardium and heart, causing massive bleeding.

Functions

Regulates the flow of Qi to relieve asthma, relieves cough and resolves Phlegm.

Clinical indications

Chest pain, cough, asthma, bronchitis, pleuritis, mastitis, gastritis, gastric ulcer.

7.

(YUTANG) YUTANG, CV 18, CONCEPTION VESSEL

Location

In a supine position, the point is located on the anterior midline of the chest, level with the third intercostal space.

Needle and moxibustion method

Inferior horizontal insertion 0.3–0.5 inch.
— *Needle sensation:* local numbness and distension.
— *Moxibustion dosage:* 3–5 cones; stick 15 minutes.

Cross-sectional anatomy of the needle passage

a. *Skin:* the medial cutaneous branches containing fibers from the anterior rami of the third intercostal nerve innervate the skin.
b. *Subcutaneous tissue:* includes the previously described skin nerve branches, and the anterior perforating branch of the internal thoracic artery and vein. The internal thoracic artery is a branch of the subclavicular artery. The internal thoracic vein drains into the brachiocephalic vein.
c. *Pectoralis major muscle:* the medial and lateral pectoralis nerves containing fibers from the brachial plexus of the fifth cervical to first thoracic nerves (C5–T1) innervate the muscle.
d. The needle reaches the body of the sternum.

Warning

Don't insert the needle deeply, as it may puncture through the thoracic cavity into the pericardium and heart, causing massive bleeding.

Functions

Regulates the flow of Qi to relieve asthma, and descends the Qi to arrest vomiting.

Clinical indications

Hematemesis, chest pain, cough, asthma, vomiting.

8.

(TACHUI) DAZHUI, GV 14, GOVERNING VESSEL

Location
In a prone or seated position and bending the head forward, the point is located on the midline of the back in the inferior fossa of the seventh cervical vertebra, between the spinous processes of the seventh cervical and first thoracic vertebrae.

Needle and moxibustion method
Slightly oblique superior insertion 0.5–1.0 inch.
— *Needle sensation:* local distension and soreness, and radiating inferiorly or bilaterally to the shoulder.
— *Moxibustion dosage:* 3–7 cones; stick 5–15 minutes.

Cross-sectional anatomy of the needle passage
(Fig. 5.2)
a. *Skin:* the cutaneous branches containing fibers from the posterior division of the eighth cervical nerve (C8) innervate the skin.
b. *Subcutaneous tissue:* includes the previously described skin nerve branches.
c. *Tendon of trapezius muscle:* the branches containing fibers from the spinal accessory nerve (CN XI) and the ventral primary division containing fibers from the third and fourth cervical nerves (C3, C4) innervate the muscle.
d. *Supraspinal ligament:* the medial branches containing fibers from the dorsal rami of the eighth cervical nerve (C8) innervate the ligament.
e. *Interspinal ligament:* between the spinous process of the seventh cervical and first thoracic vertebra. The medial branches containing fibers from the dorsal rami of the eighth cervical nerve (C8) innervate the ligament.
f. *Ligamentum flavum:* between the seventh cervical and first thoracic vertebral arches. If the needle is inserted deeply, it will puncture through the ligamentum flavum into the spinal canal.

Warning
Don't insert the needle deeply, as it may puncture the spinal cord. When the needle is inserted through the ligamentum flavum, resistance may suddenly cease. Stop inserting the needle, or it may puncture the spinal cord. If the needle punctures the spinal cord, a strong electrical sensation will be felt and panic may be shown. Extract the needle immediately. No lifting, thrusting and twirling are permitted.

Functions
Regulates the flow of Qi, nourishes Blood, reduces fever and relieves mental stress.

Clinical indications
Fever, heat stroke, schizophrenia, convulsions, bronchitis, asthma, tuberculosis, pneumothorax, eczema, hemiparalysis, shoulder pain.

9.

(SHENCHU) SHENZHU, GV 12, GOVERNING VESSEL

Location
In a seated or prone position and bending the head forward, the point is located on the midline of the back, in the inferior fossa of the spinous process of the third thoracic vertebra, between the spinous processes of the third and fourth thoracic vertebrae.

Needle and moxibustion method
Superior oblique insertion 0.5–1.0 inch.
— *Needle sensation:* distension and soreness, or heaviness radiating inferiorly.
— *Moxibustion dosage:* 3–5 cones; stick 20 minutes.

Cross-sectional anatomy of the needle passage
a. *Skin:* the medial branches containing fibers from the dorsal rami of the third thoracic nerve (T3) innervate the skin.
b. *Subcutaneous tissue:* includes the previously described skin nerve branches.
c. *Thoracolumbar fascia:* consists of superficial and deep layers, and encircles the sacrospinalis muscle.
d. *Supraspinalis ligament and sacrospinalis muscle:* the dorsal branches containing fibers from the second lumbar nerve (L2) innervate the supraspinal ligament. The dorsal branches from the spinal nerves innervate the sacrospinalis muscle.
e. *Interspinal ligament:* between the spinous process of the third and fourth thoracic vertebrae. The dorsal branches containing fibers from the third thoracic nerve (T3) innervate the ligament.
f. *Ligamentum flavum:* between the third and fourth thoracic vertebral arches. If the needle is inserted deeply, it will puncture through the ligamentum flavum into the spinal canal.

Warning
Don't insert the needle deeply, as it may puncture the spinal cord. When the needle is inserted through the ligamentum flavum, resistance may suddenly cease. If the needle punctures the spinal cord, a strong electrical sensation may be felt and panic may be shown. Extract

the needle immediately. No lifting, thrusting and twirling are permitted.

Functions

Facilitates the flow of Lung Qi to relieve asthma, and tranquilizes and calms over-excitement.

Clinical indications

Convulsions, epilepsy, hysteria, schizophrenia, lower lumbar pain, hematemesis, cough, asthma, bronchitis, fever.

10.

(SHENTAO) SHENDAO, GV 11, GOVERNING VESSEL

Location

In a seated or prone position, the point is located on the midline of the back, in the inferior fossa of the spinous process of the fifth thoracic vertebra between the spinous processes of the fifth and sixth thoracic vertebrae.

Needle and moxibustion method

Superior oblique insertion 0.5–1.0 inch.
— *Needle sensation:* local numbness and distension.
— *Moxibustion dosage:* 3–7 cones; stick 10 minutes.

Cross-sectional anatomy of the needle passage

a. *Skin:* the medial branches containing fibers from the dorsal rami of the fifth thoracic nerve (T5) innervate the skin.
b. *Subcutaneous tissue:* includes the previously described skin nerve branches.
c. *Thoracolumbar fascia:* consists of superficial and deep layers, and encircles the sacrospinalis muscle.
d. *Suprapinalis ligament and sacrospinalis muscle:* the dorsal branches containing fibers from the second lumbar nerve (L2) innervate the supraspinal ligament. The dorsal branches from the spinal nerve innervate the sacrospinalis muscle.
e. *Interspinal ligament:* between the spinous process of the fifth and sixth thoracic vertebrae. The dorsal branches containing fibers from the fifth thoracic nerve (T5) innervate the ligament.
f. *Ligamentum flavum:* between the fifth and sixth thoracic vertebral arches. If the needle is inserted deeply, it will pass through the ligamentum flavum into the spinal canal.

Warning

Don't insert the needle deeply, as it may puncture the spinal cord. When the needle is inserted through the ligamentum flavum, resistance may suddenly cease. If

the needle punctures the spinal cord, a strong electrical sensation may be felt and panic may be shown. Extract the needle immediately. No lifting, thrusting and twirling are permitted.

Functions

Reduces fever and dispels Wind, tranquilizes the Mind and calms over-excitement.

Clinical indications

Fever, headache, cough, amnesia, hysteria, infantile convulsion, back pain, precordial pain, hypertension, cerebrovascular disease.

11.

(CHUNGTING) ZHONGTING, CV 16, CONCEPTION VESSEL

Location

In a supine position, the point is located on the anterior midline of the chest, and at the same height as the fifth intercostal space.

Needle and moxibustion method

Horizontal inferior insertion 0.3–0.5 inch.
— *Needle sensation:* local numbness and distension.
— *Moxibustion dosage:* 3–5 cones; stick 10 minutes.

Cross-sectional anatomy of the needle passage

a. *Skin:* the medial cutaneous branches containing fibers from the anterior rami of the sixth intercostal nerve innervate the skin.
b. *Subcutaneous tissue:* includes the previously described skin nerve branches and the anterior perforating branch of the internal thoracic artery and vein. The internal thoracic artery is a branch of the subclavicular artery. The internal thoracic vein joins the brachiocephalic vein.
c. The needle reaches the junction of the sternum and xiphoid process.

Warning

Don't insert the needle deeply, as it may pass through the through the thoracic cavity into the pericardium and the heart, causing massive bleeding.

Functions

Regulates the flow of Qi to soothe chest oppression, and descends the flow of Qi to arrest vomiting.

Clinical indications

Tonsillitis, esophageal stricture, esophageal diverticulum, esophageal cancer, cardiac spasm, fullness of the heart, vomiting, sore throat.

12.

(CHIUWEI) JIUWEI, CV 15, CONCEPTION VESSEL, CONNECTING POINT

Location
In a supine position, the point is located on the mid abdominal line, 7 inches above the umbilicus, or just below the xiphoid process.

Needle and moxibustion method
Inferior oblique insertion 0.4–0.6 inch.
— *Needle sensation:* local distension and heaviness.
— *Moxibustion dosage:* 3–5 cones; stick 10 minutes.

Cross-sectional anatomy of the needle passage
a. *Skin:* the medial cutaneous branches containing fibers from the anterior divisions of the seventh intercostal nerve innervate the skin.
b. *Subcutaneous tissue:* includes the previously described skin nerve branches and the superficial thoracoepigastric artery and vein. The superficial thoracoepigastric vein drains into the axillary vein.
c. *Linea alba and rectus abdominis muscle:* the linea alba, which extends from the xiphoid process to the pubic symphysis, is in the middle of the abdomen. The rectus abdominis muscles are encircled by the rectus sheath. The intercostal nerve containing fibers from the seventh to twelfth thoracic nerves (T7–T12) innervate the muscle.

Warning
Don't insert the needle deeply, as it may puncture through the rectus sheath, the adipose tissue and the peritoneum to the abdominal cavity and into the liver. Lifting, thrusting and twirling of the needle may damage the liver, causing massive bleeding.

Functions
Soothes chest oppression to alleviate diaphragm pain, and refreshes the Mind.

Clinical indications
Chest pain, convulsions, hematemesis, fullness of the chest, asthma, precordial pain, abdominal distension, psychosis, hysteria.

13.

(CHUCHUEH) JUQUE, CV 14, CONCEPTION VESSEL, FRONT-MU POINT OF THE HEART

Location
In a supine position, the point is located on the mid abdominal line, 6 inches above the umbilicus.

Needle and moxibustion method
Perpendicular insertion 0.3–0.8 inch.
— *Needle sensation:* local distension and heaviness.
— *Moxibustion dosage:* 5–9 cones; stick 15 minutes.

Cross-sectional anatomy of the needle passage
a. *Skin:* the medial cutaneous branches containing fibers from the anterior divisions of the seventh intercostal nerve innervate the skin.
b. *Subcutaneous tissue:* includes the previously described skin nerve branches, and the superficial thoracoepigastric artery and vein. The superficial thoracoepigastric vein drains into the axillary vein.
c. *Linea alba and rectus abdominis muscle:* the linea alba, which extends from the xiphoid process to the pubic symphysis, is in the middle of the abdomen. The rectus abdominis muscles are encircled by the rectus sheath. The branches from the intercostal nerve containing fibers from the seventh to twelfth thoracic nerves (T7–T12) innervate the muscle.

Warning
Don't insert the needle deeply, as it may puncture through the rectus sheath, the adipose tissue and the peritoneum to the abdominal cavity and into the liver. Lifting, thrusting and twirling of the needle may damage the liver, causing massive bleeding.

Functions
Reinforces the Middle Jiao (Middle Warmer) to remove abdominal masses, and clears away Heat from the Heart to arrest mental anxiety.

Clinical indications
Fullness of the chest, cough, hematemesis, precordial pain, abdominal distension, convulsions, schizophrenia, syncope.

14.

(SHANGWAN) SHANGWAN, CV 13, CONCEPTION VESSEL

Location
In a supine position, the point is located on the mid abdominal line, 5 inches above the umbilicus.

Needle and moxibustion method
Perpendicular insertion 0.5–1.2 inches.
— *Needle sensation:* epigastric fullness and a sensation of heaviness.
— *Moxibustion dosage:* 5–7 cones; stick 10 minutes.

Cross-sectional anatomy of the needle passage
a. *Skin:* the medial cutaneous branches containing

fibers from the anterior divisions of the intercostal nerve innervate the skin.

b. *Subcutaneous tissue:* includes the previously described skin nerve branches, and the superficial thoracoepigastric artery and vein. The superficial thoracoepigastric vein drains into the axillary vein.

c. *Linea alba and rectus abdominis muscle:* the linea alba, which extends from the xiphoid process to the pubis symphysis, is in the middle of the abdomen. The rectus abdominis muscles are encircled by the rectus sheath. The branches from the intercostal nerve containing fibers from the seventh to twelfth thoracic nerves (T7–T12) innervate the muscle.

Warning

Don't insert the needle deeply, as it may puncture through the rectus sheath, the adipose tissue and the peritoneum into the liver and the pylorus of the stomach on the right and left, respectively. If the needle is lifted, thrust and twirled, the gastric contents may enter the abdominal cavity and cause peritonitis. If the needle is directed superiorly and deeply, it may puncture the liver, causing massive bleeding.

Functions

Regulates and promotes the function of the Stomach and the Spleen, and reinforces the Middle Jiao (Middle Warmer) to remove Dampness.

Clinical indications

Stomach pain, abdominal distention, vomiting, convulsions, amnesia, hypertension, angina pectoris, gastritis, gastric ulcer, gastric spasm, hepatitis, cholecystitis.

15.

(CHUNGWAN) ZHONGWAN, CV 12, CONCEPTION VESSEL, FRONT-MU POINT OF THE STOMACH

Location

In a supine position, the point is located on the mid abdominal line at the midpoint between the xiphisternal joint and the umbilicus.

Needle and moxibustion method

Perpendicular or oblique insertion 0.3–0.5 inch.
— *Needle sensation:* fullness and heaviness at the epigastric region or contracting sensation in the stomach.
— *Moxibustion dosage:* 5–9 cones; stick 5–10 minutes.

Cross-sectional anatomy of the needle passage
(Fig. 5.3)
a. *Skin:* the medial cutaneous branches containing

---

fibers from the anterior divisions of the eighth intercostal nerve innervate the skin.

b. *Subcutaneous tissue:* includes the previously described skin nerve branches, and the superficial thoracoepigastric artery and vein. The superficial thoracoepigastric vein drains into the axillary vein.

c. *Linea alba and rectus abdominis muscle:* the linea alba, which extends from the xiphoid process to the pubic symphysis, is in the middle line of the abdomen. The rectus abdominis muscles are encircled by the rectus sheath. The branches from the intercostal nerve containing fibers from the seventh to twelfth thoracic nerves (T7–T12) innervate the rectus abdominis muscle.

Warning

Don't insert the needle deeply, as it may puncture through the rectus sheath, the adipose tissue and the peritoneum to the abdominal cavity and into the stomach. If the needle is lifted, thrust and twirled, the gastric contents may enter the abdominal cavity, causing peritonitis. If the direction of the needle is upwards, deep insertion may penetrate into the liver, causing massive bleeding.

Functions

Regulates the function of the Stomach to strengthen the function of the Spleen, and warms the Middle Jiao (Middle Warmer) to remove Dampness.

Clinical indications

Stomach pain, abdominal distention, diarrhea, nausea, vomiting, gastroptosia, indigestion, syncope, convulsions, hysteria, schizophrenia, heat stroke, cerebrovascular disease, hypertension, bronchial asthma.

16.

(CHIENLI) JIANLI, CV 11, CONCEPTION VESSEL

Location

In a supine position, the point is located on the mid abdominal line, 3 inches above the umbilicus.

Needle and moxibustion method

Perpendicular insertion 0.5–1.0 inch.
— *Needle sensation:* local heaviness and distension.
— *Moxibustion dosage:* 5–7 cones; stick 10 minutes.

Cross-sectional anatomy of the needle passage
a. *Skin:* the medial cutaneous branches containing fibers from the anterior divisions of the eighth intercostal nerve innervate the skin.

b. *Subcutaneous tissue:* includes the previously described skin nerve branches, and the superficial epigastric artery and vein. The femoral artery gives rise to the superficial epigastric artery. The superficial epigastric vein joins the greater saphenous vein.

c. *Linea alba and rectus abdominis muscle:* the linea alba, which extends from the xiphoid process to the pubic symphysis is in the middle line of the abdomen. The rectus abdominis muscles are encircled by the rectus sheath. The branches from the intercostal nerve containing fibers from the seventh to twelfth thoracic nerves (T7–T12) innervate the rectus abdominis muscle.

Warning

If the needle is inserted deeply into the linea alba and the rectus abdominis muscle, it may puncture through the rectus sheath, the · adipose tissue and the peritoneum into the transverse colon. If the needle is lifted, thrust and twirled, the colonic contents may enter the abdominal cavity, causing peritonitis.

Functions

Strengthens the function of the Spleen to regulate the flow of Qi, and reinforces the function of the Stomach to eliminate undigested food.

Clinical indications

Stomach pain, vomiting, abdominal distension, edema, gastritis, gastric ulcer, indigestion.

17.

(HSIAWAN) XIAWAN, CV 10, CONCEPTION VESSEL

Location

In a supine position, the point is located on the mid abdominal line, 2 inches above the umbilicus.

Needle and moxibustion method

Perpendicular insertion 0.8–1.0 inch.
— *Needle sensation:* local distension and heaviness.
— *Moxibustion dosage:* 5–7 cones; stick 10 minutes.

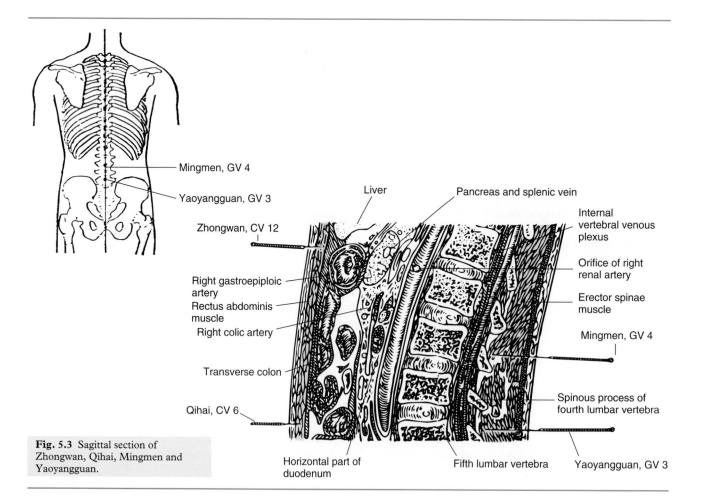

Fig. 5.3 Sagittal section of Zhongwan, Qihai, Mingmen and Yaoyangguan.

Mingmen, GV 4

Yaoyangguan, GV 3

Zhongwan, CV 12

Right gastroepiploic artery

Rectus abdominis muscle

Right colic artery

Transverse colon

Qihai, CV 6

Horizontal part of duodenum

Liver

Pancreas and splenic vein

Internal vertebral venous plexus

Orifice of right renal artery

Erector spinae muscle

Mingmen, GV 4

Spinous process of fourth lumbar vertebra

Fifth lumbar vertebra

Yaoyangguan, GV 3

Cross-sectional anatomy of the needle passage

a. *Skin:* the medial cutaneous branches containing fibers from the anterior divisions of the eighth intercostal nerve innervate the skin.

b. *Subcutaneous tissue:* includes the previously described skin nerve branches, and the superficial epigastric artery and vein. The femoral artery gives rise to the superficial epigastric artery. The superficial epigastric vein joins the greater saphenous vein.

c. *Linea alba and rectus abdominis muscle:* the linea alba, which extends from the xiphoid process to the pubic symphysis, is in the middle line of the abdomen. The rectus abdominis muscles are encircled by the rectus sheath. The branches from the intercostal nerve containing fibers from the seventh to twelfth thoracic nerves (T7–T12) innervate the rectus abdominis muscle.

Warning

If the needle is inserted deeply into the linea alba and the rectus abdominis muscle, it may puncture through the rectus sheath, the adipose tissue and the peritoneum into the transverse colon. If the needle is lifted, thrust and twirled, the colonic contents may enter the abdominal cavity, causing peritonitis.

Functions

Strengthens the function of the Spleen and Stomach, removes abdominal masses and eliminates undigested food.

Clinical indications

Abdominal pain, abdominal distension, cardiac spasm, gastritis, gastric ulcer, indigestion, vomiting, dysentery.

18.

(SHUIFEN) SHUIFEN, CV 9, CONCEPTION VESSEL

Location

In a supine position, the point is located on the midline of the abdomen, 1 inch above the umbilicus.

Needle and moxibustion method

Perpendicular insertion 0.5–1.0 inch.
— *Needle sensation:* local distension and heaviness.
— *Moxibustion dosage:* 5–7 cones; stick 15 minutes.

Cross-sectional anatomy of the needle passage

a. *Skin:* the medial cutaneous branches containing fibers from the anterior divisions of the ninth intercostal nerve innervate the skin.

b. *Subcutaneous tissue:* includes the previously described skin nerve branches, and the superficial epigastric artery and vein. The femoral artery gives rise to the superficial epigastric artery. The superficial epigastric vein joins the greater saphenous vein.

c. *Linea alba and rectus abdominis muscle:* the linea alba, which extends from the xiphoid process to the pubic symphysis, is in the middle line of the abdomen. The rectus abdominis muscles are encircled by the rectus sheath. The branches from the intercostal nerve containing fibers from the seventh to twelfth thoracic nerves (T7–T12) innervate the rectus abdominis muscle.

Warning

If the needle is inserted deeply into the linea alba and the rectus abdominis muscle, it may puncture through the rectus sheath, the adipose tissue and the peritoneum into the the small intestine. If the needle is lifted, thrust and twirled, the intestinal contents may enter the abdominal cavity, causing peritonitis.

Functions

Strengthens the function of the Spleen, induces enuresis, and regulates the water passage.

Clinical indications

Abdominal pain, edema, urinary tract obstruction, nephritis, ascites, dysentery.

19.

(LINGTAI) LINGTAI, GV 10, GOVERNING VESSEL

Location

In a seated or prone position, the point is located on the midline of the back, in the inferior fossa of the spinous process of the sixth thoracic vertebra between the spinous processes of the sixth and seventh thoracic vertebrae.

Needle and moxibustion method

Superior oblique insertion 0.5–1.0 inch.
— *Needle sensation:* distension and soreness sometimes radiating to the inferior region of the back or the anterior chest.
— *Moxibustion dosage:* 3–5 cones; stick 15 minutes.

Cross-sectional anatomy of the needle passage

a. *Skin:* the medial branches containing fibers from the dorsal rami of the sixth thoracic nerve (T6) innervate the skin.

b. *Subcutaneous tissue:* includes the previously described skin nerve branches.

c. *Thoracolumbar fascia:* consists of superficial and deep layers, and encircles the sacrospinalis muscle.

d. *Supraspinal ligament and sacrospinalis muscle:* the dorsal branches containing fibers from the second lumbar nerve (L2) innervate the supraspinal ligament. The dorsal branches from the spinal nerves innervate the sacrospinalis muscle.

e. *Interspinal ligament:* between the spinous process of the sixth and seventh thoracic vertebrae. The dorsal branches containing fibers from the sixth thoracic nerve (T6) innervate the ligament.

f. *Ligamentum flavum:* between the sixth and seventh thoracic vertebral arches. If the needle is inserted deeply, it will puncture through the ligamentum flavum into the spinal canal.

Warning

Don't insert the needle deeply, as it may puncture into the spinal cord. When the needle is inserted through the ligamentum flavum, resistance will suddenly cease. Do not continue to insert the needle. If the needle is inserted into the spinal cord, a strong electrical sensation will be felt and panic will be shown. Extract the needle immediately. No lifting, thrusting and twirling of the needle are permitted.

Functions

Reduces fever, activates the collaterals, and relieves cough and asthma.

Clinical indications

Common cold, wheezing and cough, bronchial asthma, pneumonia, bronchitis, back pain, neck stiffness.

20.

(CHIHYANG) ZHIYANG, GV 9, GOVERNING VESSEL

Location

In a seated or prone position, the point is located on the midline of the back, in the inferior fossa of the spinous process of the seventh thoracic vertebra between the spinous process of the seventh and eight thoracic vertebrae.

Needle and moxibustion method

Superior oblique insertion 0.5–1.0 inch.
— *Needle sensation:* distension and soreness radiating to the lumbar back or the anterior chest.
— *Moxibustion dosage:* 3–5 cones; stick 15 minutes.

Cross-sectional anatomy of the needle passage

a. *Skin:* the medial cutaneous branches containing fibers from the dorsal rami of the seventh thoracic

nerve (T7) innervate the skin.

b. *Subcutaneous tissue:* includes the previously described skin nerve branches.

c. *Thoracolumbar fascia:* consists of superficial and deep layers, and encircles the sacrospinalis muscle.

d. *Supraspinal ligament and sacrospinalis muscle:* the dorsal branches containing fibers from the second lumbar nerve (L2) innervate the supraspinal ligament. The dorsal branches containing fibers from the spinal nerves innervate the sacrospinalis muscle.

e. *Interspinal ligament:* between the spinous process of the seventh and eighth thoracic vertebrae. The dorsal branches of the seventh thoracic nerve (T7) innervate the ligament.

f. *Ligamentum flavum:* between the seventh and eighth thoracic vertebral arches. If the needle is inserted deeply, it will puncture through the ligamentum flavum into the spinal canal.

Warning

Don't insert the needle deeply, as it may puncture the spinal cord. When the needle is inserted through the ligamentum flavum, resistance will suddenly cease. Do not continue to insert the needle. If the needle is inserted into the spinal cord, a strong electrical sensation will be felt and panic will be shown. Extract the needle immediately. No lifting, thrusting and twirling of the needle are permitted.

Functions

Facilitates the flow of Lung Qi to arrest cough, reduces fever and removes Dampness.

Clinical indications

Cough, bronchitis, bronchial asthma, pleuritis, cholecystitis, hepatitis, jaundice, back stiffness, thoracic back pain.

21.

(CHINSO) JINSUO, GV 8, GOVERNING VESSEL

Location

In a seated or prone position, the point is located on the midline of the back, in the inferior fossa of the spinous process of the ninth thoracic vertebra between the spinous processes of the ninth and tenth thoracic vertebrae.

Needle and moxibustion method

Perpendicular insertion 0.5–1.0 inch.
— *Needle sensation:* local numbness and distension.
— *Moxibustion dosage:* 3–7 cones; stick 10 minutes.

Cross-sectional anatomy of the needle passage

a. *Skin:* the medial cutaneous branches containing fibers from the dorsal rami of the ninth thoracic nerve (T9) innervate the skin.

b. *Subcutaneous tissue:* includes the previously described skin nerve branches.

c. *Thoracolumbar fascia:* consists of superficial and deep layers, and encircles the sacrospinalis muscle.

d. *Supraspinal ligament and sacrospinalis muscle:* the dorsal branches containing fibers from the second lumbar nerve (L2) innervate the supraspinal ligament. The dorsal branches containing fibers from the spinal nerves innervate the sacrospinalis muscle.

e. *Interspinal ligament:* between the spinous process of the ninth and tenth thoracic vertebrae. The dorsal branches containing fibers from the ninth thoracic nerve (T9) innervate the interspinal ligament.

f. *Ligamentum flavum:* between the ninth and tenth thoracic vertebral arches. If the needle is inserted deeply, it will puncture through the ligamentum flavum into the spinal canal.

Warning

Don't insert the needle deeply, as it may puncture into the spinal cord. When the needle is inserted through the ligamentum flavum, resistance will suddenly cease. Do not continue to insert the needle. If the needle is inserted into the spinal cord, a strong electrical sensation will be felt and panic will be shown. Extract the needle immediately. No lifting, thrusting and twirling of the needle are permitted.

Functions

Relieves rigidity of muscles and tendons, activates the collaterals, and refreshes the Mind.

Clinical indications

Convulsions, tetanus, infantile convulsions, hysteria, schizophrenia, back stiffness, stomach pain, gastritis, gastric spasm, dizziness.

22.

(CHUNGSHU) ZHONGSHU, GV 7, GOVERNING VESSEL

Location

In a seated or prone position, the point is located on the midline of the back, in the inferior fossa of the spinous process of the tenth thoracic vertebra between the spinous processes of the tenth and eleventh thoracic vertebrae.

Needle and moxibustion method

Superior oblique insertion 0.5–1.0 inch.
— *Needle sensation:* local numbness and distension.
— *Moxibustion dosage:* 3–5 cones; stick 10 times.

Cross-sectional anatomy of the needle passage

a. *Skin:* the medial cutaneous branches containing fibers from the dorsal rami of the tenth thoracic nerve (T10) innervate the skin.

b. *Subcutaneous tissue:* includes the previously described skin nerve branches.

c. *Thoracolumbar fascia:* consists of superficial and deep layers, and encircles the sacrospinalis muscle.

d. *Supraspinal ligament and sacrospinalis muscle:* the dorsal branches containing fibers from the second lumbar nerve (L2) innervate the supraspinal ligament. The dorsal branches of the spinal nerves innervate the sacrospinalis muscle.

e. *Interspinal ligament:* between the spinous process of the tenth and eleventh thoracic vertebrae. The dorsal branches containing fibers from the tenth thoracic nerve (T10) innervate the ligament.

f. *Ligamentum flavum:* between the tenth and eleventh thoracic vertebral arches. If the needle is inserted deeply, it will puncture through the ligamentum flavum into the spinal canal.

Warning

Don't insert the needle deeply, as it may puncture into the spinal cord. When the needle is inserted through the ligamentum flavum, resistance will suddenly cease. Do not continue to insert the needle. If the needle is inserted into the spinal cord, a strong electrical sensation will be felt and panic will be shown. Extract the needle immediately. No lifting, thrusting and twirling of the needle are permitted.

Functions

Strengthens the spinal column, tonifies the function of the Kidney, and regulates the function of the Stomach to alleviate pain.

Clinical indications

Epigastric pain, lower back pain, myopia, optic neuritis, jaundice, liver cirrhosis, hepatitis, gastritis, abdominal distension.

23.

(CHICHUNG) JIZHONG, GV 6, GOVERNING VESSEL

Location

In a seated or prone position, the point is located on the midline of the back, in the inferior fossa of the spinous process of the eleventh thoracic vertebra between the spinous process of the eleventh and twelfth thoracic vertebrae.

Needle and moxibustion method
Superior oblique insertion 0.5–1.0 inch.
— *Needle sensation:* local numbness and distension.
— *Moxibustion dosage:* 3–7 cones; stick 10 minutes.

Cross-sectional anatomy of the needle passage
a. *Skin:* the medial cutaneous branches containing fibers from the dorsal rami of the eleventh thoracic nerve (T11) innervate the skin.
b. *Subcutaneous tissue:* includes the previously described skin nerve branches.
c. *Thoracolumbar fascia:* consists of superficial and deep layers, and encircles the sacrospinalis muscle.
d. *Supraspinal ligament and sacrospinalis muscle:* the dorsal branches containing fibers from the second lumbar nerve (L2) innervate the supraspinal ligament. The dorsal branches containing fibers from the spinal nerves innervate the sacrospinalis muscle.
e. *Interspinal ligament:* between the spinous process of the eleventh and twelfth thoracic vertebrae. The dorsal branches containing fibers from the eleventh thoracic nerve innervate the ligament.
f. *Ligamentum flavum:* between the eleventh and twelfth thoracic vertebral arches. If the needle is inserted deeply, it will puncture through the ligamentum flavum into the spinal canal.

Warning
Don't insert the needle deeply, as it may puncture into the spinal cord. When the needle is inserted through the ligamentum flavum, resistance will suddenly cease. Do not continue to insert the needle. If the needle is inserted into the spinal cord, a strong electrical sensation will be felt and panic will be shown. Extract the needle immediately. No lifting, thrusting and twirling of the needle are permitted.

Functions
Strengthens the function of the Spleen to remove Dampness, arrests convulsions and alleviates prostration.

Clinical indications
Common cold, hematemesis, jaundice, diarrhea, convulsions, hernia, prolapse of the anus, lower back pain.

24.
(HSUANSHU) XUANSHU, GV 5, GOVERNING VESSEL

Location
In a seated or prone position, the point is located on the midline of the back, in the inferior fossa of the spinous process of the first lumbar vertebra between the spinous processes of the first and second lumbar vertebrae.

Needle and moxibustion method
Superior oblique insertion 0.5–1.0 inch.
— *Needle sensation:* local numbness and distension.
— *Moxibustion dosage:* 3–5 cones; stick 15 minutes.

Cross-sectional anatomy of the needle passage
a. *Skin:* the medial cutaneous branches containing fibers from the dorsal rami of the first lumbar nerve (L1) innervate the skin.
b. *Subcutaneous tissue:* includes the previously described skin nerve branches.
c. *Thoracolumbar fascia:* consists of superficial and deep layers, and encircles the sacrospinalis muscle.
d. *Supraspinal ligament and sacrospinalis muscle:* the dorsal branches containing fibers from the second lumbar nerve (L2) innervate the supraspinal ligament. The dorsal branches containing fibers from the spinal nerves innervate the sacrospinalis muscle.
e. *Interspinal ligament:* between the spinous process of the first and second lumbar vertebrae. The dorsal branches containing fibers from the first lumbar nerve innervate the ligament.
f. *Ligamentum flavum:* between the first and second lumbar vertebral arches. If the needle is inserted deeply, it will puncture through the ligamentum flavum into the spinal canal.

Warning
Don't insert the needle deeply, as it may puncture into the spinal cord. When the needle is inserted through the ligamentum flavum, resistance will suddenly cease. Do not continue to insert the needle. If the needle is inserted into the spinal cord, a strong electrical sensation will be felt and panic will be shown. Extract the needle immediately. No lifting, thrusting and twirling of the needle are permitted.

Functions
Strengthens the spinal column and tonifies the function of the Kidney, astringes the intestines to correct diarrhea and alleviates prostration.

Clinical indications

Abdominal pain, diarrhea, prolapse of the anus, constipation, lower back pain.

25.

(MINGMEN) MINGMEN, GV 4, GOVERNING VESSEL

Location

In a seated or prone position, the point is located on the midline of the back, in the inferior fossa of the spinous process of the second lumbar vertebra, between the spinous processes of the second and third lumbar vertebrae.

Needle and moxibustion method

Slightly oblique superior insertion 0.5–1.0 inch.
— *Needle sensation:* local distension, and an electrical sensation radiating to the lower extremities.
— *Moxibustion dosage:* 3–7 cones; stick 5–20 minutes.

Cross-sectional anatomy of the needle passage

(Fig. 5.3)
a. *Skin:* the medial cutaneous branches containing fibers from the dorsal rami of the second lumbar nerve (L2) innervate the skin.
b. *Subcutaneous tissue:* includes the previously described skin nerve branches.
c. *Thoracolumbar fascia:* consists of superficial and deep layers, and encircles the sacrospinalis muscle.
d. *Supraspinal ligament and sacrospinalis muscle:* the dorsal branches containing fibers from the second lumbar nerve (L2) innervate the supraspinal ligament. The dorsal branches containing fibers from the spinal nerves innervate the sacrospinalis muscle.
e. *Interspinal ligament:* between the spinous process of the second and third lumbar vertebrae. The dorsal branches containing fibers from the second lumbar nerve (L2) innervate the ligament.
f. *Ligamentum flavum:* between the second and third lumbar vertebral arches. If the needle is inserted deeply, it will puncture through the ligamentum flavum into the spinal canal.

Warning

Don't insert the needle deeply, as it may puncture into the spinal cord. When the needle is inserted through the ligamentum flavum, resistance will suddenly cease. Do not continue to insert the needle. If the needle is inserted into the spinal cord, a strong electrical sensation will be felt and panic will be shown. Extract the needle immediately. No lifting, thrusting and twirling of the needle are permitted.

Functions

Dredges the channels and regulates the flow of Qi, strengthens the essence of life and reinforces the Yang.

Clinical indications

Lower back pain, lower back sprain, leukorrhea, enuresis, nocturnal emission, premature ejaculation, endometritis, pelvic inflammatory disease, sciatic pain, nephritis, sequelae of poliomyelitis.

26.

(YAOYANGKUAN) YAOYANGGUAN, GV 3, GOVERNING VESSEL

Location

In a prone position, the point is located on the midline of the back, in the inferior fossa of the spinous process of the fourth lumbar vertebra between the spinous processes of the fourth and fifth lumbar vertebrae, or at the same height as the iliac crest of the hip.

Needle and moxibustion method

Slightly oblique superior insertion 1.0–2.0 inches.
— *Needle sensation:* local distension or an electrical sensation radiating to the lower extremities.
— *Moxibustion dosage:* 3–7 cones; stick 5–20 minutes.

Cross-sectional anatomy of the needle passage

(Fig. 5.3)
a. *Skin:* the medial cutaneous branches containing fibers from the second dorsal rami of the lumbar nerve innervate the skin.
b. *Subcutaneous tissue:* includes the previously described skin nerve branches.
c. *Superficial layer of thoracolumbar fascia.*
d. *Supraspinal ligament and sacrospinalis muscle:* a thick, wide and very strong ligament. When it is punctured, a very strong needle resistance may be felt. The dorsal branches containing fibers from the second lumbar nerve (L2) innervate the supraspinal ligament. The dorsal branches containing fibers from the spinal nerves innervate the sacrospinalis muscle.
e. *Interspinal ligament:* a thin ligament located between the spinous process of the fourth and fifth lumbar vertebrae. The dorsal branches containing fibers from the fourth lumbar nerve (L4) innervate the ligament.
f. *Ligamentum flavum:* an elastic fiber between the fourth and fifth lumbar vertebral arches. On deep insertion the needle may puncture through the ligamentum flavum, and a strong needle resistance may be felt.

Functions

Regulates and tonifies the Kidney Qi, and strengthens the spinal column.

Clinical indications

Lumbosacral pain, paralysis of the lower extremities, nocturnal emission, impotence, chronic enteritis, irregular menstruation.

27.
(YAOSHU) YAOSHU, GV 2, GOVERNING VESSEL

Location

In a prone position, the point is located on the midline of the back, in the inferior fossa of the spinous process of the fourth sacral vertebra between the spinous process of the fourth and fifth sacral vertebrae; or at the sacral hiatus.

Needle and moxibustion method

Superior oblique insertion 0.5–1.0 inch.
— *Needle sensation:* local distension and numbness.
— *Moxibustion dosage:* 3–7 cones; stick 15 minutes.

Cross-sectional anatomy of the needle passage

a. *Skin:* the cutaneous branches containing fibers from the coccygeal nerve innervate the skin.
b. *Subcutaneous tissue:* includes the previously described skin nerve branches.
c. *Superficial layer of thoracolumbar fascia.*
d. *Sacrospinalis (erector spinae) muscle:* the dorsal branches containing fibers from the spinal nerves innervate the muscle.
e. *Interspinal ligament:* between the spinous process of the fourth and fifth sacral vertebrae. The dorsal branches containing fibers from the fourth sacral nerve innervate the ligament.

Functions

Tonifies the function of the Kidney to regulate menstruation, strengthens the bone and reinforces the muscles and tendons.

Clinical indications

Irregular menstruation, hernia, leukorrhea, lumbar pain, paralysis of the lower extremities, fever.

28.
(SHENCHUEH) SHENQUE, CV 8, CONCEPTION VESSEL

Location

In a supine position, the point is located in the umbilicus.

Needle and moxibustion method

No needle insertion permitted.
— *Moxibustion dosage:* 7–14 cones; stick 20–30 minutes. (Generally direct moxibustion is done on salt.)

Cross-sectional anatomy of the needle passage (Fig. 5.4)

a. *Skin:* the medial cutaneous branches containing fibers from the anterior divisions of the tenth intercostal nerve innervate the skin.
b. *Subcutaneous tissue:* includes the previously described skin nerve branches, and the superficial epigastric artery and vein. The femoral artery gives rise to the superficial epigastric artery. The superficial epigastric vein joins the greater saphenous vein.
c. *Linea alba and rectus abdominis muscle:* the linea alba, which extends from the xiphoid process to the pubic symphysis, is in the middle line of the abdomen. The rectus abdominis muscle is encircled by the rectus sheath. The branches containing fibers from the intercostal nerve of the sixth to twelfth thoracic nerves (T6–T12) innervate the rectus abdominis muscle.

Functions

Rescues the Yang, relieves prostration, and regulates the flow of Qi and the function of the Kidney.

Clinical indications

Stroke, heat stroke, abdominal pain, prolapse of the anus, dysentery, abdominal distention.

29.
(YINCHIAO) YINJIAO, CV 7, CONCEPTION VESSEL

Location

In a supine position, the point is located on the midline of the abdomen, 1 inch below the umbilicus.

Needle and moxibustion method

Perpendicular insertion 0.8–1.2 inches.
— *Needle sensation:* local numbness and distension.
— *Moxibustion dosage:* 3–5 cones; stick 10 minutes.

Cross-sectional anatomy of the needle passage

a. *Skin:* the medial cutaneous branches containing

fibers from the anterior divisions of the tenth intercostal nerve innervate the skin.

b. *Subcutaneous tissue:* includes the previously described skin nerve branches, and the superficial epigastric artery and vein. The femoral artery gives rise to the superficial epigastric artery. The superficial epigastric vein joins the greater saphenous vein.

c. *Linea alba and rectus abdominis muscle:* the linea alba, which extends from the xiphoid process to the pubic symphysis, is in the midline of the abdomen. The rectus abdominis muscle is encircled by the rectus sheath. The branches containing fibers from the intercostal nerve of the sixth to twelfth thoracic nerves (T6–T12) innervate the rectus abdominis muscle.

Warning

If the needle is inserted deeply into the linea alba and the rectus abdominis muscle, it may puncture through the rectus sheath, the adipose tissue and the peritoneum into the small intestine. If the needle is lifted, thrust and twirled, the intestinal contents may enter the abdominal cavity, causing peritonitis.

Functions

Regulates menstruation, reinforces the Chong meridian, reduces fever and removes Dampness.

Clinical indications

Abdominal distension, edema, hernia, irregular menstruation, periumbilical pain, perineal itching.

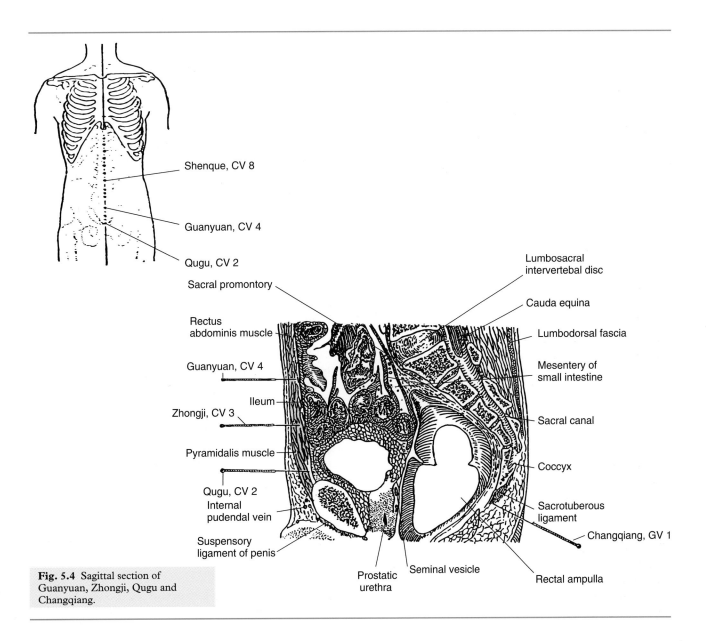

Fig. 5.4 Sagittal section of Guanyuan, Zhongji, Qugu and Changqiang.

30.

(CHIHAI) QIHAI, CV 6, CONCEPTION VESSEL

Location

In a supine position, the point is located on the midline of the abdomen, 1.5 inches below the umbilicus.

Needle and moxibustion method

Perpendicular insertion 0.5–1.0 inch or inferior oblique insertion 2.0–3.0 inches.
— *Needle sensation:* local soreness, distension and numbness radiating to the external genital region.
— *Moxibustion dosage:* 3–7 cones; stick 10–30 minutes.

Cross-sectional anatomy of the needle passage
(Fig. 5.3)
a. *Skin:* the medial cutaneous branches containing fibers from the anterior divisions of the eleventh intercostal nerve innervate the skin.
b. *Subcutaneous tissue:* includes the previously described skin nerve branches, and the superficial epigastric artery and vein. The femoral artery gives rise to the superficial epigastric artery. The superficial epigastric vein joins the greater saphenous vein.
c. *Linea alba and rectus abdominis muscle:* the linea alba, which extends from the xiphoid process to the pubic symphysis, is in the midline of the abdomen. The rectus abdominis muscle is encircled by the rectus sheath. The branches containing fibers from the intercostal nerve of the sixth to twelfth thoracic nerves (T6–T12) innervate the muscle.

Warning

1. If the needle is inserted deeply into the linea alba and the rectus abdominis muscle, it may puncture through the rectus sheath, the adipose tissue and the peritoneum into the small intestine in the male and the uterine fundus in the female. If the needle is lifted, thrust and twirled, the intestinal contents may enter the abdominal cavity, causing peritonitis.

2. No deep insertion of the needle is permitted during menstruation and pregnancy.

Functions

Tonifies the function of the Kidney, induces enuresis, and warms and reinforces the Lower Jiao (Lower Warmer) and Original Qi.

Clinical indications

Hypochondriasis, abdominal pain, abdominal distension, irregular menstruation, dysmenorrhea, enuresis, urine retention, nocturnal emission, impotence, frequency of urination.

31.

(SHIHMEN) SHIMEN, CV 5, CONCEPTION VESSEL, FRONT-MU POINT OF TRIPLE BURNER

Location

In a supine position, the point is located on the midline of the abdomen, 2 inches below the umbilicus.

Needle and moxibustion method

Perpendicular insertion 0.5–1.0 inch.
— *Needle sensation:* distension and numbness radiating inferiorly.
— *Moxibustion dosage:* 3–7 cones; stick 10 minutes.

Cross-sectional anatomy of the needle passage
a. *Skin:* the medial cutaneous branches containing fibers from the anterior divisions of the eleventh intercostal nerve innervate the skin.
b. *Subcutaneous tissue:* includes the previously described skin nerve branches, and the superficial epigastric artery and vein. The femoral artery gives rise to the superficial epigastric artery. The superficial epigastric vein joins the greater saphenous vein.
c. *Linea alba and rectus abdominis muscle:* the linea alba, which extends from the xiphoid process to the pubic symphysis, is in the midline of the abdomen. The rectus abdominis muscle is encircled by the rectus sheath. The branches containing fibers from the intercostal nerve of the sixth to twelfth thoracic nerves (T6–T12) innervate the rectus abdominis muscle.

Warning

1. If the needle is inserted deeply into the linea alba and the rectus abdominis muscle, it may puncture through the rectus sheath, the adipose tissue and the peritoneum into the small intestine. If the needle is lifted, thrust and twirled, the intestinal contents may enter the abdominal cavity, causing peritonitis.

2. Deep needle insertion in pregnant women is contraindicated.

Functions

Clears the Lower Jiao (Lower Warmer), tonifies the function of the Kidney and strengthens the function of the Spleen.

Clinical indications

Abdominal pain, dysentery, edema, hernia, urinary tract obstruction, amenorrhea, metrorrhagia.

32.

(KUANYUAN) GUANYUAN, CV 4, CONCEPTION VESSEL, FRONT-MU POINT OF THE SMALL INTESTINE

Location
In a supine position, the point is located on the midline of the abdomen, 3 inches below the umbilicus.

Needle and moxibustion method
Perpendicular insertion 0.5–1.0 inch or inferior oblique insertion 1.5–2.0 inches.
— *Needle sensation:* local soreness, swelling and numbness, sometimes radiating to the external genital region or the umbilical region.
— *Moxibustion dosage:* 3–9 cones; stick 10–30 minutes.

Cross-sectional anatomy of the needle passage
(Fig. 5.4)
a. *Skin:* the medial cutaneous branches containing fibers from the anterior divisions of the twelfth intercostal nerve innervate the skin.
b. *Subcutaneous tissue:* includes the previously described skin nerve branches, and the superficial epigastric artery and vein. The femoral artery gives rise to the superficial epigastric artery. The superficial epigastric vein joins the greater saphenous vein.
c. *Linea alba and rectus abdominis muscle:* the linea alba, which extends from the xiphoid process to the pubic symphysis, is in the midline of the abdomen. The rectus abdominis muscle is encircled by the rectus sheath. The branches containing fibers from the intercostal nerve of the sixth to twelfth thoracic nerves (T6–T12) innervate the rectus abdominis muscle.

Warning
1. If the needle is inserted deeply into the linea alba and the rectus abdominis muscle, it may puncture through the rectus sheath, the adipose tissue and the peritoneum into the small intestine. If the urinary bladder is filled with urine, the needle may puncture into the bladder. Before treatment, urinate and empty the urinary bladder.
2. Needle insertion in pregnant women is contraindicated.

Functions
Tonifies the function of the Kidney, reinforces the Original Qi, reduces Heat and removes Dampness.

Clinical indications
Enuresis, nocturnal emission, urine retention, impotence, premature ejaculation, dysmenorrhea, leukor- rhea, female infertility, pelvic inflammatory disease, nephritis, urinary tract inflammation, irregular menstruation.

33.

(CHUNGCHI) ZHONGJI, CV 3, CONCEPTION VESSEL, FRONT-MU POINT OF THE BLADDER

Location
In a supine position, the point is located on the midline of the abdomen, 4 inches below the umbilicus.

Needle and moxibustion method
Perpendicular insertion 0.5–1.0 inch.
— *Needle sensation:* local distension and soreness, and radiating to the external genital organs and the pubic region.
— *Moxibustion dosage:* 3–7 cones; stick 15–30 minutes.

Cross-sectional anatomy of the needle passage
(Fig. 5.4)
a. *Skin:* the branches containing fibers from the iliohypogastric nerve containing fibers from the lumbar plexus innervate the skin.
b. *Subcutaneous tissue:* includes the previously described skin nerve branches, and the superficial epigastric artery and vein. The femoral artery gives rise to the superficial epigastric artery. The superficial epigastric vein joins the greater saphenous vein.
c. *Linea alba and rectus abdominis muscle:* the linea alba, which extends from the xiphoid process to the pubic symphysis, is at the midline of the abdomen. The rectus abdominis muscle is encircled by the rectus sheath. The branches from the intercostal nerve of the sixth to twelfth thoracic nerves (T6–T12) innervate the rectus abdominis muscle.

Warning
1. If the needle is inserted deeply into the linea alba and the rectus abdominis muscle, it may puncture through the rectus sheath, the adipose tissue and the peritoneum into the small intestine or the urinary bladder. If the needle is lifted, thrust or twirled, the intestinal contents may enter the abdominal cavity, causing peritonitis. If the urinary bladder is filled with urine, the needle may puncture into the bladder. Before treatment, urinate and empty the urinary bladder.
2. Needle insertion in pregnant women is contraindicated.

Functions
Regulates the Chong and Ren meridians, and promotes urination.

Clinical indications

Enuresis, nocturnal emission, urine retention, impotence, premature ejaculation, irregular menstruation, leukorrhea, female infertility, pelvic inflammatory disease, nephritis, urinary tract inflammation, sciatic pain.

34.

(CHUKU) QUGU, CV 2, CONCEPTION VESSEL

Location

In a supine position, the point is located on the midline of the abdomen, in the superior fossa of the pubic symphysis.

Needle and moxibustion method

Perpendicular insertion 0.5–1.5 inches.
— *Needle sensation:* local distension and soreness, or radiating to the external genital organs.
— *Moxibustion dosage:* 3–7 cones; stick 20–30 minutes.

Cross-sectional anatomy of the needle passage

(Fig. 5.4)
a. *Skin:* the branches containing fibers from the iliohypogastric nerve containing fibers from the lumbar plexus innervate the skin.
b. *Subcutaneous tissue:* includes the previously described skin nerve branches, and the superficial epigastric artery and vein. The femoral artery gives rise to the superficial epigastric artery. The superficial epigastric vein joins the greater saphenous vein.
c. *Linea alba and rectus abdominis muscle:* the linea alba, which extends from the xiphoid process to the pubic symphysis, is in the midline of the abdomen. The rectus abdominis muscle is encircled by the rectus sheath. The branches containing fibers from the intercostal nerve of the sixth to twelfth thoracic nerves (T6–T12) innervate the rectus abdominis muscle.

Warning

If the needle is inserted deeply into the linea alba and rectus abdominis muscle, it may puncture through the rectus sheath, adipose tissue and peritoneum into the urinary bladder. If the urinary bladder is filled with urine, the needle may puncture the bladder. Before treatment, urinate and empty the urinary bladder. No deep needle insertion is permitted.

Functions

Tonifies the function of the Kidney, regulates menstruation, reduces Heat and induces enuresis.

Clinical indications

Enuresis, seminal emission, urine retention, impotence, premature ejaculation, leukorrhea, female infertility, pelvic inflammatory disease, dysmenorrhea, nephritis.

35.

(HUIYIN) HUIYIN, CV 1, CONCEPTION VESSEL

Location

In a lateral recumbent position, the point is located in the centre of the perineum at the midpoint between the male's scrotum and the anus, and between the female's posterior commissure of the vagina and the anus.

Needle and moxibustion method

Perpendicular insertion 0.3–0.7 inch.
— *Needle sensation:* local numbness and distension.
— *Moxibustion dosage:* 3–5 cones; stick 10 minutes.

Cross-sectional anatomy of the needle passage

a. *Skin:* the branches containing fibers from the perineal nerve innervate the skin.
b. *Subcutaneous tissue:* includes the previously described skin nerve branches, and the perineal artery and vein. The perineal artery arises from the internal pudendal artery.
c. *External anal sphincter muscle:* the branches containing fibers from the fourth sacral nerve (S4) innervate the muscle.
d. *Superficial and deep transverse perineal muscle:* the branches containing fibers from the pudendal nerve innervate the muscle.

Functions

Tonifies the function of the Kidney, regulates menstruation, and refreshes the Mind.

Clinical indications

Itching of perineum, hemorrhoids, seminal emission, enuresis, irregular menstruation, prolapse of uterus, infantile convulsions, convulsions, schizophrenia.

36.

(CHANGCHIANG) CHANGQIANG, GV 1, GOVERNING VESSEL, CONNECTING POINT

Location

In a prone position or with the knees to the chest, the point is located at the midpoint between the apex of the coccyx and the anus.

Needle and moxibustion method

Perpendicular insertion between the coccyx and the rectum 0.5–1.0 inch.

— *Needle sensation:* local distension and soreness radiating to the anus.

— *Moxibustion dosage:* 3–7 cones; stick 5–20 minutes.

Cross-sectional anatomy of the needle passage
(Fig. 5.4)

a. Skin: the branches containing fibers from the coccygeal nerve and the perineal branch of the pudendal nerve innervate the skin.

b. Subcutaneous tissue: includes the previously described skin nerve branches.

c. Anococcygeal and sacrotuberous ligaments: the anococcygeal ligament is between the anus and the coccyx, and the sacrotuberous ligament runs from the lateral margin of the sacral and the coccygeal bone to the ischial tuberosity.

d. Coccygeus and levator ani muscles: the coccygeus muscle is located posterior to the levator ani muscle. The branches containing fibers from the pudendal plexus of the fourth and fifth sacral nerves (S4, S5) innervate the coccygeus muscle. The branches containing fibers from the pudendal plexus of the third, fourth, and fifth sacral nerves (S3, S4, S5) innervate the levator ani muscle.

e. Posterior wall of the rectum: the needle is inserted between the sacral bone and the rectum. Don't puncture deeply through the rectal wall.

Functions

Nourishes Yin to suppress the hyperfunction of Yang, and invigorates Qi to restore consciousness after prostrational collapse.

Clinical indications

Hemorrhoids, prolapse of the anus, scrotal eczema, diarrhea, impotence, schizophrenia, inducing labor.

37.

(CHIMEN) QIMEN, LIV 14, FOOT JUE YIN LIVER MERIDIAN, FRONT-MU POINT OF THE LIVER

Location

In a supine position, the point is located in the sixth intercostal space, and on the mid-clavicular line.

Needle and moxibustion method

Oblique insertion 0.5–0.8 inch.

— *Needle sensation:* slightly sore, and radiating to the posterior abdomen.

— *Moxibustion dosage:* 5 cones; stick 5–15 minutes.

Cross-sectional anatomy of the needle passage
(Fig. 5.5)

a. Skin: the branches containing fibers from the sixth intercostal nerve innervate the skin.

b. Subcutaneous tissue: includes the previously described skin nerve branches, and the sixth intercostal artery

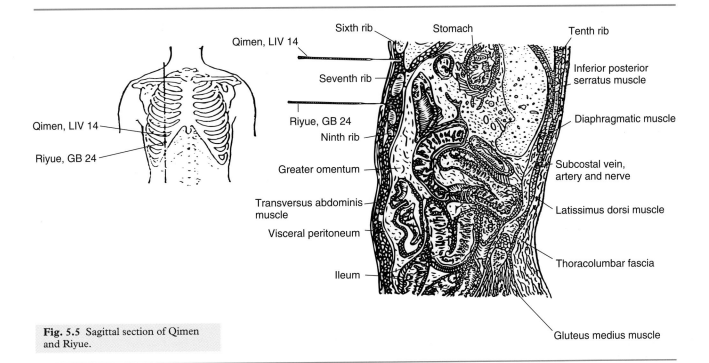

Fig. 5.5 Sagittal section of Qimen and Riyue.

Labels: Qimen, LIV 14; Riyue, GB 24; Sixth rib; Qimen, LIV 14; Seventh rib; Riyue, GB 24; Ninth rib; Greater omentum; Transversus abdominis muscle; Visceral peritoneum; Ileum; Stomach; Tenth rib; Inferior posterior serratus muscle; Diaphragmatic muscle; Subcostal vein, artery and nerve; Latissimus dorsi muscle; Thoracolumbar fascia; Gluteus medius muscle and vein. Their relative positions, from superior to inferior, are the intercostal vein, artery and nerve.

c. *External oblique muscle:* the muscular portion is lateral, and the aponeurosis is medial. The branches containing fibers from the eighth to twelfth intercostal, the iliohypogastric and the ilioinguinal nerves innervate the muscle.

Warning

If the needle is inserted through the intercostal external and internal muscles, the diaphragmatic muscle and the peritoneum into the abdominal cavity, it may puncture into the liver, and the transverse colon or the stomach on right and left, respectively. Vigorous lifting, thrusting or twirling of the needle may tear the liver, causing massive bleeding.

Functions

Clears away Heat from the Liver and the Gallbladder, and promotes Blood circulation to remove Blood Stasis.

Clinical indications

Pleurisy, hepatitis, hepatomegaly, liver cirrhosis, cholecystitis, pleuritis, myocarditis, angina pectoris, cystitis, enuresis, urine retention.

38.

(CHANGMEN) ZHANGMEN, LIV 13, FOOT JUE YIN LIVER MERIDIAN, FRONT-MU POINT OF THE SPLEEN

Location

In a lateral recumbent position, the point is located at the inferior margin of the tip of the eleventh rib.

Needle and moxibustion method

Inferior anterior oblique insertion 0.5–0.8 inch.
— *Needle sensation:* lateral abdominal distention, radiating to the posterior wall of the abdomen.
— *Moxibustion dosage:* 3 cones; stick 10–30 minutes.

Cross-sectional anatomy of the needle passage

a. *Skin:* the branches containing fibers from the tenth intercostal nerve innervate the skin.
b. *Subcutaneous tissue:* includes the previously described skin nerve branches, and the tenth intercostal artery and vein. Their relative positions, from superior to inferior, are the intercostal vein, artery and nerve.
c. *External oblique, internal oblique and transversus muscles:* the external oblique muscle is located at the deep layer of subcutaneous tissue of the inferior part of the chest and the lateral part of the abdomen. The internal oblique muscle is at the deep layer of the

external oblique muscle and the transversus muscle is at a deeper layer of the internal oblique muscle. The branches containing fibers from the eighth to twelfth intercostal, the iliohypogastric and the ilioinguinal nerves innervate the muscles.

Warning

If the needle is inserted through the transversal fascia, the adipose tissue and the peritoneum into the peritoneal cavity, it may puncture the liver and spleen to the right and left, respectively. Vigorous lifting, thrusting or twirling of the needle may tear the liver or spleen, causing massive bleeding.

Functions

Clears away Heat from the Liver, regulates the function of the Spleen, and descends the flow of Qi to relieve asthma.

Clinical indications

Hepatosplenomegaly, hepatitis, liver cirrhosis, enteritis, vomiting, abdominal distension, pleurisy, bronchial asthma.

39.

(CHIMAI) JIMAI, LIV 12, FOOT JUE YIN LIVER MERIDIAN

Location

In a supine position, the point is located 2.5 inches lateral to the anterior midline level with the inferior margin of the pubic symphysis; or in the inguinal groove lateral and inferior to Qichong [ST 30].

Needle and moxibustion method

Perpendicular insertion 0.5–1.0 inch.
— *Needle sensation:* local distension and numbness radiating to the external genital region.
— *Moxibustion dosage:* 3–5 cones; stick 10 minutes.

Cross-sectional anatomy of the needle passage

a. *Skin:* the branches containing fibers from the ilioinguinal nerve innervate the skin.
b. *Subcutaneous tissue:* includes the previously described skin nerve branches, the external pudendal artery and vein, the inferior epigastric artery and vein, and the femoral vein. The needle passes on the medial side of the femoral vein. The femoral and inferior epigastric veins join the external iliac vein. The inferior epigastric and external pudendal arteries arise from the femoral artery.
c. *Cremaster muscle (male) and round ligament of the uterus (female):* the branches containing fibers from

the genitofemoral nerve innervate the cremaster muscle and the round ligament.

Functions
Strengthens the function of the Liver, tonifies the function of the Kidney, clears Heat and removes Dampness.

Clinical indications
Penile pain, hernia, lower abdominal pain, orchitis, eczema of the external genital region, prolapse of the uterus.

40.

(SHUITU) SHUITU, ST 10, FOOT YANG MING STOMACH MERIDIAN

Location
In a seated position, the point is located on the anterior margin of the sternocleidomastoid muscle, at the midpoint between Renying [ST 9] and Qishe [ST 11].

Needle and moxibustion method
Perpendicular insertion 0.3–0.5 inch.
— *Needle sensation:* local numbness and distension.
— *Moxibustion dosage:* 3–5 cones; stick 15 minutes.

Cross-sectional anatomy of the needle passage
a. *Skin:* the transverse nerve of the neck containing fibers from the cervical plexus of the second and third cervical nerves (C2, C3) innervates the skin.
b. *Subcutaneous tissue:* includes the previously described skin nerve branches, and the platysma muscle. The cervical branches containing fibers from the facial nerve (CN VII) innervate the platysma muscle.
c. *Sternocleidomastoid and infrahyoid muscles:* the needle is inserted at the intersection of the sternocleidomastoid and infrahyoid muscles. The branches containing fibers from the spinal accessory nerve (CN XI) innervate the sternocleidomastoid muscle. The branches containing fibers from the hypoglossal nerve (CN XII) innervate the infrahyoid muscle.
d. *Common carotid artery:* the needle is inserted medial to the common carotid artery.
e. *Superior cardiac nerve and sympathetic trunk of the sympathetic nerve.*

Functions
Reduces fever to relieve sore throat, and relieves asthma.

Clinical indications
Sore throat, asthma, cough, tonsillitis, pertussis, tuber-

culosis of the cervical lymph nodes, sternocleido-mastoid muscle paralysis.

41.

(CHISHE) QISHE, ST 11, FOOT YANG MING STOMACH MERIDIAN

Location
In a seated position, the point is located 1.5 inches lateral to Tiantu [CV 22], at the superior margin of the medial clavicle, in the fossa between the sternal and clavicular heads of the sternocleidomastoid muscle.

Needle and moxibustion method
Perpendicular insertion 0.3–0.5 inch.
— *Needle sensation:* local numbness and distension.
— *Moxibustion dosage:* 3–5 cones; stick 15 minutes.

Cross-sectional anatomy of the needle passage
a. *Skin:* the anterior branches containing fibers from the supraclavicular nerve of the third and fourth cervical nerves (C3, C4) innervate the skin.
b. *Subcutaneous tissue:* includes the previously described skin nerve branches, the platysma muscle, and the anterior jugular vein pass. The cervical branches containing fibers from the facial nerve (CN VII) innervate the platysma muscle. The anterior jugular vein joins the external jugular vein.
c. *Sternocleidomastoid muscle:* the needle is inserted between the sternal and clavicular heads of the sterno-cleidomastoid muscle. The branches containing fibers from the spinal accessory nerve (CN XI) innervate the muscle.
d. *Common carotid artery:* the deep layer of the point is the common carotid artery.

Functions
Removes Heat from the Lung, resolves Phlegm, and regulates the flow of Qi to remove Blood Stasis.

Clinical indications
Sore throat, cough with dyspnea, bronchitis, tonsillitis, indigestion, hiccough.

42.

(CHIHU) QIHU, ST 13, FOOT YANG MING STOMACH MERIDIAN

Location
In a seated or supine position, the point is located 4 inches lateral to the anterior midline in the middle of

the infraclavicular fossa, directly above the nipples in men.

Needle and moxibustion method
Perpendicular insertion 0.3–0.5 inch.
— *Needle sensation:* local distension and heaviness.
— *Moxibustion dosage:* 3–5 cones; stick 15 minutes.

Cross-sectional anatomy of the needle passage
a. *Skin:* the supraclavicular branch of the third and fourth clavicle nerves and the anterior thoracic nerves innervate the skin.
b. *Subcutaneous tissue:* includes the previously described skin nerve branches.
c. *Pectoralis major muscle:* the medial and lateral anterior thoracic branches of the brachial plexus of the fifth cervical to first thoracic nerves (C5–T1) innervate the muscle.
d. *Thoracoacromial artery and vein, and subclavian vein:* the thoracoacromial artery, together with the thoracoacromial vein, is a branch of the subclavian artery. The subclavian vein joins the brachiocephalic vein.
e. *Subclavius muscle:* the lateral trunk of the brachial plexus containing fibers from the fifth and sixth cervical nerves (C5, C6) innervates the muscle.

Functions
Regulates the flow of Qi to soothe chest oppression, and relieves cough and asthma.

Clinical indications
Asthma, cough, fullness in the chest, hypochondriasis, pain in chest and back, edema of the limbs, hiccough.

43.

(KUFANG) KUFANG, ST 14, FOOT YANG MING STOMACH MERIDIAN

Location
In a supine position, the point is located 4 inches lateral to the anterior midline, and in the first intercostal space.

Needle and moxibustion method
Oblique insertion 0.3–0.5 inch.
— *Needle sensation:* local numbness and distension.
— *Moxibustion dosage:* 3–5 cones; stick 15 minutes.

Cross-sectional anatomy of the needle passage
a. *Skin:* the branches containing fibers from the anterior thoracic nerve innervate the skin.
b. *Subcutaneous tissue:* includes the previously described skin nerve branches.
c. *Pectoralis major and minor muscle:* the medial and

lateral anterior thoracic branches of the fifth cervical to first thoracic nerves (C5–T1) innervate the pectoralis major muscle. The medial anterior thoracic branch of the eighth cervical and first thoracic nerves (C8, T1) innervates the pectoralis minor muscle.
d. *Thoracoacromial artery and vein, and lateral thoracic artery:* the thoracoacromial artery, together with the thoracoacromial vein, is a branch of the subclavian artery. The lateral thoracic artery is a branch of the axillary artery.
e. *External and internal intercostal muscle:* at the intercostal space between the first and second ribs. The branches containing fibers from the intercostal nerve innervate the muscles. The deep layer of the internal and external intercostal muscles is the fascia and lung. Don't insert the needle through the intercostal muscles.

Warning
Underneath the point is the lung and the needle may puncture this, causing pneumothorax. Mild symptoms are cough, chest tightness and chest pain. Mild pneumothorax may heal spontaneously, but severe pneumothorax causes progressive respiratory difficulty and cyanosis. Tension pneumothorax may cause tachycardia, hypotension and shock.

Functions
Reduces fever, soothes chest oppression, and regulates the flow of Qi to resolve Phlegm.

Clinical indications
Fullness of the chest and hypochondrium, chest pain, difficulty in breathing, hematemesis, cough with dyspnea.

44.

(WUYI) WUYI, ST 15, FOOT YANG MING STOMACH MERIDIAN

Location
In a supine position, the point is located 4 inches lateral to the anterior midline, and in the second intercostal space.

Needle and moxibustion method
Oblique insertion 0.3–0.5 inch.
— *Needle sensation:* local distension and pain.
— *Moxibustion dosage:* 3–5 cones; stick 15 minutes.

Cross-sectional anatomy of the needle passage
a. *Skin:* the muscular branches containing fibers from the anterior thoracic nerve innervate the skin.

b. *Subcutaneous tissue:* includes the previously described skin nerve branches.

c. *Pectoralis major and minor muscles:* the medial and lateral anterior thoracic branches of the fifth cervical to first thoracic nerves (C5–T1) innervate the pectoralis major muscle. The medial anterior thoracic branch of the eighth cervical and first thoracic nerves (C8, T1) innervates the pectoralis minor muscle.

d. *Thoracoacromial artery and vein, and lateral thoracic artery and vein:* the thoracoacromial artery, together with the thoracoacromial vein, is a branch of the subclavian artery. The lateral thoracic artery, together with the lateral thoracic vein, is a branch of the axillary artery.

e. *External and internal intercostal muscles:* at the intercostal space between the second and third ribs. The branches containing fibers from the intercostal nerve innervate the external and internal intercostal muscles.

Warning
Underneath the point is the lung and the needle may puncture this, causing pneumothorax. Mild symptoms are cough, chest tightness and chest pain. Mild pneumothorax may heal spontaneously but severe symptoms are progressive respiratory difficulty and cyanosis. Tension pneumothorax may cause tachycardia, hypotension and shock.

Functions
Reduces fever, subdues swelling, and relieves cough and asthma.

Clinical indications
Cough with dyspnea, fullness of chest and hypochondrium, asthma, bronchitis, mastitis.

45.

(YINGCHUANG) YINGCHUANG, ST 16, FOOT YANG MING STOMACH MERIDIAN

Location
In a supine position, the point is located 4 inches lateral to the anterior midline, and in the third intercostal space.

Needle and moxibustion method
Oblique insertion 0.3–0.5 inch.
— *Needle sensation:* local distension and pain.
— *Moxibustion dosage:* 3–6 cones; stick 15 minutes.

Cross-sectional anatomy of the needle passage
a. *Skin:* the branches containing fibers from the anterior thoracic nerve innervate the skin.

b. *Subcutaneous tissue:* includes the previously described skin nerve branches.

c. *Pectoralis major muscle:* the medial and lateral anterior thoracic branches of the fifth cervical to first thoracic nerves (C5–T1) innervate the muscle.

d. *Thoracoacromial artery and vein:* the thoracoacromial artery and vein, are branches of the subclavian artery.

e. *External and internal intercostal muscles:* at the intercostal space between the third and fourth ribs. The branches containing fibers from the intercostal nerve innervate the external and internal intercostal muscles. At a deeper layer than the internal and external intercostal muscles is the fascia and lung. So don't puncture through these intercostal muscles.

Warning
Underneath the point is the lung and the needle may puncture this, causing pneumothorax. Mild symptoms are cough, chest pain and chest tightness. Mild pneumothorax may heal spontaneously but severe symptoms are progressive respiratory difficulty and cyanosis. Tension pneumothorax may cause tachycardia, hypotension and shock.

Functions
Reduces fever to alleviate mental depression, and regulates the flow of Qi to promote Blood circulation.

Clinical indications
Asthma, cough with dyspnea, fullness of the chest, shortness of breath, mastitis, costalgia, pain of enterocele.

46.

(JUCHUNG) RUZHONG, ST 17, FOOT YANG MING STOMACH MERIDIAN

Location
In a supine position, the point is located in the centre of the nipple. No needle puncture and moxibustion permitted.

Cross-sectional anatomy of the needle passage
a. *Skin:* the anterior cutaneous branches containing fibers from the lateral division of the fourth intercostal nerve innervate the skin.

b. *Subcutaneous tissue:* includes the previously described skin nerve branches.

c. *Pectoralis major muscle:* the medial and lateral anterior thoracic branches of the fifth cervical to first thoracic nerves (C5–T1) innervate the muscle.

d. *External and internal intercostal muscles:* at the intercostal space between fourth and fifth ribs. The branches containing fibers from the intercostal nerve innervate the external and internal intercostal muscles.

47.

(PUJUNG) BURONG, ST 19, FOOT YANG MING STOMACH MERIDIAN

Location
In a supine position, the point is located 2 inches lateral to the anterior midline of the abdomen 6 inches above the umbilicus, or 2 inches lateral to Juque [CV 14].

Needle and moxibustion method
Perpendicular insertion 0.5–0.8 inch.
— *Needle sensation:* local distension and heaviness.
— *Moxibustion dosage:* 3–5 cones; stick 15 minutes.

Cross-sectional anatomy of the needle passage
a. *Skin:* the branches containing fibers from the seventh intercostal nerve innervate the skin.
b. *Subcutaneous tissue:* includes the previously described skin nerve branches, and the superficial epigastric artery and vein. The femoral artery gives rise to the superficial epigastric artery. The superficial epigastric vein joins the greater saphenous vein.
c. *Rectus sheath:* the rectus sheath encircles the rectus abdominis muscle.
d. *Rectus abdominis muscle and inferior epigastric artery and vein:* the branches containing fibers from the seventh to twelfth intercostal nerves innervate the rectus abdominis muscle. The external iliac artery gives rise to the inferior epigastric artery. The inferior epigastric vein joins the external iliac vein.
e. *Transversus muscle:* the branches containing fibers from the seventh to twelfth intercostal nerves innervate the transversus muscle. The seventh intercostal nerve supplies the point.

Warning
Directly beneath the point is the liver. If the needle is inserted deeply, it will puncture through the posterior wall of the rectus sheath, the transverse muscle, the external peritoneal adipose tissue and the peritoneum into the liver. Usually the patient will feel nothing, or only slight pain. Lifting, thrusting, and twirling of the needle may damage the liver. The complications are pain in the liver area, and a small amount of swelling from hematoma or bile stasis. If the liver capsule is damaged, a small amount of blood or bile may drain into the peritoneal cavity and irritate the peritoneum, causing tension and pain.

Functions
Regulates the function of the Middle Jiao (Middle Warmer) and Stomach, and relieves flatulence and asthma.

Clinical indications
Fullness of the abdomen, vomiting, hematemesis, cough and dyspnea, chest and back pain, accumulation of Phlegm and Heat in the Lung.

48.

(CHENGMAN) CHENGMAN, ST 20, FOOT YANG MING STOMACH MERIDIAN

Location
In a supine position, the point is located 5 inches above the umbilicus, and 2 inches lateral to Shangwan [CV 13] on the abdominal midline.

Needle and moxibustion method
Perpendicular insertion 0.5–0.8 inches.
— *Needle sensation:* local distension and heaviness.
— *Moxibustion dosage:* 3–5 cones; stick 15 minutes.

Cross-sectional anatomy of the needle passage
a. *Skin:* the branches containing fibers from the seventh intercostal nerve innervate the skin.
b. *Subcutaneous tissue:* includes the previously described skin nerve branches, and the superficial epigastric artery and vein. The femoral artery gives rise to the superficial epigastric artery. The superficial epigastric vein joins the greater saphenous vein.
c. *Rectus sheath:* the rectus sheath encircles the rectus abdominis muscle.
d. *Rectus abdominis muscle, inferior epigastric artery and vein:* the branches containing fibers from the seventh to twelfth intercostal nerves innervate the rectus abdominis muscle. The external iliac artery gives rise to the inferior epigastric artery. The inferior epigastric vein joins the external iliac vein.
e. *Transversus muscle:* the branches containing fibers from the seventh and twelfth intercostal nerves innervate the transversus muscle. The seventh intercostal nerve supplies the point.

Warning
Directly beneath the point is the liver. If the needle is inserted deeply, it will puncture through the posterior wall of the rectus sheath, the transversus muscle, the external peritoneal adipose tissue and the peritoneum into the liver. Usually the patient will feel nothing, or only slight pain. Lifting, thrusting and twirling of the needle may damage the liver. The complications are

pain in the liver area, and a small amount of swelling from hematoma or bile stasis. If the liver capsule is damaged, a small amount of blood or bile may drain into the peritoneal cavity and irritate the peritoneum, causing tension and pain.

Functions
Strengthens the Spleen and Stomach, and regulates the Stomach to eliminate undigested food.

Clinical indications
Borborygmus, hernia pain, tympanites, diarrhea, jaundice, pain in the hypochondrium, hematemesis, cough and dyspnea.

49.

(LIANGMEN) LIANGMEN, ST 21, FOOT YANG MING STOMACH MERIDIAN

Location
In a supine position, the point is located 4 inches above the umbilicus, and 2 inches lateral to the anterior midline, level with Zhongwan [CV 12].

Needle and moxibustion method
Perpendicular insertion 0.5–0.8 inch.
— *Needle sensation:* epigastric pressure and fullness.
— *Moxibustion dosage:* 3–5 cones; stick 15 minutes.

Cross-sectional anatomy of the needle passage
a. *Skin:* the branches containing fibers from the seventh and eighth intercostal nerves innervate the skin.
b. *Subcutaneous tissue:* includes the previously described skin nerve branches, and the superficial epigastric artery and vein. The femoral artery gives rise to the superficial epigastric artery. The superficial epigastric vein joins the greater saphenous vein.
c. *Rectus sheath:* the rectus sheath encircles the rectus abdominis muscle.
d. *Rectus abdominis muscle, inferior epigastric artery and vein:* the branches containing fibers from the seventh to twelfth intercostal nerves innervate the rectus abdominis muscle. The external iliac artery gives rise to the inferior epigastric artery. The inferior epigastric vein joins the external iliac vein.
e. *Transversus muscle:* the branches containing fibers from the eleventh and twelfth intercostal nerves innervate the transversus muscle. The seventh intercostal nerve supplies the point.

Warning
Directly beneath the right and left points are the liver and pylorus of stomach, respectively. If the needle is inserted deeply, it will puncture through the posterior wall of the rectus sheath, the transversus muscle, the external peritoneal adipose tissue and the peritoneum into the liver or the pylorus of the stomach. Usually the patient will feel nothing, or only slight pain. Lifting, thrusting and twirling the needle may damage the liver or the pylorus of the stomach. The complications of liver are pain in the liver area, and a small amount of swelling from hematoma or bile stasis. If the liver capsule is damaged, a small amount of blood or bile drains into the peritoneal cavity and irritates the peritoneum, causing tension and pain. The severe complications of damaging the pylorus of the stomach are a small amount of stomach content draining into the peritoneal cavity, irritating the peritoneum and causing the tension and rebound pain of peritonitis.

Functions
Strengthens the Spleen, regulates the flow of Qi, and regulates the Stomach and Middle Jiao (Middle Warmer).

Clinical indications
Prolapse of the anus, stomach pain, gastric ulcer, acute gastritis, hernia pain.

50.

(KUANMEN) GUANMEN, ST 22, FOOT YANG MING STOMACH MERIDIAN

Location
In a supine position, the point is located 3 inches above the umbilicus, and 2 inches lateral to the abdominal midline level with Jianli [CV 11].

Needle and moxibustion method
Perpendicular insertion 0.5–0.8 inch.
— *Needle sensation:* local distension and heaviness.
— *Moxibustion dosage:* 3–5 cones; stick 15 minutes.

Cross-sectional anatomy of the needle passage
a. *Skin:* the branches containing fibers from the eighth intercostal nerve innervate the skin.
b. *Subcutaneous tissue:* includes the previously described skin nerve branches, and the superficial epigastric artery and vein. The femoral artery gives rise to the superficial epigastric artery. The superficial epigastric vein joins the greater saphenous vein.
c. *Rectus sheath:* the rectus sheath encircles the rectus abdominis muscle.
d. *Rectus abdominis muscle, inferior epigastric artery and vein:* the branches containing fibers from the seventh to twelfth intercostal nerves innervate the muscle.

The eighth intercostal nerve supplies the point. The external iliac artery gives rise to the inferior epigastric artery. The inferior epigastric vein joins the external iliac vein.

Warning

Directly beneath the point is the transverse colon. If the needle is inserted deeply, it will puncture through the posterior wall of the rectus sheath, the transversus muscle, the external peritoneal adipose tissue and the peritoneum into the transverse colon. Lifting, thrusting and twirling the needle may damage the transverse colon. Complications can arise if a small amount of intestinal contents drains into the peritoneal cavity, irritating the peritoneum and causing the tension and rebound pain of peritonitis.

Functions

Regulates the function of the Intestine and Stomach, and regulates the flow of Qi to eliminate undigested food.

Clinical indications

Fullness of the chest, dysentery, edema, constipation, gastric ulcer, gastric spasm, abdominal distension, abdominal pain.

51.

(TAIYI) TAIYI, ST 23, FOOT YANG MING STOMACH MERIDIAN

Location

In a supine position, the point is located 2 inches above the umbilicus, and 2 inches lateral to the anterior midline, level with Xiawan [CV 10].

Needle and moxibustion method

Perpendicular insertion 0.5–0.8 inch.
— *Needle sensation:* local distension and heaviness.
— *Moxibustion dosage:* 3–5 cones; stick 15 minutes.

Cross-sectional anatomy of the needle passage

a. *Skin:* the branches containing fibers from the eighth intercostal nerve innervate the skin.
b. *Subcutaneous tissue:* includes the previously described skin nerve branches, and the superficial epigastric artery and vein. The femoral artery gives rise to the superficial epigastric artery. The superficial epigastric vein joins the greater saphenous vein.
c. *Rectus sheath:* the rectus sheath encircles the rectus abdominis muscle.
d. *Rectus abdominis muscle, inferior epigastric artery and vein:* the branches containing fibers from the seventh to twelfth intercostal nerves innervate the rectus

---

abdominis muscle. The eighth intercostal nerve supplies the point. The external iliac artery gives rise to the inferior epigastric artery. The inferior epigastric vein joins the external iliac vein.

Warning

Directly beneath the point is the transverse colon. If the needle is inserted deeply, it will puncture through the posterior wall of the rectus sheath, the transversus muscle, the external peritoneal adipose tissue and the peritoneum into the transverse colon. Lifting, thrusting and twirling the needle may damage the transverse colon. Complications can arise if a small amount of intestinal contents drain into the peritoneal cavity, irritating the peritoneum and causing the tension and rebound pain of peritonitis.

Functions

Eliminates Phlegm to awaken and clear the Mind, relieves flatulence and eliminates undigested food.

Clinical indications

Stomach pain, gastritis, gastric ulcer, indigestion, epilepsy, enuresis, beriberi, nervousness, intestinal hernia.

52.

(HUAJOUMEN) HUAROUMEN, ST 24, FOOT YANG MING STOMACH MERIDIAN

Location

In a supine position, the point is located 1 inch above the umbilicus, and 2 inches lateral to the abdominal midline, level with Shuifen [CV 9].

Needle and moxibustion method

Perpendicular insertion 0.7–1.0 inch.
— *Needle sensation:* local distension and heaviness radiating inferiorly.
— *Moxibustion dosage:* 3–5 cones; stick 15 minutes.

Cross-sectional anatomy of the needle passage

a. *Skin:* the branches containing fibers from the ninth intercostal nerve innervate the skin.
b. *Subcutaneous tissue:* includes the previously described skin nerve branches, and the superficial epigastric artery and vein. The femoral artery gives rise to the superficial epigastric artery. The superficial epigastric vein joins the greater saphenous vein.
c. *Rectus sheath:* the rectus sheath encircles the rectus abdominis muscle.
d. *Rectus abdominis muscle, inferior epigastric artery and vein:* the branches containing fibers from the seventh to twelfth intercostal nerves innervate the rectus

abdominis muscle. The ninth intercostal nerve supplies the point. The external iliac artery gives rise to the inferior epigastric artery. The inferior epigastric vein joins the external iliac vein.

Warning
Directly beneath the point is the small intestine. If the needle is inserted deeply, it will puncture through the posterior wall of the rectus sheath, the transversus muscle, the external peritoneal adipose tissue and the peritoneum into the small intestine. Lifting, thrusting and twirling the needle may damage the small intestine. Severe complications can arise if a small amount of the intestinal contents drains into the peritoneal cavity, irritating the peritoneum and causing the tension and rebound pain of peritonitis.

Functions
Strengthens the Stomach to arrest vomiting, and regulates the function of the Middle Jiao (Middle Warmer) to remove Dampness.

Clinical indications
Stomach pain, vomiting, manic depressive syndrome, convulsions, schizophrenia, ascites, hematemesis, stiffness of the tongue.

53.

(TIENCHU) TIANSHU, ST 25, FOOT YANG MING STOMACH MERIDIAN, FRONT-MU POINT OF THE LARGE INTESTINE

Location
In a supine position, the point is located 2 inches lateral to the umbilicus.

Needle and moxibustion method
Perpendicular insertion 1.0–1.5 inches.
— *Needle sensation:* local distension and soreness, and radiating to the ipsilateral abdomen.
— *Moxibustion dosage:* 5–9 cones; stick 10–15 minutes.

Cross-sectional anatomy of the needle passage
a. *Skin:* the cutaneous branches containing fibers from the tenth intercostal nerve innervate the skin.
b. *Subcutaneous tissue:* includes the previously described skin nerve branches, and the superficial epigastric artery and vein. The femoral artery gives rise to the superficial epigastric artery. The superficial epigastric vein joins the greater saphenous vein.
c. *Rectus sheath:* the rectus sheath encircles the rectus abdominis muscle.
d. *Rectus abdominis muscle, inferior epigastric artery and vein:* the branches containing fibers from the seventh

to twelfth intercostal nerves innervate the rectus abdominis muscle. The tenth intercostal nerve supplies the point. The external iliac artery gives rise to the inferior epigastric artery. The inferior epigastric vein joins the external iliac vein.

Warning
If the needle is inserted deeply through the posterior wall of the rectus sheath, the transversus muscle, the external peritoneal adipose tissue and the peritoneum into the peritoneal cavity, it may puncture into the small intestine. Lifting, thrusting and twirling the needle may damage the small intestine. Severe complications can result if a small amount of the intestinal contents drain into the peritoneal cavity, irritating the peritoneum and causing tension and rebound pain.

Functions
Regulates the function of the Middle Jiao (Middle Warmer) and Stomach, and regulates the flow of Qi to strengthen the function of the Spleen and the Large Intestine.

Clinical indications
Acute and chronic dysentery, acute and chronic diarrhea, acute and chronic enteritis, appendicitis, abdominal distension, constipation, ascites, irregular menstruation.

54.

(WAILING) WAILING, ST 26, FOOT YANG MING STOMACH MERIDIAN

Location
In a supine position, the point is located 1 inch below the umbilicus and 2 inches lateral to the anterior midline.

Needle and moxibustion method
Perpendicular insertion 0.5–1.0 inch.
— *Needle sensation:* Local distension and numbness radiating inferiorly.
— *Moxibustion dosage:* 7–15 cones; stick 10–20 minutes.

Cross-sectional anatomy of the needle passage
a. *Skin:* the branches containing fibers from the tenth intercostal nerve innervate the skin.
b. *Subcutaneous tissue:* includes the previously described skin nerve branches, and the superficial epigastric artery and vein. The femoral artery gives rise to the superficial epigastric artery. The superficial epigastric vein joins the greater saphenous vein.
c. *Rectus sheath:* the rectus sheath encircles the rectus abdominis muscle.

d. *Rectus abdominis muscle, inferior epigastric artery and vein:* the branches containing fibers from the seventh to twelfth intercostal nerves innervate the rectus abdominis muscle. The external iliac artery gives rise to the inferior epigastric artery. The inferior epigastric vein joins the external iliac vein.

Warning

If the needle is inserted deeply through the posterior rectus sheath, the transversus muscle, the external peritoneal adipose tissue and the peritoneum into the peritoneal cavity, it will puncture the small intestine. Strong thrusting and twirling of the needle may damage the small intestine and a small amount of intestinal contents may drain into the peritoneal cavity, irritating the peritoneum and causing tension and rebound pain.

Functions

Regulates the function of the Stomach to remove Dampness, and regulates the flow of Qi to promote Blood circulation.

Clinical indications

Abdominal pain, acute and chronic enteritis, appendicitis, constipation, hernia, dysmenorrhea, irregular menstruation.

55.

(TACHU) DAJU, ST 27, FOOT YANG MING STOMACH MERIDIAN

Location

In a supine position, the point is located 2 inches below the umbilicus and 2 inches lateral to the anterior midline.

Needle and moxibustion method

Perpendicular insertion 0.5–1.0 inch.
— *Needle sensation:* local distension and heaviness radiating inferiorly.
— *Moxibustion dosage:* 7–15 cones; stick 15 minutes.

Cross-sectional anatomy of the needle passage

a. *Skin:* the branches containing fibers from the eleventh intercostal nerve innervate the skin.
b. *Subcutaneous tissue:* includes the previously described skin nerve branches, and the superficial epigastric artery and vein. The femoral artery gives rise to the superficial epigastric artery. The superficial epigastric vein joins the greater saphenous vein.
c. *Rectus sheath:* the rectus sheath encircles the rectus abdominis muscle.
d. *Rectus abdominis muscle, inferior epigastric artery and vein:* the branches containing fibers from the seventh

---

to twelfth intercostal nerves innervate the muscle. The external iliac artery gives rise to the inferior epigastric artery. The inferior epigastric vein joins the external iliac vein.

Warning

Directly beneath the point is the small intestine. If the needle is inserted through the posterior rectus sheath, the transversus muscle, the external peritoneal adipose tissue and the peritoneum into the peritoneal cavity, it will puncture the small intestine. A small amount of the intestinal contents may drain into the peritoneal cavity, irritating the peritoneum and causing tension and rebound pain.

Functions

Strengthens the body's resistance, removes Dampness, and regulates the flow of Qi to eliminate undigested food.

Clinical indications

Distension of the lower abdomen, enteritis, appendicitis, constipation, hemiplegia, insomnia, enuresis, impotence, tiredness and heaviness of the limbs.

56.

(SHUITAO) SHUIDAO, ST 28, FOOT YANG MING STOMACH MERIDIAN

Location

In a supine position, the point is located 3 inches below the umbilicus and 2 inches lateral to the abdominal midline level with Guanyuan [CV 4].

Needle and moxibustion method

Perpendicular insertion 0.5–1.0 inch.
— *Needle sensation:* local distension radiating to the external genital region.
— *Moxibustion dosage:* 7–15 cones; stick 15 minutes.

Cross-sectional anatomy of the needle passage

a. *Skin:* the branches containing fibers from the twelfth intercostal nerve innervate the skin.
b. *Subcutaneous tissue:* includes the previously described skin nerve branches, and the superficial epigastric artery and vein. The femoral artery gives rise to the superficial epigastric artery. The superficial epigastric vein joins the greater saphenous vein.
c. *Rectus sheath:* the rectus sheath encircles the rectus abdominis muscle.
d. *Rectus abdominis muscle, inferior epigastric artery and vein:* the branches containing fibers from the seventh to twelfth intercostal nerves innervate the muscle. The external iliac artery gives rise to the inferior

epigastric artery. The inferior epigastric vein joins the external iliac vein.

Warning
Directly beneath the point is the small intestine. If the needle is inserted through the posterior sheath, the transversus muscle, the external peritoneal adipose tissue and the peritoneum into the peritoneal cavity, it will puncture into the small intestine. A small amount of the intestinal contents may drain into the peritoneal cavity, irritating the peritoneum and causing tension and rebound pain.

Functions
Reduces fever, removes Dampness, and clears and regulates the water passages.

Clinical indications
Distension of the lower abdomen, cystitis, nephritis, enuresis, edema, hernia, dysmenorrhea, infertility.

57.

(KUEILAI) GUILAI, ST 29, FOOT YANG MING STOMACH MERIDIAN

Location
In a supine position, the point is located 4 inches below the umbilicus and 2 inches lateral to the abdominal midline level with Zhongji [CV 3].

Needle and moxibustion method
Perpendicular insertion or oblique insertion towards the pubic symphysis 1.0–1.5 inches.
— *Needle sensation:* lower abdominal soreness and distension, and radiating to the external genital organs.
— *Moxibustion dosage:* 5–7 cones; stick 10–20 minutes.

Cross-sectional anatomy of the needle passage
a. *Skin:* the ilioepigastric branch of the lumbar plexus of the twelfth thoracic and first lumbar nerves (T12, L1) innervates the skin.
b. *Subcutaneous tissue:* includes the previously described skin nerve branches, and the superficial epigastric artery and vein. The femoral artery gives rise to the superficial epigastric artery. The superficial epigastric vein joins the greater saphenous vein.
c. *Lateral margin of rectus abdominis muscle, external oblique and internal oblique muscles, and tendon of transversus muscle:* the lateral part of the external oblique, the internal oblique and the transversus muscle forms the local musculature; the medial part is aponeurosis which becomes the rectus sheath at the lateral margin of the rectus abdominis muscle. The branches containing fibers from the seventh to

twelfth thoracic nerves (T7–T12) innervate the external oblique muscle. The branches containing fibers from the seventh thoracic to first lumbar nerves (T7–L1) innervate the the internal oblique and transversus muscles. The branches containing fibers from the twelfth thoracic and first lumbar (T12, L1) nerves supply the point.

Functions
Regulates the flow of Qi to promote Blood circulation, and strengthens the function of the Liver and Kidney.

Clinical indications
Irregular menstruation, orchitis, endometritis, adnexa inflammation, infertility, dysmenorrhea, prolapse of the uterus, impotence, hernia.

58.

(TZUKUNGXUE) ZIGONGXUE, EX-CA 1, EXTRA POINT OF THE CHEST AND ABDOMEN

Location
In a supine position, the point is located 4 inches below the umbilicus and 3 inches lateral to the abdominal midline level with Zhongji [CV 3].

Needle and moxibustion method
Perpendicular insertion or oblique insertion to the pubic symphysis 1.5–2.0 inches.
— *Needle sensation:* lower abdominal distension and soreness, or radiating to the external genital organs.
— *Moxibustion dosage:* 5–7 cones; stick 10–20 minutes.

Cross-sectional anatomy of the needle passage
a. *Skin:* the ilioepigastric branch of the lumbar plexus of the twelfth thoracic and first lumbar nerves (T12, L1) innervates the skin.
b. *Subcutaneous tissue:* includes the previously described skin nerve branches, and the superficial epigastric artery and vein. The femoral artery gives rise to the superficial epigastric artery. The superficial epigastric vein joins the greater saphenous vein.
c. *External oblique, internal oblique and transversus muscles:* the layers of these three muscles from superficial to deep are the external oblique, the internal oblique and the transversus. The branches containing fibers from the seventh to twelfth thoracic nerves (T7–T12) innervate the external oblique muscle. The branches containing fibers from the seventh thoracic to first lumbar nerves (T7–L1) innervate the internal oblique and transversus muscles.

Warning

If the needle is inserted through the transversus muscle, the posterior wall of the rectus sheath, the external peritoneal adipose tissue and the peritoneum into the peritoneal cavity, it may puncture into internal organs.

Functions

Tonifies the function of the Kidney.

Clinical indications

Prolapse of the uterus, irregular menstruation, dysmenorrhea, pelvic inflammatory disease, female infertility, pyelonephritis, cystitis, orchitis, appendicitis.

59.

(CHICHUNG) QICHONG, ST 30, FOOT YANG MING STOMACH MERIDIAN

Location

In a supine position the point is located 5 inches below the umbilicus, and 2 inches lateral to the midline of the abdomen, or at the superior margin of the inguinal ligament and medial to the inferior epigastric artery.

Needle and moxibustion method

Perpendicular insertion 0.5–1.0 inch.
— *Needle sensation:* local heaviness and distension.

Medial inferior oblique insertion 1.0–2.0 to the external genital organs.
— *Needle sensation:* distension and soreness radiating to the external genital organs.
— *Moxibustion dosage:* 3–5 cones; stick 5–10 minutes.

Cross-sectional anatomy of the needle passage

a. *Skin:* the ilioinguinal branch of the lumbar plexus of the anterior division of the twelfth thoracic and first lumbar nerve (T12, L1) innervates the skin.
b. *Subcutaneous tissue:* includes the previously described skin nerve branches, and the superficial epigastric artery and vein. The femoral artery gives rise to the superficial epigastric artery. The superficial epigastric vein joins the greater saphenous vein.
c. *Tendon sheath of external oblique muscle:* the lateral part is muscular and the medial part is the aponeurosis. The inferior margin of the aponeurosis thickens to become the inguinal ligament. The aponeurosis of the rectus abdominis muscle divides at the superior lateral pubic tubercle to become a triangular fissure, called the subcutaneous inguinal ring. The needle is inserted at the superior lateral part of the subcutaneous inguinal ring. The branches containing fibers from the seventh to twelfth thoracic nerves (T7–T12) innervate the muscle.
d. *Internal oblique and inferior part of transversus muscles:*

the internal oblique muscle is the deep layer of the external oblique muscle, and the transversus muscle is the deeper layer of the internal oblique muscle. The branches containing fibers from the seventh thoracic to first lumbar nerves (T7–L1) innervate the muscles.
e. The needle is inserted on the medial side of the inferior epigastric artery and vein. The external iliac artery gives rise to the inferior epigastric artery. The inferior epigastric vein joins the external iliac vein.

Warning

If the needle is inserted deeply, it may puncture into the inguinal canal which consists of the spermatic cord in the male and the round ligament of uterus in the female.

Functions

Reduces fever, removes Dampness, and tonifies the function of the Stomach to regulate the adverse flow of Qi.

Clinical indications

Hernia, male and female genital organ disease, cystitis, orchitis, enuresis, impotence, emission, irregular menstruation.

60.

(TINGCHUAN) DINGCHUAN, EX-B 1, EXTRA POINT OF THE BACK

Location

In a prone or seated positions and bending the head forward, the point is located 0.5 inch lateral to Dazhui [GV 14].

Needle and moxibustion method

Medial oblique insertion 0.5–1.0 inch.
— *Needle sensation:* local distension and soreness, or radiating to the shoulder or the chest.
— *Moxibustion dosage:* 3–5 cones; stick 5–15 minutes.

Cross-sectional anatomy of the needle passage

a. *Skin:* the branches containing fibers from the posterior cutaneous nerve of the eighth cervical nerve (C8) innervate the skin.
b. *Subcutaneous tissue:* includes the previously described skin nerve branches.
c. *Tendon of trapezius muscle:* the branches containing fibers from the spinal accessory nerve (CN XI) and the ventral primary division of the third and fourth cervical nerves (C3, C4) innervate the muscle.
d. *Rhomboid muscle:* the branches containing fibers from the dorsal scapular branch of the fourth and fifth cervical nerves (C4, C5) innervate the muscle.

e. *Splenius cervicis muscle:* the lateral branches containing fibers from the dorsal division of the second to fifth cervical nerves (C2–C5) innervate the muscle.

f. *Superior posterior serratus muscle:* the branches containing fibers from the first to fourth intercostal nerves innervate the muscle.

g. *Sacrospinalis (erector spinae) muscle:* the branches containing fibers from the dorsal divisions of the spinal nerves innervate the muscle. The lateral branches containing fibers from the dorsal divisions of the eighth cervical and first thoracic nerves (C8, T1) innervate the point.

Functions
Expels exterior Wind and descends Lung Qi.

Clinical indications
Cough, bronchitis, asthma, urticaria, neck stiffness.

containing fibers from the dorsal primary division of the spinal nerves innervate the muscle. The lateral branches of the dorsal divisions of the first and second thoracic nerves (T1, T2) innervate the point.

Warning
The needle should be inserted in a medially oblique direction. If the needle is inserted deeply in a perpendicular or laterally oblique direction, it may puncture through the thoracic wall, causing pneumothorax.

Functions
Expels Wind to relieve Exterior syndrome, regulates the Blood and relieves rigidity of the joints.

Clinical indications
Fever, headache, cough, common cold, shoulder pain, neck stiffness, knee pain, sore throat, lower back pain, malaria.

61.

(TACHU) DAZHU, BL 11, FOOT TAI YANG BLADDER MERIDIAN

Location
In a prone position, the point is located 1.5 inches lateral and inferior to the spinous process of the first thoracic vertebra.

Needle and moxibustion method
Medial oblique insertion 0.5–1.0 inch.
— *Needle sensation:* local distension, soreness and numbness, or sometimes radiating to the intercostal region.
— *Moxibustion dosage:* 3–7 cones; stick 10 minutes.

Cross-sectional anatomy of the needle passage
a. *Skin:* the medial branches containing fibers from the posterior divisions of the first thoracic nerve (T1) innervate the skin.

b. *Subcutaneous tissue:* includes the previously described skin nerve branches.

c. *Trapezius muscle:* the branches containing fibers from the spinal accessory nerve (CN XI) and the ventral division of the third and fourth cervical nerves (C3, C4) innervate the muscle.

d. *Rhomboid muscle:* the scapular branch of the fourth and fifth cervical nerves (C4, C5) innervates the muscle.

e. *Tendon of superior posterior serratus muscle:* the branches of the first to fourth intercostal nerves innervate the muscle.

f. *Sacrospinalis (erector spinae) muscle:* the branches

62.

(FENGMEN) FENGMEN, BL 12, FOOT TAI YANG BLADDER MERIDIAN

Location
In a prone position, the point is located 1.5 inches lateral and inferior to the spinous process of the second thoracic vertebra.

Needle and moxibustion method
Medial oblique insertion 0.5–1.0 inch.
— *Needle sensation:* local distension and soreness, or sometimes radiating to the intercostal region.
— *Moxibustion dosage:* 3–5 cones; stick 15 minutes.

Cross-sectional anatomy of the needle passage
(Fig. 5.6)
a. *Skin:* the medial branches containing fibers from the posterior divisions of the second thoracic nerve (T2) innervate the skin.

b. *Subcutaneous tissue:* includes the previously described skin nerve branches.

c. *Trapezius muscle:* the branches containing fibers from the spinal accessory (CN XI) and the ventral primary division of the third and fourth cervical nerves (C3, C4) innervate the muscle.

d. *Rhomboid muscle:* the branches containing fibers from the dorsal scapular nerve of the fourth and fifth cervical nerves (C4, C5) innervate the muscle.

e. *Tendon of superior posterior serratus muscle:* the branches containing fibers from the first to fourth intercostal nerves innervate the muscle.

f. *Sacrospinalis (erector spinae) muscle:* the branches

containing fibers from the dorsal primary divisions of the spinal nerves innervate the muscle. The branches containing fibers from the lateral branches of the dorsal divisions of the second and third thoracic nerves (T2, T3) innervate the point.

g. The transversospinal muscle is located deep and posterior to the sacrospinalis muscle.

Warning

The needle should be inserted in a medially oblique direction. If the needle is inserted deeply in a perpendicular or laterally oblique direction, it may puncture through the thoracic wall, causing pneumothorax.

Functions

Expels Wind, regulates the function of the Lung, and reduces Heat to remove swelling.

Clinical indications

Common cold, bronchitis, pneumonia, pleurisy, asthma, urticaria, shoulder and surrounding soft tissue disease.

63.

(FEISHU) FEISHU, BL 13, FOOT TAI YANG BLADDER MERIDIAN, BACK-SHU POINT OF THE LUNG

Location

In a prone position, the point is located 1.5 inches lateral and inferior to the spinous process of the third thoracic vertebra.

Needle and moxibustion method

Medial oblique insertion 0.5–1.0 inch.
— *Needle sensation:* local distension and soreness, or sometimes radiating to the intercostal region.
— *Moxibustion dosage:* 3–5 cones; stick 5–15 minutes.

Cross-sectional anatomy of the needle passage
(Fig. 5.6)

a. Skin: the medial cutaneous branches containing fibers from the posterior division of the third thoracic nerve (T3) innervate the skin.

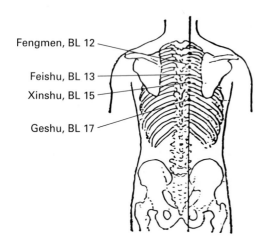

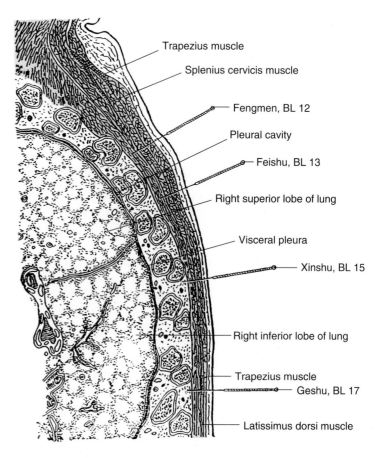

Fengmen, BL 12
Feishu, BL 13
Xinshu, BL 15
Geshu, BL 17

Trapezius muscle
Splenius cervicis muscle
Fengmen, BL 12
Pleural cavity
Feishu, BL 13
Right superior lobe of lung
Visceral pleura
Xinshu, BL 15
Right inferior lobe of lung
Trapezius muscle
Geshu, BL 17
Latissimus dorsi muscle

Fig. 5.6 Sagittal section of Fengmen, Feishu, Xinshu and Geshu.

b. *Subcutaneous tissue:* includes the previously described skin nerve branches.

c. *Trapezius muscle:* the branches containing fibers from the spinal accessory nerve (CN XI) and the ventral primary division of the third and fourth cervical nerves (C3, C4) innervate the muscle.

d. *Rhomboid muscle:* the dorsal scapular branch of the fourth and fifth cervical nerves (C4, C5) innervates the muscle.

e. *Tendon of superior posterior serratus muscle:* the branches containing fibers from the first to fourth intercostal nerves innervate the muscle.

f. *Sacrospinalis (erector spinae) muscle:* the branches containing fibers from the dorsal primary divisions of the spinal nerves innervate the muscle. The lateral branches containing fibers from the dorsal divisions of the third and fourth thoracic nerves (T3, T4) innervate the point.

g. The transversospinal muscle is located deep and posterior to the sacrospinalis muscle.

Warning

The needle should be inserted in a medially oblique direction. If the needle is inserted deeply in a perpendicular or laterally oblique direction, it may puncture through the thoracic wall, causing pneumothorax.

Functions

Regulates the Lung Qi, reduces fever and nourishes the Yin.

Clinical indications

Bronchitis, asthma, pneumonia, tuberculosis, pleuritis, spontaneous sweating, night sweating.

64.

(CHUEYINSHU) JUEHYINSHU, BL 14, FOOT TAI YANG BLADDER MERIDIAN

Location

In a prone position, the point is located 1.5 inches lateral and inferior to the spinous process of the fourth thoracic vertebra.

Needle and moxibustion method

Medial oblique insertion 0.5–1.0 inch.

— *Needle sensation:* local distension and soreness, or sometimes radiating to the intercostal region.

— *Moxibustion dosage:* 3–5 cones; stick 10–20 minutes.

Cross-sectional anatomy of the needle passage

a. *Skin:* the medial cutaneous branches containing fibers from the posterior division of the fourth

thoracic nerve (T4) innervate the skin.

b. *Subcutaneous tissue:* includes the previously described skin nerve branches.

c. *Trapezius muscle:* the branches containing fibers from the spinal accessory nerve (CN XI) and the ventral primary division of the third and fourth cervical nerves (C3, C4) innervate the muscle.

d. *Rhomboid muscle:* the dorsal scapular branch of the fourth and fifth cervical nerves (C4, C5) innervates the muscle.

e. *Tendon of superior posterior serratus muscle:* the branches containing fibers from the first to fourth intercostal nerves innervate the muscle.

f. *Sacrospinalis (erector spinae) muscle:* the branches containing fibers from the dorsal primary division of the spinal nerves innervate the muscle. The lateral branches containing fibers from the dorsal divisions of the fourth and fifth thoracic nerves (T4, T5) innervate the point.

g. The transversospinal muscle is located deep and posterior to the sacrospinalis muscle.

Warning

The needle should be inserted in a medially oblique direction. If the needle is inserted deeply in a perpendicular or laterally oblique direction, it may puncture through the thoracic cavity, causing pneumothorax.

Functions

Regulates the function of the Lung and Heart Qi, and regulates the function of the Stomach to arrest vomiting.

Clinical indications

Cough, tachycardia, myocarditis, pericarditis, angina pectoris, vomiting, precordial pain, gastric ulcer, gastric spasm, gastritis.

65.

(TUSHU) DUSHU, BL 16, FOOT TAI YANG BLADDER MERIDIAN

Location

In a prone position, the point is located 1.5 inches lateral and inferior to the spinous process of the sixth thoracic vertebra.

Needle and moxibustion method

Medial oblique insertion 0.5–0.7 inch.

— *Needle sensation:* local distension and soreness, or sometimes radiating to the lateral or anterior part of the chest.

— *Moxibustion dosage:* 3–5 cones; stick 10–20 minutes.

Cross-sectional anatomy of the needle passage
(Fig. 5.6)

a. *Skin:* the medial cutaneous branches of the posterior division of the sixth thoracic nerve (T6) innervate the skin.

b. *Subcutaneous tissue:* includes the previously described skin nerve branches.

c. *Trapezius muscle:* the branches containing fibers from the spinal accessory nerve (CN XI) and the ventral primary division of the third and fourth cervical nerves (C3, C4) innervate the muscle.

d. *Latissimus dorsi muscle:* the thoracodorsal branches of the sixth, seventh, and eighth cervical nerves (C6, C7, C8) innervate the muscle.

e. *Sacrospinalis (erector spinae) muscle:* the branches containing fibers from the dorsal primary division of the spinal nerves innervate the muscle. The lateral branches containing fibers from the dorsal divisions of the sixth and seventh thoracic nerves (T6, T7) innervate the point.

f. The transversospinal muscle is located deep and posterior to the sacrospinalis muscle.

Warning

The needle should be inserted in a medially oblique direction. If the needle is punctured deeply in a perpendicular or laterally oblique direction, it may penetrate through the thoracic wall, causing pneumothorax.

Functions

Regulates the flow of Qi, improves Blood circulation, and regulates the function of the Heart.

Clinical indications

Precordial pain, hypertension, myocarditis, pericarditis, angina pectoris, tachycardia, dyspnea, stomach pain, gastric ulcer, gastritis, gastric spasm.

66.

(KESHU) GESHU, BL 17, FOOT TAI YANG BLADDER MERIDIAN

Location

In a prone position, the point is located 1.5 inches lateral and inferior to the spinous process of the seventh thoracic vertebra.

Needle and moxibustion method

Medial oblique insertion 0.5–1.0 inch.
— *Needle sensation:* local distension and soreness, or sometimes radiating to the intercostal region.
— *Moxibustion dosage:* 3–5 cones; stick 5–15 minutes.

Cross-sectional anatomy of the needle passage
(Fig. 5.6)

a. *Skin:* the medial cutaneous branches containing fibers from the posterior division of the seventh thoracic nerve (T7) innervate the skin.

b. *Subcutaneous tissue:* includes the previously described skin nerve branches.

c. *Trapezius muscle:* the branches containing fibers from the spinal accessory nerve (CN XI) and the ventral primary divisions of the third and fourth cervical nerves (C3, C4) innervate the muscle.

d. *Latissimus dorsi muscle:* the thoracodorsal branches of the sixth, seventh, and eighth cervical nerves (C6, C7, C8) innervate the muscle.

e. *Sacrospinalis (erector spinae) muscle:* the branches containing fibers from the dorsal primary divisions of the spinal nerves innervate the muscle. The lateral branches containing fibers from the seventh thoracic nerve and the medial branches containing fibers from the seventh and eighth thoracic nerves (T7, T8) innervate the muscle.

f. The transversospinal muscle is located deep and posterior to the sacrospinalis muscle.

Warning

The needle should be inserted in a medially oblique direction. If the needle is punctured deeply in a perpendicular or laterally oblique direction, it may penetrate through the thoracic wall, causing pneumothorax.

Functions

Regulates Blood circulation and the flow of Qi, eliminates Phlegm and promotes resuscitation.

Clinical indications

Chronic anemia, chronic hemorrhagic disease, diaphragmatic muscle spasm, neurogenic vomiting, urticaria, tuberculosis of the lymph nodes, stomach cancer, esophageal stenosis.

67.

(CHIENCHUNGSHU) JIANZHONGSHU, SI 15, HAND TAI YANG SMALL INTESTINE MERIDIAN

Location

In a seated position, the point is located 2 inches lateral to the inferior border of the spinous process of the seventh cervical vertebra, or 2 inches lateral to Dazhui [GV 14]; or in the fossa medial to the superior angle of the scapula.

Needle and moxibustion method
Oblique insertion 0.3–0.6 inch.
— *Needle sensation:* local numbness and distension.
— *Moxibustion dosage:* 5–10 cones; stick 15 minutes.

Cross-sectional anatomy of the needle passage
a. *Skin:* the medial cutaneous branches containing fibers from the dorsal division of the seventh and eighth cervical nerves (C7, C8) innervate the skin.
b. *Subcutaneous tissue:* includes the previously described skin nerve branches.
c. *Trapezius muscle:* the branches containing fibers from the spinal accessory nerve (CN XII) and the branches containing fibers from the ventral rami of the third and fourth cervical nerves (C3, C4) innervate the muscle.
d. *Transverse cervical artery and dorsal scapular nerve:* the transverse cervical artery arises from the thyrocervical artery.
e. *Levator scapulae muscle:* the branches containing fibers from the cervical plexus of the third and fourth cervical nerves (C3, C4) innervate the muscle.

Functions
Reduces fever, improves acuity of vision, and relieves cough and asthma.

Clinical indications
Cough and dyspnea, bronchitis, bronchial asthma, hematemesis, pain of the shoulder and back, chills and fever, myopia, optic neuritis.

68.

(CHIENWAISHU) JIANWAISHU, SI 14, HAND TAI YANG SMALL INTESTINE MERIDIAN

Location
In a seated position, the point is located 3 inches lateral to the spinous process of the first thoracic vertebra level with Taodao [GV 13], and at the medial superior margin of the scapula.

Needle and moxibustion method
Oblique insertion 0.3–0.7 inch.
— *Moxibustion dosage:* 3–7 cones.

Cross-sectional anatomy of the needle passage
a. *Skin:* the medial cutaneous branches containing fibers from the dorsal divisions of the eighth cervical and first thoracic nerves (C8, T1) innervate the skin.
b. *Subcutaneous tissue:* includes the previously described skin nerve branches.
c. *Trapezius muscle:* the branches containing fibers from

the spinal accessory nerve (CN XI) and the branches containing fibers from the ventral rami of the third and fourth cervical nerves (C3, C4) innervate the muscle.
d. *Transverse cervical artery and dorsal scapular nerve:* the transverse cervical artery arises from the thyrocervical artery.
e. *Levator scapulae muscle:* the branches containing fibers from the cervical plexus of the third and fourth cervical nerves (C3, C4) innervate the muscle.
f. *Rhomboid muscle:* the dorsal scapular branch of the brachial plexus of the fifth cervical nerve (C5) innervates the muscle.

Functions
Clears the channels to relieves rigidity of the joints, dispels Cold and alleviates pain.

Clinical indications
Pain of the shoulder and back, neck stiffness, paralysis of the upper extremities.

69.

(CHUYUAN) QUYUAN, SI 13, HAND TAI YANG SMALL INTESTINE MERIDIAN

Location
In a seated position, the point is located at the medial border of the supraspinatous fossa of the scapula, at the midpoint between Naoshu (SI 10) and the spinous process of the second thoracic vertebra.

Needle and moxibustion method
Perpendicular insertion 0.5–0.8 inch.
— *Needle sensation:* local distension and soreness.
— *Moxibustion dosage:* 3–5 cones; stick 5–15 minutes.

Cross-sectional anatomy of the needle passage
(Fig. 5.7)
a. *Skin:* the cutaneous branches containing fibers from the dorsal division of the first, second, and third thoracic nerves (T1, T2, T3) innervate the skin.
b. *Subcutaneous tissue:* includes the previously described skin nerve branches.
c. *Trapezius muscle:* the branches containing fibers from the spinal accessory nerve (CN XI) and the ventral primary divisions of the third and fourth cervical nerves (C3, C4) innervate the muscle.
d. *Supraspinatus muscle:* the branches containing fibers from the suprascapular nerve of the fifth and sixth cervical nerves (C5, C6) innervate the muscle.

Functions

Expels Wind, activates the collaterals, relaxes rigidity of the muscles and tendons and removes Blood Stasis.

Clinical indications

Tendinitis of supraspinatus muscle, shoulder joint and surrounding soft tissue disease, neck stiffness.

70.

(PINGFENG) BINGFENG, SI 12, HAND TAI YANG SMALL INTESTINE MERIDIAN

Location

In a seated position, the point is located in the middle of the suprascapular fossa while raising the hand, or at the midpoint between Quyuan [SI 13] and Jugu [LI 16].

Needle and moxibustion method

Perpendicular insertion 0.5–0.7 inch.
— *Moxibustion doseage:* 3–5 cones.

Cross-sectional anatomy of the needle passage

a. *Skin:* the suprascapular branch of the fifth and sixth cervical nerves (C5, C6) innervates the skin.
b. *Subcutaneous tissue:* includes the previously described skin nerve branches.
c. *Trapezius muscle:* the branches containing fibers from the spinal accessory nerve (CN XI) and the ventral primary divisions of the third and fourth cervical nerves (C3, C4) innervate the muscle.
d. *Suprascapular artery, vein and nerve:* the suprascapular artery, together with the suprascapular vein, arises from the thyrocervical artery.
e. *Supraspinatus muscle:* the suprascapular branch of the brachial plexus of the fifth cervical nerve (C5) innervates the muscle.

Functions

Clears and activates the channels and collaterals, regulates the flow of Qi and expels Wind.

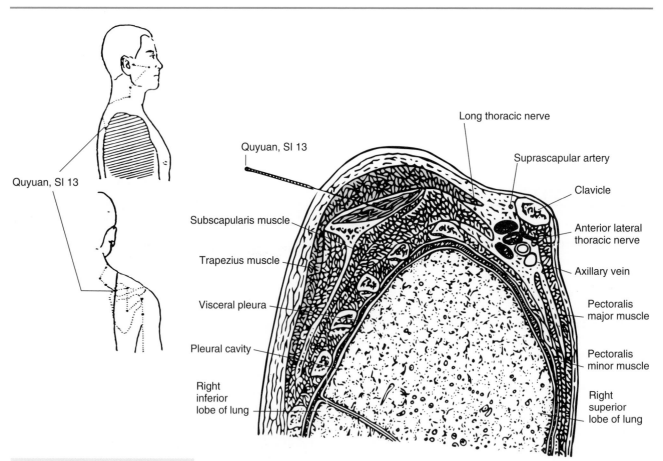

Fig. 5.7 Sagittal section of Quyuan.

Clinical indications

Shoulder pain, numbness of the upper extremities, neck stiffness, rheumatoid arthritis.

71.

(TIENTSUNG) TIANZONG, SI 11, HAND TAI YANG SMALL INTESTINE MERIDIAN

Location

In a seated position, the point is located in the infraspinatous fossa of the scapula. Draw a vertical line from the inferior angle of the scapula to the inferior margin of the spine of the scapula, the point is located at the superior third of this line, midway between the medial and lateral borders of the scapula.

Needle and moxibustion method

Perpendicular insertion 0.5–0.7 inch.
— *Needle sensation:* local distension and soreness.
— *Moxibustion dosage:* 3–5 cones; stick 5–15 minutes.

Cross-sectional anatomy of the needle passage

(Fig. 5.8)

a. *Skin:* the cutaneous branches of the dorsal divisions of the third, fourth, and fifth thoracic nerves (T3, T4, T5) innervate the skin.

b. *Subcutaneous tissue:* includes the previously described skin nerve branches.

c. *Inferior margin of trapezius muscle:* the branches containing fibers from the spinal accessory nerve (CN XI) and the ventral primary divisions of the third and fourth cervical nerves (C3, C4) innervate the muscle.

d. *Infraspinatus muscle:* the suprascapular branch of the fifth and sixth cervical nerves (C5, C6) innervates the muscle. Deep needling reaches the bony structure below the infraspinatous fossa of the scapula.

Functions

Reduces fever, disperses accumulation of masses, soothes chest oppression and regulates Qi and alleviates mental depression.

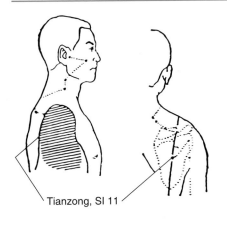

Tianzong, SI 11

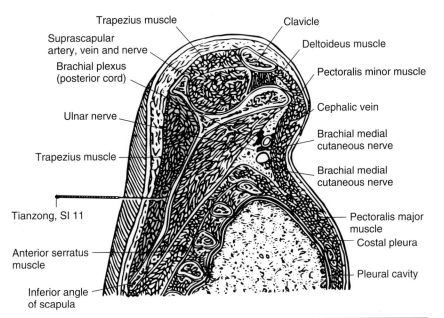

Trapezius muscle
Clavicle
Suprascapular artery, vein and nerve
Deltoideus muscle
Brachial plexus (posterior cord)
Pectoralis minor muscle
Ulnar nerve
Cephalic vein
Brachial medial cutaneous nerve
Trapezius muscle
Brachial medial cutaneous nerve
Tianzong, SI 11
Pectoralis major muscle
Costal pleura
Anterior serratus muscle
Pleural cavity
Inferior angle of scapula

Fig. 5.8 Sagittal section of Tianzong.

Clinical indications

Shoulder and surrounding soft tissue pain, mumps, bronchitis, mastitis, lower back sprain.

72.

(KANSHU) GANSHU, BL 18, FOOT TAI YANG BLADDER MERIDIAN, BACK-SHU POINT OF THE LIVER

Location

In a prone position, the point is located 1.5 inches lateral and inferior to the spinous process of the ninth thoracic vertebra.

Needle and moxibustion method

Medial oblique insertion 0.5–1.0 inch.
— *Needle sensation:* local distension and soreness, or sometimes radiating to the intercostal region.
— *Moxibustion dosage:* 3–5 cones; stick 5–15 minutes.

Cross-sectional anatomy of the needle passage

(Fig. 5.9)

a. *Skin:* the medial cutaneous branches containing fibers from the posterior division of the ninth thoracic nerve (T9) innervate the skin.

b. *Subcutaneous tissue:* includes the previously described skin nerve branches.

c. *Trapezius muscle:* the branches containing fibers from the spinal accessory nerve (CN XI) and the ventral primary divisions of the third and fourth cervical nerves (C3, C4) innervate the muscle.

d. *Latissimus dorsi muscle:* the thoracodorsal branches of the sixth, seventh, and eighth cervical nerves (C6, C7, C8) innervate the muscle.

e. *Sacrospinalis (erector spinae) muscle:* the branches containing fibers from the dorsal primary division of the spinal nerves innervate the muscle. The medial branches containing fibers from the dorsal division of the ninth and tenth thoracic nerves (T9, T10) innervate the point.

f. The transversospinalis muscle is located in the deep layer of the sacrospinalis muscle.

Warning

The needle should be inserted in a medially oblique direction. If the needle is punctured deeply perpendicularly or in a laterally oblique direction, it may penetrate through the thoracic wall, causing pneumothorax.

Functions

Regulates the function of the Liver, regulates Qi and

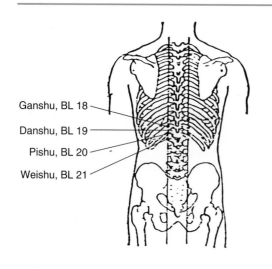

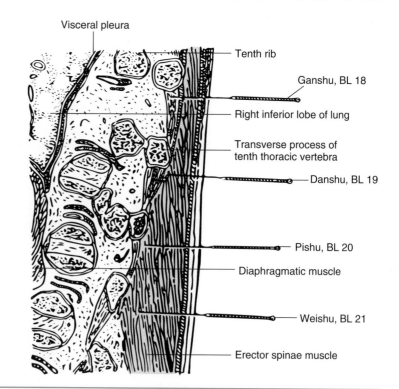

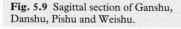
Fig. 5.9 Sagittal section of Ganshu, Danshu, Pishu and Weishu.

alleviates mental depression, and regulates Blood circulation to tranquilize the Mind.

Clinical indications
Acute and chronic hepatitis, cholecystitis, gastric disease, eye diseases, irregular menstruation, neurasthenia, intercostal neuralgia, hysteria, schizophrenia, convulsions, dizziness, cerebrovascular disease.

73.

(TANSHU) DANSHU, BL 19, FOOT TAI YANG BLADDER MERIDIAN, BACK-SHU POINT OF THE GALLBLADDER

Location
In a prone position, the point is located 1.5 inches lateral and inferior to the spinous process of the tenth thoracic vertebra.

Needle and moxibustion method
Medial oblique insertion 0.5–1.0 inch.
— *Needle sensation:* local soreness and distension.
— *Moxibustion dosage:* 3–5 cones; stick 5–15 minutes.

Cross-sectional anatomy of the needle passage
(Fig. 5.9)
a. *Skin:* the cutaneous branches containing fibers from the dorsal divisions of the tenth thoracic nerve (T10) innervate the skin.
b. *Subcutaneous tissue:* includes the previously described skin nerve branches.
c. *Inferior margin of trapezius muscle:* the branches containing fibers from the spinal accessory nerve (CN XI) and the ventral primary division of the third and fourth cervical nerves (C3, C4) innervate the muscle.
d. *Latissimus dorsi muscle:* the thoracodorsal branches of the sixth, seventh, and eighth cervical nerves (C6, C7, C8) innervate the muscle.
e. *Sacrospinalis (erector spinae) muscle:* the branches containing fibers from the dorsal primary divisions of the spinal nerves innervate the muscle. The medial branches of the dorsal divisions of the tenth and eleventh thoracic nerves (T10, T11) innervate the point.
f. The transversospinalis muscle is located in the deep layer of the sacrospinalis muscle.

Warning
The needle should be inserted in a medially oblique direction. If the needle is deeply inserted perpendicularly or in a laterally oblique direction, it may penetrate through the thoracic wall, causing pneumothorax.

Functions
Reduces Heat, removes Dampness, and regulates the function of the Middle Jiao.

Clinical indications
Hepatitis, cholecystitis, gastritis, gallbladder ascariasis, tuberculosis of lymph node, pleurisy, sciatic pain, abdominal distension.

74.

(PISHU) PISHU, BL 20, FOOT TAI YANG BLADDER MERIDIAN, BACK-SHU POINT OF THE SPLEEN

Location
In a prone position, the point is located 1.5 inches lateral and inferior to the spinous process of the eleventh thoracic vertebra.

Needle and moxibustion method
Medial oblique insertion 0.5–1.5 inches.
— *Needle sensation:* local distension, soreness and numbness, and radiating to the lumbar region.
— *Moxibustion dosage:* 3–7 cones; stick 5–20 minutes.

Cross-sectional anatomy of the needle passage
(Fig. 5.9)
a. *Skin:* the cutaneous branches containing fibers from the dorsal divisions of the eleventh thoracic nerve (T11) innervate the skin.
b. *Subcutaneous tissue:* includes the previously described skin nerve branches.
c. *Latissimus dorsi muscle:* the thoracodorsal branches of the sixth, seventh, and eighth cervical nerves (C6, C7, C8) innervate the muscle.
d. *Tendon of inferior posterior serratus muscle:* the branches containing fibers from the ninth, tenth, and eleventh intercostal and subcostal nerves innervate the muscle.
e. *Sacrospinalis (erector spinae) muscle:* the branches containing fibers from the dorsal primary divisions of the spinal nerve innervate the muscle. The medial branches containing fibers from the dorsal divisions of the eleventh and twelfth thoracic nerves (T11, T12) innervate the point.
f. The transversospinal muscle is located in the deep layer of the sacrospinalis muscle.

Warning
The needle should be inserted in a medially oblique direction. If the needle is deeply inserted perpendicularly or in a laterally oblique direction, it may puncture through the thoracic wall into the costophrenic sinus, damaging the liver and kidney.

Functions

Regulates the function of the Spleen to remove Dampness, and regulates the function of the Stomach and Middle Jiao (Middle Warmer).

Clinical indications

Gastritis, peptic ulcer, gastric prolapse, neurogenic vomiting, indigestion, hepatitis, enteritis, edema, anemia, uterine prolapse, chronic hemorrhagic disease, splenohepatomegaly, urticaria.

75.

(WEISHU) WEISHU, BL 21, FOOT TAI YANG BLADDER MERIDIAN, BACK-SHU POINT OF THE STOMACH

Location

In a prone position, the point is located 1.5 inches lateral to the posterior midline, lateral and inferior to the spinous process of the twelfth thoracic vertebra.

Needle and moxibustion method

Slightly medially perpendicular insertion 1.0–1.5 inches.
— *Needle sensation:* local soreness, distension and numbness, and radiating to the lumbar region.
— *Moxibustion dosage:* 3–7 cones; stick 5–20 minutes.

Cross-sectional anatomy of the needle passage
(Fig. 5.9)

a. *Skin:* the cutaneous branches containing fibers from the dorsal division of the twelfth thoracic nerve (T12) innervate the skin.
b. *Subcutaneous tissue:* includes the previously described skin nerve branches.
c. *Superficial layer of thoracolumbar fascia, tendon of latissimus dorsi muscle, and tendon of inferior posterior serratus muscle:* the superficial layer of the thoracolumbar fascia is the superficial part of the sacrospinalis muscle. The thoracodorsal branches of the sixth, seventh, and eighth cervical nerves (C6, C7, C8) and the posterior branches of the lumbar nerve innervate these fascias.
d. *Sacrospinalis (erector spinae) muscle:* the branches containing fibers from the dorsal primary divisions of the spinal nerve innervate the muscle. The medial branches containing fibers from the dorsal divisions of the twelfth thoracic and first lumbar nerves (T12, L1) innervate the point.
e. The transversospinalis muscle is located in the deep layer of the sacrospinalis muscle.

Warning

The point is located on the posterior wall of the abdomen. If the needle is inserted deeply or in a later-

ally oblique direction, it may puncture into and damage the liver and kidney.

Functions

Regulates the function of the Stomach and Middle Jiao (Middle Warmer), removes Dampness and eliminates undigested food.

Clinical indications

Gastric pain, gastritis, gastric prolapse, gastric ulcer, pancreatitis, hepatitis, liver cirrhosis, enteritis, insomnia, lower back pain.

76.

(SANCHIAOSHU) SANJIAOSHU, BL 22, FOOT TAI YANG BLADDER MERIDIAN, BACK-SHU POINT OF THE TRIPLE BURNER

Location

In a prone position, the point is located 1.5 inches lateral to the posterior midline, lateral and inferior to the spinous process of the first lumbar vertebra.

Needle and moxibustion method

Perpendicular insertion 0.5–1.0 inch.
— *Needle sensation:* local distension, soreness and numbness, and radiating to the lumbar region.
— *Moxibustion dosage:* 3–7 cones; stick 15 minutes.

Cross-sectional anatomy of the needle passage

a. *Skin:* the cutaneous branches containing fibers from the dorsal divisions of the first lumbar nerve (L1) innervate the skin.
b. *Subcutaneous tissue:* includes the previously described skin nerve branches.
c. *Superficial layer of thoracolumbar fascia, tendon of latissimus dorsi muscle, and tendon of inferior posterior serratus muscle:* the superficial layer of the thoracolumbar fascia is the superficial part of the sacrospinalis muscle. The thoracodorsal branch of the sixth, seventh, and eighth cervical nerves (C6, C7, C8) and the posterior branches of the lumbar nerve innervate these fascias.
d. *Sacrospinalis (erector spinae) muscle:* the branches of the dorsal primary division of the spinal nerve innervate the muscle. The medial branches containing fibers from the dorsal divisions of the first and second lumbar nerves (L1, L2) innervate the point.
e. The transversospinalis muscle is located in the deep layer of the sacrospinalis muscle.

Warning

The point is located on the posterior wall of the

abdomen. If the needle is inserted deeply or in a laterally oblique direction, it may puncture into and damage the liver and kidney.

Functions
Regulates the flow of Qi to alleviate water retention, and clears and regulates the Triple Jiao (Triple Warmer).

Clinical indications
Abdominal fullness, indigestion, vomiting, dysentery, hepatitis, liver cirrhosis, nephritis, cystitis, edema, lower back pain.

77.

(SHENSHU) SHENSHU, BL 23, FOOT TAI YANG BLADDER MERIDIAN, BACK-SHU POINT OF THE KIDNEY

Location
In a prone position, the point is located 1.5 inches lateral to the posterior midline, lateral and inferior to the spinous process of the second lumbar vertebra.

Needle and moxibustion method
Slightly medial perpendicular insertion 1.0–2.0 inches.
— *Needle sensation:* local distension and soreness, or electrical sensation radiating to the buttock and the lower extremities.
— *Moxibustion dosage:* 3–7 cones; stick 5–20 minutes.

Cross-sectional anatomy of the needle passage
(Fig. 5.10)
a. *Skin:* the medial branches containing fibers from the dorsal division of the second lumbar nerve (L2) innervate the skin.
b. *Subcutaneous tissue:* includes the previously described skin nerve branches.
c. *Superficial layer of thoracolumbar fascia and tendon of latissimus dorsi muscle:* the superficial layer of the thoracolumbar fascia is the superficial part of the sacrospinalis muscle. The thoracodorsal branches of the sixth, seventh, and eighth cervical nerves (C6, C7, C8) and the posterior branches containing fibers from the lumbar nerve innervate the fascias.
d. The superior cluneal nerves of the lateral branches of the dorsal division of the first, second, and third lumbar nerves (L1, L2, L3) pass through the deep layer of the previously described fascia. If the needle is inserted into the nerves, an electrical sensation will radiate to the buttock.
e. *Sacrospinalis (erector spinae) muscle:* the branches containing fibers from the dorsal primary divisions of the spinal nerve innervate the muscle. The medial

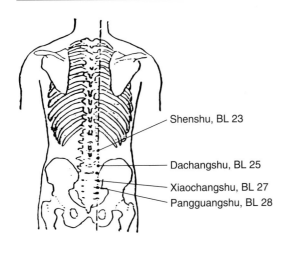

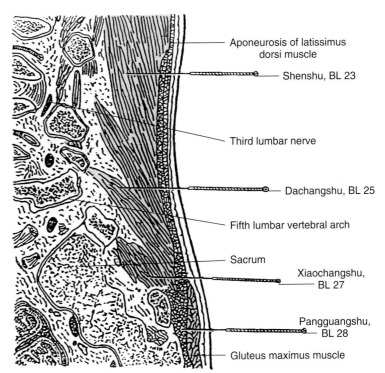

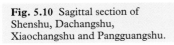

Fig. 5.10 Sagittal section of Shenshu, Dachangshu, Xiaochangshu and Pangguangshu.

Aponeurosis of latissimus dorsi muscle

Shenshu, BL 23

Third lumbar nerve

Dachangshu, BL 25

Fifth lumbar vertebral arch

Sacrum

Xiaochangshu, BL 27

Pangguangshu, BL 28

Gluteus maximus muscle

Shenshu, BL 23

Dachangshu, BL 25

Xiaochangshu, BL 27

Pangguangshu, BL 28

branches containing fibers from the dorsal divisions of the second and third lumbar nerves (L2, L3) innervate the point.

f. The transversospinalis muscle is located in the deep layer of the sacrospinalis muscle.

g. The lumbar plexus from the twelfth thoracic and first, second, and third lumbar nerves pass between the deep lumbar muscle and the posterior abdominal muscle. If the needle is inserted into the lumbar plexus, an electrical sensation radiates to the buttock and the anterior thigh.

Warning

The point is located over the posterior wall of the abdomen. If the needle is inserted deeply and in a laterally oblique direction, it may puncture into and damage the liver and kidney.

Functions

Strengthens the function of the Kidney Qi, and improves hearing and acuity of vision.

Clinical indications

Nephritis, renal colic, nephroptosis, lower back pain, seminal emission, impotence, enuresis, irregular menstruation, bronchial asthma, tinnitus, deafness. baldness, anemia, lumbar soft tissue disease, sequelae of poliomyelitis.

78.

(CHIHAISHU) QIHAISHU, BL 24, FOOT TAI YANG BLADDER MERIDIAN

Location

In a prone position, the point is located 1.5 inches lateral to the posterior midline, and lateral and inferior to the spinous process of the third lumbar vertebra.

Needle and moxibustion method

Perpendicular insertion 0.8–1.2 inches.
— *Needle sensation:* lumbar region swelling and soreness, or electrical numbness sensation radiating to the hip region.
— *Moxibustion dosage:* 3–7 cones.

Cross-sectional anatomy of the needle passage

a. *Skin:* the medial branches containing fibers from the dorsal division of the third lumbar nerve (L3) innervate the skin.

b. *Subcutaneous tissue:* includes the previously described skin nerve branches.

c. *Superficial layer of thoracolumbar fascia and tendon of latissimus dorsi muscle:* the superficial layer of the

thoracolumbar fascia is the superficial part of the sacrospinalis muscle. The thoracodorsal branches of the sixth, seventh and eighth cervical nerves (C6, C7, C8) and the posterior branches of the lumbar nerve innervate the fascia.

d. *Sacrospinalis (erector spinae) muscle:* the branches containing fibers from the dorsal divisions of the spinal nerves innervate the muscle.

e. The transversospinalis muscle is located at the deep layer of the sacrospinalis muscle.

Warning

The point is located over the posterior wall of the abdomen. If the needle is inserted deeply or in a laterally oblique direction, it may puncture into and damage the liver and kidney.

Functions

Regulates and invigorates the Qi, enriches Blood, and clears and activates the channels and collaterals.

Clinical indications

Lower back pain, hemorrhoids, cystitis, seminal emission, enuresis, impotence, premature ejaculation, dysmenorrhea, irregular menstruation.

79.

(TACHANGSHU) DACHANGSHU, BL 25, FOOT TAI YANG BLADDER MERIDIAN, BACK-SHU POINT OF THE LARGE INTESTINE

Location

In a prone position, the point is located 1.5 inches lateral and inferior to the spinous process of the fourth lumbar vertebra.

Needle and moxibustion method

Perpendicular insertion 1.0–2.0 inches.
— *Needle sensation:* lumbar distension and soreness.
  Slightly laterally oblique insertion 2.0–3.0 inches (treating sciatica).
— *Needle sensation:* numbness and electrical sensation radiating to the lower extremities.
  Oblique inferior insertion penetrating to Xiaochangshu [BL 27] (treating sacroiliitis).
— *Needle sensation:* lumbar distension and soreness radiating to the sacroiliac joint.
— *Moxibustion dosage:* 3–7 cones; stick 5–20 minutes.

Cross-sectional anatomy of the needle passage
(Fig. 5.10)

a. *Skin:* the lateral cutaneous branches of the dorsal

divisions of the fourth lumbar nerve (L4) innervate the skin.

b. *Subcutaneous tissue:* includes the previously described skin nerve branches.

c. *Superficial layer of thoracolumbar fascia:* the fascia is thickened at this region.

d. *Sacrospinalis (erector spinae) muscle:* the needle is passed between the longissimus and iliocostocervicalis divisions of the sacrospinalis muscle. The muscular branches of the dorsal divisions of the spinal nerves innervate the point.

Functions

Regulates the function of the Large and Small Intestines, and regulates the flow of Qi to relieve stagnation in the abdomen.

Clinical indications

Lumbocrural pain, lumbar sprain, enteritis, constipation, dysentery, sacroiliitis.

80.

(KUANYUANGSHU) GUANYUANSHU, BL 26, FOOT TAI YANG BLADDER MERIDIAN

Location

In a prone position, the point is located 1.5 inches lateral to the posterior midline and lateral and inferior to the spinous process of the fifth lumbar vertebra.

Needle and moxibustion method

Perpendicular insertion 0.8–1.2 inches.
— *Needle sensation:* local distension and soreness, and sometimes radiating to the lower extremities.
— *Moxibustion dosage:* 3–7 cones; stick 15 minutes.

Cross-sectional anatomy of the needle passage

a. *Skin:* the lateral cutaneous branches containing fibers from the dorsal division of the fourth and fifth lumbar nerves innervate the skin.

b. *Subcutaneous tissue:* includes the previously described skin nerve branches.

c. *Sacrospinalis (erector spinae) muscle:* the muscular branches containing fibers from the dorsal division of the spinal nerves innervate the muscle.

Functions

Tonifies the Kidney, regulates the channels, and regulates the function of the Lower Jiao (Lower Warmer).

Clinical indications

Dysentery, lower back pain, abdominal masses.

81.

(HSIAOCHANGSHU) XIAOCHANGSHU, BL 27, FOOT TAI YANG BLADDER MERIDIAN, BACK-SHU POINT OF THE SMALL INTESTINE

Location

In a prone position, the point is located 1.5 inches lateral to the posterior midline, lateral to the first sacral foramen, at the midpoint between the medial margin of the posterior superior iliac spine and the sacral foramen.

Needle and moxibustion method

Perpendicular insertion 1.0–1.5 inches.
— *Needle sensation:* local distension and soreness.

Oblique insertion penetrating to Dachangshu [BL 25] 2.0–3.0 inches (treating sacroiliitis and pelvic inflammatory disease).
— *Needle sensation:* distension and soreness radiating to whole sacroiliac articulation.
— *Moxibustion dosage:* 3–7 cones; stick 5–20 minutes.

Cross-sectional anatomy of the needle passage
(Fig. 5.10)

a. *Skin:* the lateral cutaneous branches containing fibers from the dorsal divisions of the fifth lumbar and first sacral nerves (L5, S1) innervate the skin.

b. *Subcutaneous tissue:* includes the previously described skin nerve branches.

c. *The superficial layer of the thoracolumbar fascia.*

d. *Medial margin of the gluteus maximus muscle:* the branches containing fibers from the inferior gluteal nerve of the fifth lumbar and first sacral nerves (L5, S1) innervate the muscle.

e. *Sacrospinalis (erector spinae) muscle:* the muscular branches containing fibers from the dorsal divisions of the spinal nerves innervate the muscle.

f. If the needle is penetrated to Dachangshu [BL 25], it will penetrate between the gluteus maximus and the sacrospinalis muscles.

Functions

Regulates the Small Intestine, reduces Heat and removes Dampness.

Clinical indications

Lower back pain, sacroiliac joint disease, seminal emission, enuresis, enteritis, constipation, pelvic inflammatory disease.

82.

(PANGKUANGSHU) PANGGUANGSHU, BL 28, FOOT TAI YANG BLADDER MERIDIAN, BACK-SHU POINT OF THE BLADDER

Location

In a prone position, the point is located 1.5 inches lateral to the posterior midline, lateral to the second posterior sacral foramen, at the midpoint between the medial margin of the posterior superior iliac spine and the sacral foramen.

Needle and moxibustion method

Perpendicular insertion 1.0–1.5 inches.
— *Needle sensation:* local soreness and distension.
— *Moxibustion dosage:* 3–7 cones; stick 5–20 minutes.

Cross-sectional anatomy of the needle passage

(Fig. 5.10)
a. *Skin:* the dorsal divisions of the middle cluneal nerve of the first and second sacral nerves (S1, S2) innervate the skin.
b. *Subcutaneous tissue:* includes the previously described skin nerve branches.
c. *Gluteus maximus muscle:* the branches containing fibers from the inferior gluteal nerve of the fifth lumbar to second sacral nerves (L5, S1, S2) innervate the muscle.
d. *Sacrospinalis (erector spinae) muscle:* the muscular branches of the dorsal divisions of the spinal nerves innervate the muscle.
e. The needle reaches the posterior surface of the sacrum.

Functions

Strengthens the Lower Jiao (Lower Warmer), and clears and regulates the water passages.

Clinical indications

Lumbosacral pain, sciatic pain, diarrhea, constipation, diabetes mellitus, genitourinary diseases.

83.

(CHUNGLUSHU) ZHONGLUSHU, BL 29, FOOT TAI YANG BLADDER MERIDIAN

Location

In a prone position, the point is located 1.5 inches lateral to the posterior midline, and lateral to the third sacral foramen.

Needle and moxibustion method

Perpendicular insertion 0.8–1.2 inches.
— *Needle sensation:* local numbness and distension.
— *Moxibustion dosage:* 3–7 cones; stick 15 minutes.

Cross-sectional anatomy of the needle passage

a. *Skin:* the dorsal divisions of the middle cluneal nerve of the second and third sacral nerves (S2, S3) innervate the skin.
b. *Subcutaneous tissue:* includes the previously described skin nerve branches.
c. *Gluteus maximus muscle:* the branches containing fibers from the inferior gluteal nerve of the fifth lumbar to second sacral nerves (L5, S1, S2) innervate the muscle.
d. *Sacrospinalis (erector spinae) muscle:* the muscular branches containing fibers from the dorsal divisions of the spinal nerves innervate the muscle.
e. The needle reaches the posterior surface of the sacrum.

Functions

Relieves rigidity of the muscles and tendons, improves Blood circulation, and regulates the function of the Intestines to relieve abdominal stagnation and masses.

Clinical indications

Dysentery, hernia pain, lower back pain.

84.

(PAIHUANSHU) BAIHUANSHU, BL 30, FOOT TAI YANG BLADDER MERIDIAN

Location

In a prone position, the point is located 1.5 inches lateral to the posterior midline, and lateral to the fourth sacral foramen.

Needle and moxibustion method

Perpendicular insertion 0.8–1.2 inches.
— *Needle sensation:* distension and soreness at the sacral region sometimes radiating to the lower extremities.
— *Moxibustion dosage:* 3–5 cones; stick 10 minutes.

Cross-sectional anatomy of the needle passage

a. *Skin:* the dorsal divisions of the inferior cluneal nerve of the fifth lumbar and first and second sacral nerves (L5, S1, S2) innervate the skin.
b. *Subcutaneous tissue:* includes the previously described skin nerve branches and the inferior gluteal artery and vein.
c. *Gluteus maximus muscle:* the branches containing fibers from the inferior gluteal nerve of the fifth

lumbar and first and second sacral nerves (L5, S1, S2) innervate the muscle.

d. *Internal pudendal artery, vein and nerve:* the internal pudendal artery, together with the internal pudendal vein, arises from the internal iliac artery.

e. *Inferior margin of tendon of sacrospinalis (erector spinae) muscle:* the muscular branches containing fibers from the dorsal divisions of the spinal nerve innervate the muscle.

Functions

Reduces Heat and removes Dampness, and regulates the function of the Lower Jiao (Lower Warmer).

Clinical indications

Hernia pain, leukorrhea, seminal emission, irregular menstruation, lumbago.

85.

(SHANGLIAO) SHANGLIAO, BL 31, FOOT TAI YANG BLADDER MERIDIAN

Location

In a prone position, the point is located in the first sacral foramen one finger's breadth lateral to the posterior midline, at the midpoint between the inferior margin of the first spinous process of the sacrum and the posterior superior iliac spine.

Needle and moxibustion method

Perpendicular insertion 1.0–2.0 inches.

— *Needle sensation:* sacral distension and soreness, or radiating to the lower extremities.

— *Moxibustion dosage:* 3–7 cones; stick 5–20 minutes.

Perpendicular insertion penetrating through from the posterior and anterior sacral foramina to the pelvic cavity. The needle is inserted at a 60° angle through the sacral foramen to the pubic symphysis about 2.5 inches deep into the first sacral nerve.

Cross-sectional anatomy of the needle passage
(Fig. 5.11)

a. *Skin:* the dorsal branches containing fibers from the middle cluneal nerve of the first sacral nerve (S1) innervate the skin.

b. *Subcutaneous tissue:* includes the previously described skin nerve branches.

c. *Superficial layer of the thoracolumbar fascia:* the fascia is prominently thickened at this region.

d. *Sacrospinalis (erector spinae) muscle:* the muscular branches containing fibers from the dorsal divisions of the spinal nerves innervate the muscle.

e. *First posterior sacral foramen, dorsal division of first sacral nerve, and first sacral nerve trunk:* if the needle is inserted into the nerve, a strong electrical sensation will be felt.

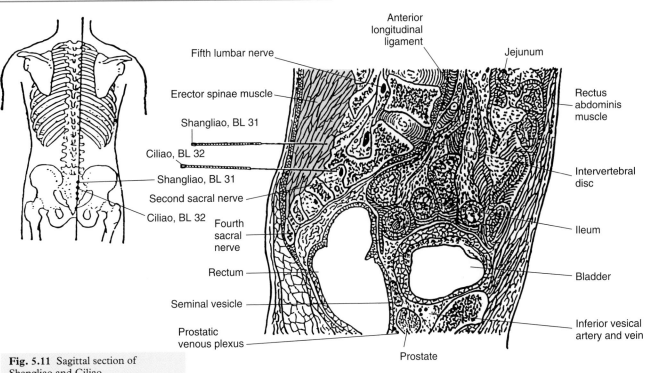

Fig. 5.11 Sagittal section of Shangliao and Ciliao.

Functions
Strengthens the Lower Jiao (Lower Warmer), strengthens the lumbar and knee joints.

Clinical indications
Genitourinary tract disease, lumbosacral pain, sciatic pain, constipation. This point induces abortion.

86.

(TZULIAO) CILIAO, BL 32, FOOT TAI YANG BLADDER MERIDIAN

Location
In a prone position, the point is located on the medial side of the posterior superior iliac spine, in the second posterior sacral foramen.

Needle and moxibustion method
Perpendicular insertion 1.0–2.0 inches.
— *Needle sensation:* sacral distension and soreness; if the needle is inserted into the sacral nerve, a strong electrical sensation will be felt.
— *Moxibustion dosage:* 3–7 cones; stick 5–20 minutes.

Cross-sectional anatomy of the needle passage
(Fig. 5.11)
a. *Skin:* the dorsal branches containing fibers from the middle cluneal nerve of the second sacral nerve (S2) innervate the skin.
b. *Subcutaneous tissue:* includes the previously described skin nerve branches.
c. *Superficial layer of thoracodorsal fascia:* the fascia is prominently thickened and covers the sacrospinalis muscle.
d. *Sacrospinalis (erector spinae) muscle:* the muscular branches containing fibers from the dorsal division of the spinal nerve innervate the muscle.
e. If the needle is inserted directly through the second posterior sacral foramen, it will puncture the dorsal branch of the second nerve.
f. If the needle is inserted through from the posterior to the anterior sacral foramen into the second sacral nerve trunk, a strong electrical sensation will be felt.

Functions
Strengthens the lumbar joint, regulates menstruation and arrests leukorrhea.

Clinical indications
Genitourinary tract disease, lumbosacral pain, sciatic pain, constipation, induces labor.

87.

(CHUNGLIAO) ZHONGLIAO, BL 33, FOOT TAI YANG BLADDER MERIDIAN

Location
In a prone position, the point is located 1.0 inch lateral to the posterior midline, in the third posterior sacral foramen.

Needle and moxibustion method
Perpendicular insertion 0.8–1.2 inches.
— *Needle sensation:* local numbness and distension, and sometimes radiating anteriorly.
— *Moxibustion dosage:* 3–7 cones; stick 10 minutes.

Cross-sectional anatomy of the needle passage
a. *Skin:* the dorsal branches containing fibers from the middle cluneal nerve of the third sacral nerve (S3) innervate the skin.
b. *Subcutaneous tissue:* includes the previously described skin nerve branches.
c. *Gluteus maximus muscle:* the branches containing fibers from the inferior gluteal nerve of the fifth lumbar and first and second sacral nerves (L5, S1, S2) innervate the muscle.
d. *Superficial layer of thoracolumbar fascia:* the fascia is prominently thickened and covers the sacrospinalis muscle.
e. *Sacrospinalis (erector spinae) muscle:* the muscular branches of the dorsal divisions of the spinal nerves innervate the muscle.
f. If the needle is inserted directly through the third posterior sacral foramen, it will puncture the dorsal branch of the third sacral nerve.
g. If the needle is inserted through from the posterior to the anterior sacral foramen into the third sacral nerve trunk, a strong electrical sensation will be felt.

Functions
Strengthens the Kidney, regulates menstruation, reduces Heat and removes Dampness.

Clinical indications
Leukorrhea, constipation, lower back pain, scanty menstruation, seminal emission, enuresis, impotence.

88.

(HSIALIAO) XIALIAO, BL 34, FOOT TAI YANG BLADDER MERIDIAN

Location
In a prone position, the point is located lateral to the

posterior midline, in the fourth posterior sacral foramen.

Needle and moxibustion method
Perpendicular insertion 0.8–1.2 inches.
— *Needle sensation:* local numbness and distension, sometimes radiating to the external genital region.
— *Moxibustion dosage:* 5–7 cones; stick 10 minutes.

Cross-sectional anatomy of the needle passage
a. Skin: the dorsal branches containing fibers from the middle cluneal nerve of the fourth sacral nerve (S4) innervate the skin.
b. Subcutaneous tissue: includes the previously described skin nerve branches.
c. Gluteus maximus muscle: the branches containing fibers from the inferior gluteal nerve of the fifth lumbar and first and second sacral nerves (L5, S1, S2) innervate the muscle.
d. Superficial layer of thoracolumbar fascia: the fascia is prominently thickened and covers the sacrospinalis muscle.
e. Sacrospinalis (erector spinae) muscle: the muscular branches containing fibers from the dorsal division of the spinal nerves innervate the muscle.
f. If the needle is inserted directly through the fourth posterior sacral foramen, it will puncture the dorsal branches of the fourth sacral nerve.
g. If the needle is inserted through from the posterior to the anterior sacral foramen into the fourth sacral nerve trunk, a strong electrical sensation will be felt.

Functions
Strengthens the Kidney, regulates menstruation, and regulates the function of the Lower Jiao (Lower Warmer).

Clinical indications
Leukorrhea, strangury with turbid urine, periumbilical colic due to invasion of Cold, pain of the lower abdomen, dysentery, hemafascia.

89.

(HUIYANG) HUIYANG, BL 35, FOOT TAI YANG BLADDER MERIDIAN

Location
In a prone position, the point is located 0.5 inch lateral to the posterior midline, and lateral to the tip of the coccyx.

Needle and moxibustion method
Perpendicular insertion 0.5–1.0 inch.

— *Needle sensation:* local distension and numbness radiating to the external genital region.
— *Moxibustion dosage:* 3–7 cones; stick 10 times.

Cross-sectional anatomy of the needle passage
a. Skin: the branches containing fibers from the coccygeal nerve innervate the skin.
b. Subcutaneous tissue: includes the previously described skin nerve branches.
c. Gluteus maximus muscle: the branches containing fibers from the inferior gluteal nerve of the fifth lumbar and first and second sacral nerves (L5, S1, S2) innervate the muscle.
d. The superficial layer of the thoracolumbar fascia.

Functions
Regulates the flow of Qi and the function of the intestines, and reduces Heat and Dampness.

Clinical indications
Leukorrhea, dysentery, abdominal pain, hemafascia.

90.

(FUFEN) FUFEN, BL 41, FOOT TAI YANG BLADDER MERIDIAN

Location
In a prone or seated position, the point is located 3.0 inches lateral to the posterior midline, or 1.5 inches lateral to Fengmen [BL 12], on the medial margin of the scapula between the second and third ribs.

Needle and moxibustion method
Oblique insertion 0.3–0.5 inch or use a triangular needle to induce bleeding.
— *Needle sensation:* local numbness and distension.
— *Moxibustion dosage:* 3–7 cones; stick 10 minutes.

Cross-sectional anatomy of the needle passage
a. Skin: the lateral cutaneous branches containing fibers from the dorsal divisions of the second thoracic nerve (T2) innervate the skin.
b. Subcutaneous tissue: includes the previously described skin nerve branches.
c. Trapezius muscle: the branches containing fibers from the spinal accessory nerve (CN XI) and the ventral primary division of the third and fourth cervical nerves (C3, C4) innervate the muscle.
d. Rhomboid muscle: the branches containing fibers from the dorsal scapular nerve of the fourth and fifth cervical nerves (C4, C5) innervate the muscle.
e. Iliocostocervicalis muscle: the branches containing fibers from the dorsal primary division of the spinal nerves innervate the muscle.

f. The dorsal and lateral branches of the second intercostal artery, vein, and nerve.

Warning
The needle should be inserted shallowly, or it may puncture through the thoracic wall, causing pneumothorax.

Functions
Expels Wind and dispels Cold, relieves rigidity of the muscles and tendons and activates the collaterals.

Clinical indications
Neck stiffness, elbow numbness, upper extremities paralysis, common cold, bronchitis, pneumonia.

91.
(POHU) POHU, BL 42, FOOT TAI YANG BLADDER MERIDIAN

Location
In a prone position, the point is located 3.0 inches lateral to the posterior midline, or 1.5 inches lateral to Feishu [BL 13], on the medial margin of the scapula between the third and fourth ribs.

Needle and moxibustion method
Oblique insertion 0.3–0.5 inch.
— *Needle sensation:* local numbness and distension.
— *Moxibustion dosage:* 3–7 cones; stick 15 minutes.

Cross-sectional anatomy of the needle passage
a. Skin: the lateral cutaneous branches containing fibers from the posterior divisions of the third thoracic nerve (T3) innervate the skin.
b. Subcutaneous tissue: includes the previously described skin nerve branches.
c. Trapezius muscle: the branches containing fibers from the spinal accessory nerve (CN XI) and the ventral primary divisions of the third and fourth cervical nerves (C3, C4) innervate the muscle.
d. Rhomboid muscle: the dorsal scapular nerve branches containing fibers from the fourth and fifth cervical nerves (C4, C5) innervate the muscle.
e. Iliocostocervicalis muscle: the branches containing fibers from the dorsal primary division of the spinal nerves innervate the muscle.
f. The dorsal and lateral branches of the third intercostal artery, vein, and nerve.

Warning
The needle can only be inserted shallowly, or it may puncture through the thoracic wall, causing pneumothorax.

Functions
Clears and regulates the Lung Qi, and relieves cough and asthma.

Clinical indications
Neck stiffness, back pain, tuberculosis, cough and dyspnea, common cold, bronchial asthma.

92.
(KAOHUANG) GAOHUANG, BL 43, FOOT TAI YANG BLADDER MERIDIAN

Location
In a seated and prone position, the point is located 3.0 inches lateral to the posterior midline, 1.5 inches lateral to Chuehyinshu [BL 14], on the medial margin of the scapula between the fourth and fifth ribs.

Needle and moxibustion method
Oblique insertion 0.3–0.5 inch.
— *Needle sensation:* local distension and soreness, sometimes radiating to the scapula.
— *Moxibustion dosage:* 7–15 cones; stick 15–30 minutes.

Cross-sectional anatomy of the needle passage
a. Skin: the lateral cutaneous branches containing fibers from the posterior divisions of the fourth thoracic nerve (T4) innervate the skin.
b. Subcutaneous tissue: includes the previously described skin nerve branches.
c. Trapezius muscle: the branches containing fibers from the spinal accessory nerve (CN XI) and the ventral primary divisions of the third and fourth cervical nerves (C3, C4) innervate the muscle.
d. Rhomboid muscle: the branches containing fibers from the dorsal scapular nerve of the fourth and fifth cervical nerves (C4, C5) innervate the muscle.
e. Iliocostocervicalis muscle: the branches containing fibers from the dorsal primary divisions of the spinal nerves innervate the muscle.
f. The dorsal and lateral branches containing fibers from the intercostal artery, vein, and nerve.

Warning
The needle should be inserted shallowly, or it may puncture through the thoracic wall, causing pneumothorax.

Functions
Strengthens the function of the Lung and Spleen, and invigorates and restores Qi.

Clinical indications

Tuberculosis, hematemesis, cough and dyspnea, bronchial asthma, impotence, nocturnal emission.

93.

(SHENTANG) SHENTANG, BL 44, FOOT TAI YANG BLADDER MERIDIAN

Location

In a prone position, the point is located 3.0 inches lateral to the posterior midline, or 1.5 inches lateral to Xinshu [BL 15], on the medial margin of the scapula between the fifth and sixth ribs.

Needle and moxibustion method

Oblique insertion 0.3–0.5 inch.
— *Needle sensation:* local numbness and distension.
— *Moxibustion dosage:* 7–15 cones; stick 10 minutes.

Cross-sectional anatomy of the needle passage

a. *Skin:* the lateral cutaneous branches containing fibers from the posterior divisions of the fifth thoracic nerve (T5) innervate the skin.
b. *Subcutaneous tissue:* includes the previously described skin nerve branches.
c. *Trapezius muscle:* the branches containing fibers from the spinal accessory nerve (CN XI) and the ventral primary divisions of the third and fourth cervical nerves (C3, C4) innervate the muscle.
d. *Rhomboid muscle:* the branches containing fibers from the dorsal scapular nerve of the fourth and fifth cervical nerves (C4, C5) innervate the muscle.
e. *Iliocostocervicalis muscle:* the branches containing fibers from the dorsal primary divisions of the spinal nerves innervate the muscle.
f. The dorsal and lateral branches of the fifth intercostal artery, vein, and nerve.

Warning

The needle can only be inserted shallowly, or it may puncture through the thoracic wall, causing pneumothorax.

Functions

Regulates the function of the Lung, relieves asthma, and regulates the flow of Qi and the function of the Stomach.

Clinical indications

Cough and dyspnea, asthma, lower back pain, precordial pain, tachycardia, choking sensation in chest.

94.

(YIHSI) YIXI, BL 45, FOOT TAI YANG BLADDER MERIDIAN

Location

In a prone position, the point is located 3.0 inches lateral to the posterior midline, or 1.5 inches lateral to Dushu [BL 16], on the medial margin of the scapula between the sixth and seventh ribs.

Needle and moxibustion method

Oblique insertion 0.3–0.5 inch.
— *Needle sensation:* local numbness and distension.
— *Moxibustion dosage:* 3–7 cones; stick 10 minutes.

Cross-sectional anatomy of the needle passage

a. *Skin:* the lateral cutaneous branches of the posterior divisions of the sixth thoracic nerve (T6) innervate the skin.
b. *Subcutaneous tissue:* includes the previously described skin nerve branches.
c. *Trapezius muscle:* the branches containing fibers from the spinal accessory nerve (CN XI) and the ventral primary division of the third and fourth cervical nerves (C3, C4) innervate the muscle. The needle is passed on the lateral margin of the muscle.
d. *Iliocostocervicalis muscle:* the branches of the dorsal primary divisions of the spinal nerves innervate the muscle.
e. The dorsal and lateral branches of the sixth intercostal artery, vein, and nerve.

Warning

The needle should be inserted shallowly, or it may puncture through the thoracic wall, causing pneumothorax.

Functions

Reduces fever, expels Wind, and relieves cough and asthma.

Clinical indications

Cough and dyspnea, asthma, shoulder pain, bronchitis, bronchial asthma, pericarditis, angina pectoris.

95.

(KEKUAN) GEGUAN, BL 46, FOOT TAI YANG BLADDER MERIDIAN

Location

In a prone position, the point is located 3.0 inches lateral to the posterior midline, or 1.5 inches lateral to Geshu [BL 17], on the medial margin of the scapula between the seventh and eighth ribs.

Needle and moxibustion method

Oblique insertion 0.3–0.5 inches.
— *Needle sensation:* local numbness and distension.
— *Moxibustion dosage:* 3–7 cones; stick 15 minutes.

Cross-sectional anatomy of the needle passage

a. *Skin:* the lateral cutaneous branches of the posterior divisions of the seventh thoracic nerve (T7) innervate the skin.
b. *Subcutaneous tissue:* includes the previously described skin nerve branches.
c. *Latissimus dorsi muscle:* the thoracodorsal branches of the sixth, seventh, and eighth cervical nerves (C6, C7, C8) innervate the muscle.
d. *Iliocostocervicalis muscle:* the branches containing fibers from the dorsal primary divisions of the spinal nerve innervate the muscle.
e. The dorsal and lateral branches of the seventh intercostal artery, vein, and nerve.

Warning

The needle should be inserted shallowly, or it may puncture through the thoracic wall, causing pneumothorax.

Functions

Promotes and regulates Blood circulation, regulates the function of the Stomach and descends rebellious stomach Qi.

Clinical indications

Nausea, vomiting, belching, gastritis, gastric ulcer, esophageal spasm, cardiac spasm, back pain.

96.

(HUNMEN) HUNMEN, BL 47, FOOT TAI YANG BLADDER MERIDIAN

Location

In a prone position, the point is located 3.0 inches lateral to the posterior midline, or 1.5 inches lateral to Ganshu [BL 18], between the ninth and tenth ribs.

Needle and moxibustion method

Oblique insertion 0.3–0.5 inch.
— *Needle sensation:* local numbness and distension.
— *Moxibustion dosage:* 3–7 cones; stick 15 minutes.

Cross-sectional anatomy of the needle passage

a. *Skin:* the lateral cutaneous branches of the posterior divisions of the ninth thoracic nerve (T9) innervate the skin.
b. *Subcutaneous tissue:* includes the previously described skin nerve branches.

c. *Latissimus dorsi muscle:* the thoracodorsal branches of the sixth, seventh, and eighth cervical nerves (C6, C7, C8) innervate the muscle.
d. *Iliocostocervicalis muscle:* the branches of the dorsal primary divisions of the spinal nerve innervate the muscle.
e. The dorsal and lateral branches of the ninth intercostal artery, vein, and nerve.

Warning

The needle should be inserted shallowly, or it may puncture through the thoracic wall, causing pneumothorax.

Functions

Removes Heat from the Liver and Gallbladder, regulates Blood flow and tranquilizes the Mind.

Clinical indications

Back pain, chest pain, vomiting, gastritis, diarrhea, shock, hysteria, insomnia, cholecystitis.

97.

(YANGKANG) YANGGANG, BL 48, FOOT TAI YANG BLADDER MERIDIAN

Location

In a prone position, the point is located 3.0 inches lateral to the posterior midline, or 1.5 inches lateral to Danshu [BL 19], between the tenth and eleventh ribs.

Needle and moxibustion method

Oblique insertion 0.3–0.5 inch.
— *Needle sensation:* local numbness and distension.
— *Moxibustion dosage:* 3–7 cones; stick 15 minutes.

Cross-sectional anatomy of the needle passage

a. *Skin:* the lateral cutaneous branches containing fibers from the posterior divisions of the tenth thoracic nerve (T10) innervate the skin.
b. *Subcutaneous tissue:* includes the previously described skin nerve branches.
c. *Latissimus dorsi muscle:* the thoracodorsal branches of the sixth, seventh, and eighth cervical nerves (C6, C7, C8) innervate the muscle.
d. *Iliocostocervicalis muscle:* the branches containing fibers from the dorsal primary division of the spinal nerves innervate the muscle.
e. The dorsal and lateral branches containing fibers from the tenth intercostal artery, vein, and nerve.

Warning

The needle should be inserted shallowly, or it may

puncture through the thoracic wall, causing pneumothorax.

Functions
Reduces Heat from the Gallbladder, and regulates the function of the Middle Jiao (Middle Warmer) to resolve Dampness.

Clinical indications
Dysentery, jaundice, hepatitis, cholecystitis, gastritis, gastric spasm, enteritis, abdominal pain, bloody urine.

98.

(YISHE) YISHE, BL 49, FOOT TAI YANG BLADDER MERIDIAN

Location
In a prone position, the point is located 3.0 inches lateral to the posterior midline, or 1.5 inches lateral to Pishu [BL 20], between the eleventh and twelfth ribs.

Needle and moxibustion method
Oblique insertion 0.3–0.5 inch.
— *Needle sensation:* local numbness and distension.
— *Moxibustion dosage:* 3–7 cones; stick 15 minutes.

Cross-sectional anatomy of the needle passage
a. *Skin:* the lateral cutaneous branches containing fibers from the posterior divisions of the eleventh thoracic nerve (T11) innervate the skin.
b. *Subcutaneous tissue:* includes the previously described skin nerve branches.
c. *Latissimus dorsi muscle:* the branches containing fibers from the thoracodorsal nerve of the sixth, seventh, and eighth cervical nerves (C6, C7, C8) innervate the muscle.
d. *Iliocostocervicalis muscle:* the branches containing fibers from the dorsal primary division of the spinal nerve innervate the muscle.
e. The dorsal and lateral branches of the eleventh intercostal artery, vein, and nerve.

Warning
The point is located on the posterior wall of the abdomen. If the needle is inserted deeply, it may puncture into and damage the kidney or liver.

Functions
Regulates and strengthens Spleen Yang, and removes Damp Heat.

Clinical indications
Vomiting, diabetes mellitus, jaundice, hepatitis, cholecystitis, enteritis, abdominal pain.

99.

(WEITSANG) WEICANG, BL 50, FOOT TAI YANG BLADDER MERIDIAN

Location
In a prone position, the point is located 3.0 inches lateral to the posterior midline, or 1.5 inches lateral to Weishu [BL 21], and inferior to the twelfth rib.

Needle and moxibustion method
Oblique insertion 0.3–0.5 inch.
— *Needle sensation:* local numbness and distension.
— *Moxibustion dosage:* 3–7 cones; stick 15 minutes.

Cross-sectional anatomy of the needle passage
a. *Skin:* the lateral cutaneous branches of the posterior divisions of the twelfth thoracic nerve (T12) innervate the skin.
b. *Subcutaneous tissue:* includes the previously described skin nerve branches.
c. *Latissimus dorsi muscle:* the branches containing fibers from the thoracodorsal nerve of the sixth, seventh, and eighth cervical nerves (C6, C7, C8) innervate the muscle.
d. *Iliocostocervicalis muscle:* the branches containing fibers from the dorsal primary divisions of the spinal nerve innervate the muscle.
e. The dorsal and lateral branches of the twelfth intercostal artery, vein, and nerve.

Warning
The point is located on the posterior wall of the abdomen. If the needle is inserted deeply, it may puncture into and damage the kidney.

Functions
Regulates the function of the Stomach to remove Dampness, regulates the flow of Qi and relieves depression.

Clinical indications
Epigastric pain, abdominal distension, liver cirrhosis, cardiac spasm, gastritis, gastric spasm, gastric ulcer, enteritis, back pain, edema.

100.

(CHIHSHIH) ZHISHI, BL 52, FOOT TAI YANG BLADDER MERIDIAN

Location
In a prone position, the point is located 3.0 inches lateral to the posterior midline, 1.5 inches lateral to Shenshu [BL 23].

Needle and moxibustion method

Perpendicular insertion 0.5–1.0 inch.

— *Needle sensation:* Local numbness and distension.

— *Moxibustion dosage:* 7–15 cones; stick 15 minutes.

Cross-sectional anatomy of the needle passage

a. *Skin:* the lateral cutaneous branches containing fibers from the dorsal divisions of the second lumbar nerve (L2) innervate the skin.

b. *Subcutaneous tissue:* includes the previously described skin nerve branches.

c. *Latissimus dorsi muscle:* the thoracodorsal branches of the sixth, seventh, and eighth cervical nerves (C6, C7, C8) innervate the muscle.

d. *Iliocostocervicalis muscle:* the branches containing fibers from the dorsal primary divisions of the spinal nerves innervate the muscle.

e. The dorsal branches of the second lumbar artery and vein, and lateral branches containing fibers from the second lumbar nerve.

Warning

The point is located on the posterior wall of the abdomen. If the needle is inserted deeply, it may puncture into and damage the small intestine. Lifting, thrusting, and twirling the needle vigorously may damage the intestinal wall. The intestinal contents may drain into the peritoneal cavity, irritating the peritoneum and causing abdominal tension and pain.

Functions

Tonifies the Kidney to arrest seminal emission and removes Heat to induce diuresis.

Clinical indications

Seminal emission, impotence, frequency of urination, irregular menstruation, knee joint pain, edema, chronic gastritis, chronic enteritis, constipation.

101.

(PAOHUANG) BAOHUANG, BL 53, FOOT TAI YANG BLADDER MERIDIAN

Location

In a prone position, the point is located 3.0 inches lateral to the posterior midline, 1.5 inches lateral to Pangguangshu [BL 28].

Needle and moxibustion method

Perpendicular insertion 0.8–1.2 inches.

— *Needle sensation:* local distension and numbness radiating inferiorly.

— *Moxibustion dosage:* 7–15 cones; stick 15 minutes.

Cross-sectional anatomy of the needle passage

a. *Skin:* the branches containing fibers from the superior cluneal nerve innervate the skin.

b. *Subcutaneous tissue:* includes the previously described skin nerve branches.

c. *Gluteus maximus muscle:* the branches containing fibers from the inferior gluteal nerve of the fifth lumbar to second sacral nerves (L5, S1, S2) innervate the muscle.

d. *Gluteus medius muscle:* the branches containing fibers from the superior gluteal nerve of the fourth lumbar to first sacral nerves (L4, L5, S1) innervate the muscle.

e. *Gluteus minimus muscle:* the branches of the superior gluteal nerve of the fourth lumbar to first sacral nerves (L4, L5, S1) innervate the muscle.

f. *Superior gluteal artery, vein, and nerve:* the superior gluteal artery, together with the superior gluteal vein, arises from the internal iliac artery.

g. The needle reaches the posterior surface of the sacrum.

Functions

Strengthens the waist and the function of the Kidney, and removes Heat to induce diuresis.

Clinical indications

Constipation, abdominal pain, edema, back pain, orchitis, cystitis, urethritis, enuresis.

102.

(CHIHPIEN) ZHIBIAN, BL 54, FOOT TAI YANG BLADDER MERIDIAN

Location

In a prone position, the point is located 3.0 inches lateral to the posterior midline, at the level of the fourth spinous process of the sacrum, or 3 inches lateral to the sacral hiatus.

Needle and moxibustion method

Perpendicular insertion 3.0–3.5 inches (treating sciatica).

— *Needle sensation:* local distension and soreness, and electrical sensation radiating to the lower extremities, when punctured deeply.

Medially oblique insertion 2.0–3.0 inches at 45° (treating external genital organ disease).

— *Needle sensation:* local swelling and soreness, or an electrical sensation radiating to the external genital organ or the anus.

Medially inferior oblique insertion 2.0–3.0 inches at 45° (treating anal disease).

— *Needle sensation:* distension and soreness radiating to the anus.

Perpendicular insertion to Huantiao [GB 30] (treating overstrain of gluteal muscle).

— *Moxibustion dosage:* 5–7 cones; stick 5–20 minutes.

Cross-sectional anatomy of the needle passage

a. *Skin:* the branches containing fibers from the superior cluneal nerve of the first lumbar nerve (L1) innervate the skin.
b. *Subcutaneous tissue:* includes the previously described skin nerve branches.
c. *Gluteus maximus muscle:* the branches containing fibers from the inferior gluteal nerve of the fifth lumbar to second sacral nerves (L5, S1, S2) innervate the muscle.
d. *Sciatic nerve:* the largest peripheral nerve of the human body. The nerve contains fibers from the fourth and fifth lumbar and first, second and third sacral nerves (L4, L5, S1, S2, S3). If the needle is inserted into the nerve, an electrical sensation will radiate to the lower extremities.
e. *Quadratus femoris muscle:* the deep layer of the needle reaches the muscle. The branches containing fibers from the sacral plexus of the fourth lumbar to first sacral nerves (L4, L5, S1) innervate the muscle.
f. If the needle is inserted in a medially oblique direction, it may puncture the pudendal nerve, causing an electrical sensation radiating to the external genital organs and the anus.

Functions

Clears and activates the channels and collaterals, and strengthens the waist and knee joints.

Clinical indications

Sciatic pain, paralysis of the lower extremities, external genital organ and anal diseases, overstrain of the gluteal muscle.

103.

(TIENLIAO) TIANLIAO, TB 15, HAND TRIPLE BURNER MERIDIAN

Location

In a prone position, the point is located in the fossa superior to the spine of the scapula, at the midpoint between Jianjing [GB 21] and Quyuan [SI 13].

Needle and moxibustion method

Perpendicular insertion 0.3–0.5 inch.
— *Needle sensation:* local numbness and distension.
— *Moxibustion dosage:* 3–5 cones; stick 5–10 minutes.

Cross-sectional anatomy of the needle passage

a. *Skin:* the branches containing fibers from the suprascapular nerve innervate the skin.
b. *Subcutaneous tissue:* includes the previously described skin nerve branches.
c. *Trapezius muscle:* the branches containing fibers from the spinal accessory nerve (CN XI) and the ventral branches containing fibers from the third and fourth cervical nerves (C3, C4) innervate the muscle.
d. *Supraspinatus muscle:* the suprascapular branches of the brachial plexus of the fifth cervical nerve (C5) innervate the muscle.

Functions

Clears and activates the channels and collaterals, and relieves rigidity of the muscles, tendons and joints.

Clinical indications

Shoulder pain, neck stiffness, common cold.

104.

(TIENCHIH) TIANCHI, PC 1, HAND JUE YIN PERICARDIUM MERIDIAN

Location

In a supine or seated position, the point is located 1 inch lateral to the nipple in the fourth intercostal space.

Needle and moxibustion method

Oblique insertion 0.2–0.3 inch.
— *Needle sensation:* local numbness and distension.
— *Moxibustion dosage:* 3–5 cones; stick 10 minutes.

Cross-sectional anatomy of the needle passage

a. *Skin:* the anterior cutaneous branches containing fibers from the lateral divisions of the fourth intercostal nerve innervate the skin.
b. *Subcutaneous tissue:* includes the previously described skin nerve branches.
c. *Pectoralisis major muscle:* the medial and lateral pectoral branches from the brachial plexus containing fibers from the fifth cervical to first thoracic nerves (C5, C6, C7, C8, T1) innervate the muscle. The needle is inserted at the inferior margin of the muscle.
d. *Pectoralis minor muscle:* the needle is inserted at the inferior margin of the muscle. The medial pectoral branches from the brachial plexus of the eighth cervical and first thoracic nerves (C8, T1) innervate the muscle.
e. *External and internal intercostal muscles:* the branches containing fibers from the intercostal nerve innervate the muscles.

Warning

Directly beneath the point is the lung, so oblique insertion is preferable to perpendicular insertion. The angle between the needle and skin should be no greater than 25° as any steeper angle may puncture through the thoracic wall and damage the lung, causing pneumothorax or massive bleeding. Mild symptoms, which may heal spontaneously, are cough and chest pain. Severe symptoms are progressive respiratory difficulty and cyanosis.

Functions

Regulates the flow of Qi to soothe chest oppression, reduces fever and resolves local masses.

Clinical indications

Asthma, axillary pain and distension, choking sensation in the chest.

105.

(YUMEN) YUMEN, LU 2, HAND TAI YIN LUNG MERIDIAN

Location

In a supine or seated position, the point is located at the lateral superior part of the front of the chest in the fossa inferior to the lateral end of the clavicle and 6 inches lateral to the anterior midline.

Needle and moxibustion method

Lateral oblique insertion 0.5–0.8 inch. WARNING: No deep medial insertion, it may puncture into the lung.
— *Needle sensation:* local distension radiating to the upper extremities.
— *Moxibustion dosage:* 3–7 cones; stick 15 minutes.

Cross-sectional anatomy of the needle passage

a. *Skin:* the middle and dorsal branches containing fibers from the supraclavicular nerve of the fourth cervical nerve (C4) innervate the skin.
b. *Subcutaneous tissue:* includes the previously described skin nerve branches, and the cephalic vein pass. The cephalic vein joins the axillary vein.
c. *Deltoid muscle:* the needle is inserted at the superior lateral part of the muscle. The anterior branches containing fibers from the axillary nerve of the fifth and sixth cervical nerves (C5, C6) innervate the muscle.
d. The needle is inserted close to the superior part of the axillary and thoracoacromial artery. The thoracoacromial artery arises from the axillary artery.
e. Lateral branches of the anterior thoracic nerve and lateral cord of the brachial plexus.

Functions

Reduces fever and promotes the dispersing function of the Lung, and relieves cough and asthma.

Clinical indications

Asthma, chest pain, frozen shoulder, abdominal pain.

106.

(TAPAO) DABAO, SP 21, FOOT TAI YIN SPLEEN MERIDIAN, GREAT CONNECTING POINT

Location

In a supine or lateral position and with the arm raised, the point is located on the mid-axillary line, and 6 inches below the armpits; or on the mid-axillary line midway between the axilla and the tip of the eleventh rib.

Needle and moxibustion method

Oblique insertion 0.3–0.5 inch.
— *Needle sensation:* local numbness and distension.
— *Moxibustion dosage:* 3–5 cones; stick 10 minutes.

Cross-sectional anatomy of the needle passage

a. *Skin:* the branches containing fibers from the sixth intercostal nerve and the terminal branches of the long thoracic nerve innervate the skin.
b. *Subcutaneous tissue:* includes the previously described skin nerve branches, the sixth intercostal artery and vein, and the thoracodorsal artery and vein. The thoracodorsal artery, together with the thoracodorsal vein, arises from the subscapular artery.
c. *Anterior serratus and latissimus dorsi muscles:* the needle is passed between these two muscles. The long thoracic branches of the brachial plexus of the fifth and sixth cervical nerves (C5, C6) innervate the anterior serratus muscle. The branches containing fibers from the thoracodorsal nerve innervate the latissimus dorsi muscle.
d. *Internal and external intercostal muscles:* the branches containing fibers from the intercostal nerves innervate the muscles.

Warning

Directly beneath the point is the lung, so oblique insertion is better than perpendicular insertion. The angle between the needle and skin should be no greater than 25° as a steeper angle may puncture through the thoracic wall and damage the lung, causing pneumothorax. Mild symptoms, which may heal spontaneously, are cough, chest pain, and chest tightness. Severe symptoms are progressive respiratory difficulty and cyanosis. Tension pneumothorax may cause tachycardia, hypotension, and shock.

Functions
Expels pathogenic Cold from the channels, and regulates the collaterals.

Clinical indications
Pain in the chest and hypochondrium, asthma, whole body pain, weakness of the extremities, bronchitis, rheumatoid arthritis, pleuritis, pleurisy, pericarditis.

107.
(CHOUJUNG) ZHOURONG, SP 20, FOOT TAI YANG SPLEEN MERIDIAN

Location
In a seated or supine position, the point is located 6 inches lateral to the anterior midline, in the second intercostal space.

Needle and moxibustion method
Oblique insertion 0.3–0.5 inch.
— *Needle sensation:* local numbness and distension.
— *Moxibustion dosage:* 5 cones; stick 10 minutes.

Cross-sectional anatomy of the needle passage
a. *Skin:* the lateral cutaneous branches of the second intercostal nerve innervate the skin.
b. *Subcutaneous tissue:* includes the previously described skin nerve branches, the muscular branches of the anterior thoracic nerve, the lateral thoracic artery and vein, and the second intercostal artery and vein. The lateral thoracic artery, together with the lateral thoracic vein, arises from the axillary artery.
c. *Pectoralis major muscle:* the medial and lateral pectoral branches of the brachial plexus of the fifth cervical to first thoracic nerves (C5, C6, C7, C8, T1) innervate the muscle.
d. *Pectoralis minor muscle:* the medial pectoral branches of the brachial plexus of the eighth cervical and first thoracic nerves (C8, T1) innervate the muscle.
e. *Internal and external intercostal muscles:* the branches containing fibers from the intercostal nerve innervate the muscle.

Warning
Directly beneath the point is the lung, so oblique insertion is better than perpendicular insertion. The angle between the needle and skin should be no greater than 25° as a steeper angle may puncture through the thoracic wall and damage the lung, causing pneumothorax. Mild symptoms, which may heal spontaneously, are cough, chest pain, and chest tightness. Severe

---

symptoms are progressive respiratory difficulty and cyanosis. Tension pneumothorax may cause tachycardia, hypotension, and shock.

Functions
Removes Heat from the Lung, regulates the function of the Stomach, and relieves cough and asthma.

Clinical indications
Fullness of the chest and hypochondrium, cyanosis and dyspnea, sputum.

108.
(HSIUGHSIANG) XIONGXIANG, SP 19, FOOT TAI YIN SPLEEN MERIDIAN

Location
In a seated or supine position, the point is located 6 inches lateral to the anterior midline, in the third intercostal space.

Needle and moxibustion method
Oblique insertion 0.3–0.5 inch.
— *Needle sensation:* local numbness and distension.
— *Moxibustion dosage:* 3–5 cones; stick 15 minutes.

Cross-sectional anatomy of the needle passage
a. *Skin:* the lateral cutaneous branches containing fibers from the third intercostal nerve innervate the skin.
b. *Subcutaneous tissue:* includes the previously described skin nerve branches, the lateral thoracic artery and vein, and the third intercostal artery and vein. The lateral thoracic artery, together with the lateral thoracic vein, arises from the axillary artery.
c. *Inferior margin of pectoralis major and minor muscles:* the medial and lateral pectoral branches of the brachial plexus of the fifth cervical to first thoracic nerves (C5, C6, C7, C8, T1) innervate the pectoralis major muscle. The medial pectoral branches of the brachial plexus of the eighth cervical and first thoracic nerves (C8, T1) innervate the pectoralis minor muscle.
d. *Anterior serratus muscle:* the long thoracic branches of the brachial plexus of the fifth to seventh cervical nerves (C5, C6, C7) innervate the muscle.
e. *Internal and external intercostal muscles:* the branches containing fibers from the intercostal nerve innervate the muscles.

Warning
Directly beneath the point is the lung, so oblique insertion is better than perpendicular insertion. The angle

between the needle and skin should be no greater than 25° as a steeper angle may puncture through the thoracic wall and damage the lung, causing pneumothorax. Mild symptoms, which may heal spontaneously, are cough, chest pain, and chest tightness. Severe symptoms are progressive respiratory difficulty and cyanosis. Tension pneumothorax may cause tachycardia, hypotension, and shock.

Functions
Regulates the flow of Qi to soothe chest oppression, and clears and activates the channels and collaterals.

Clinical indications
Fullness of the chest and hypochondrium, pain in the chest and back, bronchitis, bronchial asthma, pneumonia, pleuritis.

109.
(TIENHSI) TIANXI, SP 18, FOOT TAI YIN SPLEEN MERIDIAN

Location
In a seated or supine position, the point is located 6 inches lateral to the anterior midline, in the fourth intercostal space lateral to the nipple.

Needle and moxibustion method
Oblique insertion 0.3–0.5 inch.
— *Needle sensation:* local soreness and distension.
— *Moxibustion dosage:* 3–5 cones; stick 15 minutes.

Cross-sectional anatomy of the needle passage
a. *Skin:* the lateral branches containing fibers from the fourth intercostal nerve innervate the skin.
b. *Subcutaneous tissue:* includes the previously described skin nerve branches, the lateral thoracic artery and vein, and the thoracoepigastric artery and vein. The lateral thoracic artery, together with the lateral thoracic vein, arises from the axillary artery. The thoracoepigastric vein drains into the superficial epigastric and the lateral thoracic veins.
c. *Inferior margin of pectoralis major muscle:* the medial and lateral pectoral branches of the brachial plexus of the fifth cervical to first thoracic nerves (C5, C6, C7, C8, T1) innervate the muscle.
d. *Anterior serratus muscle:* the long thoracic branches of the brachial plexus of the fifth to seventh cervical nerves (C5, C6, C7) innervate the muscle.
e. *Internal and external intercostal muscles:* the branches containing fibers from the intercostal nerve innervate the muscle.

Warning
Directly beneath the point is the lung, so oblique insertion is better than perpendicular insertion. The angle between the needle and skin should be no greater than 25° as a steeper angle may puncture through the thoracic wall and damage the lung, causing pneumothorax. Mild symptoms, which may heal spontaneously, are cough, chest pain, and chest tightness. Severe symptoms are progressive respiratory difficulty and cyanosis. Tension pneumothorax may cause tachycardia, hypotension, and shock.

Functions
Regulates the flow of Qi and Blood circulation, restores menstruation and promotes lactation.

Clinical indications
Fullness of the chest, cough and dyspnea, mastitis, insufficiency of milk, pneumonia, bronchial asthma, pleuritis, pleurisy.

110.
(SHIHTOU) SHIDOU, SP 17, FOOT TAI YIN SPLEEN MERIDIAN

Location
In a supine position, the point is located 6 inches lateral to the anterior midline, in the fifth intercostal space.

Needle and moxibustion method
Oblique insertion 0.3–0.5 inch.
— *Needle sensation:* local soreness and distension.
— *Moxibustion dosage:* 3–5 cones; stick 15 minutes.

Cross-sectional anatomy of the needle passage
a. *Skin:* the lateral cutaneous branches of the fifth intercostal nerve innervate the skin.
b. *Subcutaneous tissue:* includes the previously described skin nerve branches, the lateral thoracic artery, and the thoracoepigastric vein. The lateral thoracic artery arises from the axillary artery. The thoracoepigastric vein drains into the superficial epigastric and lateral thoracic veins.
c. *Anterior serratus muscle:* the long thoracic branches of the brachial plexus of the fifth to seventh cervical nerves (C5, C6, C7) innervate the muscle.
d. *Internal and external intercostal muscles:* at the deep layer of the anterior serratus muscle. The branches containing fibers from the intercostal nerve innervate the muscle.

Warning
Directly beneath the point is the lung, so oblique insertion is better than perpendicular insertion. The angle

between the needle and skin should be no greater than 25° as a steeper angle may puncture through the thoracic wall and damage the lung, causing pneumothorax. Mild symptoms, which may heal spontaneously, are cough, chest pain, and chest tightness. Severe symptoms are progressive respiratory difficulty and cyanosis. Tension pneumothorax may cause tachycardia, hypotension, and shock.

Functions
Regulates the function of the Spleen to remove Dampness, and descends rebellious Qi to arrest vomiting and lung disorders.

Clinical indications
Fullness and discomfort in chest and hypochondrium, pain in the hypochondrium, cough and dyspnea, neurogenic vomiting, indigestion, bronchial asthma, emphysema, pneumonia, bronchitis, pleuritis.

111.

(FUAI) FUAI, SP 16, FOOT TAI YIN SPLEEN MERIDIAN

Location
In a supine position, the point is located 4 inches lateral to the anterior midline, and 3 inches above Daheng [Sp 15].

Needle and moxibustion method
Perpendicular insertion 0.5–1.0 inch.
— *Needle sensation:* local numbness and distension.
— *Moxibustion dosage:* 3–5 cones; stick 15 minutes.

Cross-sectional anatomy of the needle passage
a. *Skin:* the branches containing fibers from the eighth intercostal nerve innervate the skin.
b. *Subcutaneous tissue:* includes the previously described skin nerve branches, the eighth intercostal artery and vein, and the superior epigastric artery.
c. *Internal and external oblique and transversus muscles:* the branches containing fibers from the eighth to twelfth intercostal nerves innervate the muscles.

Warning
Directly beneath the point is the transverse colon. If the needle is inserted deeply, it will puncture into the intestine. Vigorous thrusting and twirling of the needle may cause a small amount of the intestinal contents to drain into the peritoneal cavity, irritating the peritoneum and causing tension and rebound pain.

Functions
Regulates the function of the Stomach and Intestine, and strengthens the function of the Middle Jiao (Middle Warmer).

Clinical indications
Cold abdominal pain, umbilical pain, indigestion, constipation, dysentery, gastric ulcer, gastritis, enteritis.

112.

(TAHENG) DAHENG, SP 15, FOOT TAI YIN SPLEEN MERIDIAN

Location
In a supine position, the point is located 4 inches lateral to the umbilicus.

Needle and moxibustion method
Perpendicular insertion 0.7–1.2 inches.
— *Needle sensation:* local soreness and distension.
  Horizontal insertion 0.7–1.2 inches towards the umbilicus (treating ascariasis disease).
— *Needle sensation:* local distension and soreness, sometimes radiating to the ipsilateral abdomen.
— *Moxibustion dosage:* 5–10 cones; stick 15 minutes.

Cross-sectional anatomy of the needle passage
a. *Skin:* the branches containing fibers from the tenth intercostal nerve innervate the skin.
b. *Subcutaneous tissue:* includes the previously described skin nerve branches, the tenth intercostal artery and vein, and the superficial inferior epigastric artery and vein.
c. *External and internal oblique and transversus muscles:* the branches containing fibers from the eighth to twelfth intercostal nerves innervate the muscle.

Warning
Directly beneath the point is the small intestine. If the needle is inserted deeply, it will puncture into the intestine. Vigorous thrusting and twirling of the needle may cause a small amount of intestinal contents to drain into the peritoneal cavity, irritating the peritoneum and causing tension and rebound pain.

Functions
Warms the Middle Jiao (Middle Warmer) to reduce Cold, and eliminates undigested food.

Clinical indications
Diarrhea, constipation, abdominal pain, abdominal distension, dysentery.

113.

(FUCHIEH) FUJIE, SP 14, FOOT TAI YIN SPLEEN MERIDIAN

Location

In a supine position, the point is located 4 inches lateral to the anterior midline, and 1.3 inches below Daheng [Sp 15].

Needle and moxibustion method

Perpendicular insertion 0.5–1.0 inch.
— *Needle sensation:* local numbness and distension.
— *Moxibustion dosage:* 3–7 cones; stick 15 minutes.

Cross-sectional anatomy of the needle passage

a. *Skin:* the branches containing fibers from the eleventh intercostal nerve innervate the skin.
b. *Subcutaneous tissue:* includes the previously described skin nerve branches, the anterior cutaneous branches of the eleventh intercostal artery and vein, and the superior and inferior epigastric artery and vein.
c. *External and internal oblique and transversus muscles:* the branches containing fibers from the eighth to twelfth intercostal nerves innervate the muscles.

Warning

Directly beneath the point is the small intestine. If the needle is inserted deeply, it will puncture into the intestine. Vigorous thrusting and twirling of the needle may cause a small amount of intestinal contents to drain into the peritoneal cavity, irritating the peritoneum and causing tension and rebound pain.

Functions

Warms the Stomach and eases upset of the Stomach and Spleen, and regulates the Qi of the Fu.

Clinical indications

Umbilical pain, hernia pain, cough with dyspnea, peritonitis, appendicitis, enteritis, indigestion.

114.

(FUSHE) FUSHE, SP 13, FOOT TAI YIN SPLEEN MERIDIAN

Location

In a supine position, the point is located 4 inches lateral to the anterior midline, on the lateral part of the rectus abdominis muscle, and superior to the inguinal ligament 0.7 inch above SP 12.

Needle and moxibustion method

Perpendicular insertion 0.5–1.0 inch.
— *Needle sensation:* local distension and numbness radiating inferiorly.
— *Moxibustion dosage:* 3–5 cones; stick 10–15 minutes.

Cross-sectional anatomy of the needle passage

a. *Skin:* the ilioinguinal branches of the first lumbar nerve innervate the skin.
b. *Subcutaneous tissue:* includes the previously described skin nerve branches.
c. *Superior part of inguinal ligament:* the needle is inserted superior to the inguinal ligament.
d. *Tendons of external and internal oblique muscles:* the branches containing fibers from the iliohypogastric and ilioinguinal nerves innervate the muscles.
e. Inferior abdominal muscle.

Warning

Directly beneath the point are the cecum and sigmoid colon on the right and left, respectively. If the needle is inserted deeply, it will puncture into the intestine. Vigorous thrusting and twirling of the needle may cause a small amount of intestinal contents to drain into the peritoneal cavity, irritating the peritoneum and causing tension and rebound pain.

Functions

Warms the Middle Jiao (Middle Warmer), relieves pain, and promotes Blood circulation to remove Blood Stasis.

Clinical indications

Abdominal pain, peritonitis, appendicitis, enteritis, hernia, abdominal mass.

115.

(SHUFU) SHUFU, KI 27, FOOT SHAO YIN KIDNEY MERIDIAN

Location

In a supine position, the point is located 2 inches lateral to the anterior midline, in the depression on the inferior border of the medial head of the clavicle.

Needle and moxibustion method

Oblique insertion 0.3–0.4 inch.
— *Needle sensation:* local numbness and distension.
— *Moxibustion dosage:* 3–5 cones; stick 15 minutes.

Cross-sectional anatomy of the needle passage

a. *Skin:* the anterior branches of the supraclavicular nerve innervate the skin.

b. *Subcutaneous tissue:* includes the previously described skin nerve branches.

c. *Pectoralis major muscle:* the medial and lateral pectoral branches of the brachial plexus of the fifth cervical to first thoracic nerves (C5, C6, C7, C8, T1) innervate the muscle.

Warning

Directly beneath the point is the lung, so oblique insertion is better than perpendicular insertion. The angle between the needle and skin should be no greater than 25° as a steeper angle may puncture through and damage the lung, causing pneumothorax. Mild symptoms, which may heal spontaneously, are cough and chest pain. Severe symptoms are progressive respiratory difficulty and cyanosis.

Functions

Tonifies the function of the Kidney to improve inspiration, and expels Phlegm to relieve asthma.

Clinical indications

Cough, chest pain, bronchitis, bronchial asthma, pleuritis, pleurisy, neurogenic vomiting.

116.

(YUCHUNG) YUZHONG, KI 26, FOOT SHAO YIN KIDNEY MERIDIAN

Location

In a supine position, the point is located 2 inches lateral to the anterior midline, in the first intercostal space.

Needle and moxibustion method

Oblique insertion 0.3–0.5 inch.
— *Needle sensation:* local numbness and distension.
— *Moxibustion dosage:* 3–5 cones; stick 15 minutes.

Cross-sectional anatomy of the needle passage

a. *Skin:* the cutaneous branches of the first intercostal nerve innervate the skin.

b. *Subcutaneous tissue:* includes the previously described skin nerve branches, and the perforating branches of the first internal thoracic artery and vein.

c. *Pectoralis major muscle:* the medial and lateral pectoral branches of the brachial plexus of the fifth cervical to first thoracic nerves (C5, C6, C7, C8, T1) innervate the muscle.

d. *External intercostal ligaments.*

e. *External and internal intercostal muscles:* the branches containing fibers from the first intercostal nerve innervate the muscles. Beneath the internal and external intercostal muscles is the lung.

Warning

Directly beneath the point is the lung, so oblique insertion is better than perpendicular insertion. The angle between the needle and skin shuld be no greater than 25° as a steeper angle may puncture through and damage the lung, causing pneumothorax. Mild symptoms, which may heal spontaneously, are cough and chest pain. Severe symptoms are progressive respiratory difficulty and cyanosis.

Functions

Ventilates the Lung to relieve asthma, and regulates the flow of Qi to dissolve Phlegm.

Clinical indications

Cough, bronchial asthma, fullness of chest, bronchitis, pneumonia, tuberculosis.

117.

(SHENTSANG) SHENCANG, KI 25, FOOT SHAO YIN KIDNEY MERIDIAN

Location

In a supine position, the point is located 2 inches lateral to the anterior midline, in the second intercostal space.

Needle and moxibustion method

Oblique insertion 0.3–0.5 inch.
— *Needle sensation:* local numbness and distension.
— *Moxibustion dosage:* 3–5 cones; stick 15 minutes.

Cross-sectional anatomy of the needle passage

a. *Skin:* the cutaneous branches containing fibers from the second intercostal nerve innervate the skin.

b. *Subcutaneous tissue:* includes the previously described skin nerve branches, and the perforating branches of the second internal thoracic artery and vein.

c. *Pectoralis major muscle:* the medial and lateral pectoral branches of the brachial plexus of the fifth cervical to first thoracic nerves (C5, C6, C7, C8, T1) innervate the muscle.

d. *External and internal intercostal muscles:* the branches containing fibers from the second intercostal nerve innervate the muscles. Beneath the internal and external intercostal muscles is the lung.

Warning

Directly beneath the point is the lung, so oblique insertion is better than perpendicular. The angle between the needle and skin should be no greater than 25° as a steeper angle may puncture through and damage the lung, causing pneumothorax. Mild symptoms, which may heal spontaneously, are cough and chest pain.

Severe symptoms are progressive respiratory difficulty and cyanosis.

Functions
Clears away Heat from the Lung, regulates the function of the Stomach and relieves cough and asthma.

Clinical indications
Cough, asthma, chest pain, indigestion, gastritis, gastroptosis, neurogenic vomiting.

118.
(LINGHSU) LINGXU, KI 24, FOOT SHAO YIN KIDNEY MERIDIAN

Location
In a supine position, the point is located 2 inches lateral to the anterior midline, in the third intercostal space.

Needle and moxibustion method
Oblique insertion 0.3–0.5 inch.
— *Needle sensation:* local numbness and distension.
— *Moxibustion dosage:* 3–5 cones; stick 10 minutes.

Cross-sectional anatomy of the needle passage
a. *Skin:* the cutaneous branches containing fibers from the third intercostal nerve innervate the skin.
b. *Subcutaneous tissue:* includes the previously described skin nerve branches, and the perforating branches of the third internal thoracic artery and vein.
c. *Pectoralis major muscle:* the medial and lateral pectoral branches of the brachial plexus of the fifth cervical to first thoracic nerves (C5, C6, C7, C8,T1) innervate the muscle.
d. *External and internal intercostal muscles:* the branches containing fibers from the third intercostal nerve innervate the muscles. Beneath the internal and external intercostal muscles is the lung.

Warning
Directly beneath the point is the lung, so oblique insertion is better than perpendicular insertion. The angle between the needle and skin should be no greater than 25° as a steeper angle may puncture through and damage the lung, causing pneumothorax. Mild symptoms, which may heal spontaneously, are cough and chest pain. Severe symptoms are progressive respiratory difficulty and cyanosis.

Functions
Regulates and promotes the function of Lung Qi, and ventilates the Lung and reduces fever.

Clinical indications
Cough, asthma, mastitis, bronchitis, pleuritis, gastritis, indigestion, prolapse of the stomach.

119.
(SHENFENG) SHENFENG, KI 23, FOOT SHAO YIN KIDNEY MERIDIAN

Location
In a supine position, the point is located 2 inches lateral to the anterior midline, and in the fourth intercostal space.

Needle and moxibustion method
Oblique insertion 0.3–0.5 inch.
— *Needle sensation:* local distension and heaviness.
— *Moxibustion dosage:* 3–5 cones; stick 15 minutes.

Cross-sectional anatomy of the needle passage
a. *Skin:* the cutaneous branches containing fibers from the fourth intercostal nerve innervate the skin.
b. *Subcutaneous tissue:* includes the previously described skin nerve branches, and the perforating branches of the fourth internal thoracic artery and vein.
c. *Pectoralis major muscle:* the medial and lateral pectoral branches of the brachial plexus of the fifth cervical to first thoracic nerves (C5, C6, C7, C8, T1) innervate the muscle.
d. *External and internal intercostal muscles:* the branches containing fibers from the fourth intercostal nerve innervate the muscles. The deeper layers of the internal and external intercostal muscles are the lung and the heart on the right and left sides, respectively.

Warning
Directly beneath the point is the lung and heart at right and left, respectively so oblique insertion is better than perpendicular insertion. The angle between needle and skin should be no greater than 25° as a steeper angle may puncture through and damage the lung and the heart, causing pneumothorax or massive bleeding. Mild symptoms of pneumothorax, which may heal spontaneously, are cough and chest pain. Severe symptoms are progressive respiratory difficulty and cyanosis.

Functions
Tonifies the function of the Kidney, strengthens the function of the Spleen, and regulates the function of the Lung and relieves asthma.

Clinical indications
Cough and cyanosis, vomiting, asthma, mastitis, bronchitis, cardiac spasm, pleurisy, tachycardia.

120.

(PULANG) BULANG, KI 22, FOOT SHAO YIN KIDNEY MERIDIAN

Location
In a supine position, the point is located 2 inches lateral to the anterior midline, in the fifth intercostal space.

Needle and moxibustion method
Oblique insertion 0.3–0.5 inch.
— *Needle sensation:* local numbness and distension.
— *Moxibustion dosage:* 3–5 cones; stick 10 minutes.

Cross-sectional anatomy of the needle passage
a. *Skin:* the cutaneous branches containing fibers from the fifth intercostal nerve innervate the skin.
b. *Subcutaneous tissue:* includes the previously described skin nerve branches, and the fifth perforating branches of the internal thoracic artery and vein.
c. *Pectoralis major muscle:* the medial and lateral pectoral branches of the brachial plexus of the fifth cervical to first thoracic nerve (C5, C6, C7, C8, T1) innervate the muscle.
d. *External and internal intercostal muscles:* the branches containing fibers from the fifth intercostal nerve innervate the muscles. The deep layers of the internal and external intercostal muscles are the lung or liver and heart on the right and left sides, respectively.

Warning
Directly beneath the point are the lung or liver and heart on the right and left sides respectively, so oblique insertion is better than perpendicular insertion. The angle between the needle and skin should be no greater than 25° as a steeper angle may puncture through and damage the internal organs, causing pneumothorax or massive bleeding. Mild symptoms of pneumothorax, which may heal spontaneously, are cough and chest pain. Severe symptoms are progressive respiratory difficulty and cyanosis.

Functions
Regulates and promotes the function of Lung Qi, and relieves cough and asthma.

Clinical indications
Cough, asthma, vomiting, rhinitis, bronchitis, pleurisy, gastritis.

121.

(YOUMEN) YOUMEN, KI 21, FOOT SHAO YIN KIDNEY MERIDIAN

Location
In a supine position, the point is located 6 inches above the umbilicus, and 0.5 inch lateral to Juque [CV 14].

Needle and moxibustion method
Perpendicular insertion 0.3–0.7 inch.
— *Needle sensation:* local distension and numbness.
— *Moxibustion dosage:* 5 cones; stick 15 minutes.

Cross-sectional anatomy of the needle passage
a. *Skin:* the branches containing fibers from the seventh intercostal nerve innervate the skin.
b. *Subcutaneous tissue:* includes the previously described skin nerve branches.
c. *Rectus sheath and rectus abdominis muscle:* the branches containing fibers from the seventh to twelfth intercostal nerves innervate the muscle.
d. *Tendons of external and internal oblique muscles:* the branches containing fibers from the eighth to twelfth intercostal, the iliohypogastric, and the ilioinguinal nerves innervate the muscles.
e. *Tendon of transversus muscle:* the branches containing fibers from the seventh to twelfth intercostal, the iliohypogastric, and the ilioinguinal nerves innervate the muscle.

Warning
If the needle is inserted through the abdominal cavity, it may puncture into the liver. Vigorous lifting, thrusting, and twirling of the needle may cause massive bleeding. If the needle punctures into the liver, press the wound hard to prevent internal bleeding.

Functions
Dissipates Blood Stasis, reduces Heat, and regulates the function of the Stomach and removes Dampness.

Clinical indications
Abdominal pain, abdominal distension, indigestion, vomiting, dysentery.

122.

(FUTUNGKU) FUTONGGU, KI 20, FOOT SHAO YIN KIDNEY MERIDIAN

Location
In a supine position, the point is located 5 inches above the umbilicus, and 0.5 inch lateral to Shangwan [CV 13].

Needle and moxibustion method

Perpendicular insertion 0.5–1.0 inch.

— *Needle sensation:* local distension and heaviness.

— *Moxibustion dosage:* 3–5 cones; stick 10 minutes.

Cross-sectional anatomy of the needle passage

a. *Skin:* the branches containing fibers from the seventh intercostal nerve innervate the skin.

b. *Subcutaneous tissue:* includes the previously described skin nerve branches, and the superior epigastric artery.

c. *Rectus sheath and rectus abdominis muscle:* the branches containing fibers from the seventh to twelfth intercostal nerves innervate the muscle.

d. *Tendons of external and internal oblique muscles:* the branches containing fibers from the eighth to twelfth intercostal, the iliohypogastric and the ilioinguinal nerves innervate the muscles.

e. *Tendon of transversus muscle:* the branches containing fibers from the seventh to twelfth intercostal, the iliohypogastric, and the ilioinguinal nerves innervate the muscle.

Warning

If the needle is inserted through the abdominal cavity, it may puncture into the liver. Vigorous lifting, thrusting, and twirling of the needle may cause massive bleeding. If the needle punctures the liver, press the wound hard to prevent internal bleeding.

Functions

Clears away Heart Fire, strengthens the function of the Spleen, and descends rebellious Qi to arrest vomiting.

Clinical indications

Abdominal pain, abdominal distension, vomiting, indigestion, optic neuritis, bronchial asthma, peptic ulcer, spasm of the stomach.

123.

(YINTU) YINDU, KI 19, FOOT SHAO YIN KIDNEY MERIDIAN

Location

In a supine position, the point is located 4 inches above the umbilicus, and 0.5 inch lateral to Zhongwan [CV 12].

Needle and moxibustion method

Perpendicular insertion 0.5–1.0 inch.

— *Needle sensation:* local distension and heaviness.

— *Moxibustion dosage:* 3–5 cones; stick 10 minutes.

Cross-sectional anatomy of the needle passage

a. *Skin:* the branches containing fibers from the seventh intercostal nerve innervate the skin.

b. *Subcutaneous tissue:* includes the previously described skin nerve branches, and the superior epigastric artery.

c. *Rectus abdominis muscle and rectus sheath:* the branches containing fibers from the seventh to twelfth intercostal nerves innervate the muscle.

d. *Tendons of external and internal oblique muscles:* the branches of the eighth to twelfth intercostal, the iliohypogastric, and the ilioinguinal nerves innervate the muscles.

e. *Tendon of transversus muscle:* the branches containing fibers from the seventh to twelfth intercostal, the iliohypogastric, and the ilioinguinal nerves innervate the muscle.

Warning

If the needle is inserted through the abdominal wall, it may puncture into the liver and the stomach on the right and left sides, respectively. Vigorous lifting, thrusting, and twirling of the needle may cause massive bleeding or the stomach contents may drain into the peritoneal cavity, causing tension and pain. If the needle punctures the liver, press the wound hard to prevent internal bleeding.

Functions

Tonifies the function of the Kidney, nourishes the Liver, regulates the flow of Qi and relieves epigastric distension.

Clinical indications

Abdominal pain, epigastric pain, constipation, vomiting, epilepsy, bronchial asthma, emphysema, indigestion, infertility.

124.

(SHIHKUAN) SHIGUAN, KI 18, FOOT SHAO YIN KIDNEY MERIDIAN

Location

In a supine position, the point is located 3 inches above the umbilicus, and 0.5 inch lateral to Jianli [CV 11].

Needle and moxibustion method

Perpendicular insertion 0.5–1.0 inch.

— *Needle sensation:* local distension and heaviness.

— *Moxibustion dosage:* 3–5 cones; stick 10 minutes.

Cross-sectional anatomy of the needle passage

a. *Skin:* the branches containing fibers from the eighth

intercostal nerve innervate the skin.

b. *Subcutaneous tissue:* includes the previously described skin nerve branches, and the superior epigastric artery.

c. *Rectus abdominis muscle and rectus sheath:* the branches containing fibers from the seventh to twelfth intercostal nerve innervate the muscle.

d. *Tendons of external and internal oblique muscles:* the branches of the seventh to twelfth intercostal, the iliohypogastric, and the ilioinguinal nerves innervate the muscles.

e. *Tendon of transversus muscle:* the branches containing fibers from the seventh to twelfth intercostal, the iliohypogastric, and the ilioinguinal nerves innervate the muscle.

Warning

If the needle is inserted through the abdominal wall, it may puncture into the small intestine. Vigorous lifting, thrusting, and twirling of the needle may cause intestinal contents to drain into the peritoneal cavity, irritating the peritoneum and causing tension and rebound pain.

Functions

Nourishes the Yin to reduce empty Heat, and regulates the function of the Middle Jiao (Middle Warmer) to eliminate undigested food.

Clinical indications

Vomiting, abdominal pain, constipation, infertility, gastritis, gastric ulcer, stomach spasm, dysmenorrhea.

125.

(SHANGCHU) SHANGQU, KI 17, FOOT SHAO YIN KIDNEY MERIDIAN

Location

In a supine position, the point is located 2 inches above the umbilicus, and 0.5 inch lateral to Xiawan [CV 10].

Needle and moxibustion method

Perpendicular insertion 0.5–1.0 inch.
— *Needle sensation:* local distension and heaviness.
— *Moxibustion dosage:* 3–5 cones; stick 10 minutes.

Cross-sectional anatomy of the needle passage

a. *Skin:* the branches containing fibers from the eighth intercostal nerve innervate the skin.

b. *Subcutaneous tissue:* includes the previously described skin nerve branches, and the superior epigastric artery.

c. *Rectus abdominis muscle and rectus sheath:* the branches containing fibers from the seventh to

twelfth intercostal nerves innervate the muscle.

d. *Tendons of external and internal oblique muscles:* the branches containing fibers from the eighth to twelfth intercostal, the iliohypogastric, and the ilioinguinal nerves innervate the muscles.

e. *Tendon of transversus muscle:* the branches containing fibers from the seventh to twelfth intercostal, the iliohypogastric, and the ilioinguinal nerves innervate the muscle.

Warning

If the needle is inserted through the abdominal wall, it may puncture into the small intestine. Vigorous lifting, thrusting, or twirling of the needle may cause intestinal contents to drain into the peritoneal cavity, irritating the peritoneum and causing tension and rebound pain.

Functions

Clears and regulates the Stomach and Intestine, regulates the function of the Middle Jiao (Middle Warmer) and removes Dampness.

Clinical indications

Abdominal masses, constipation, dysentery, abdominal pain, gastritis, stomach spasm, enteritis.

126.

(HUANGSHU) HUANGSHU, KI 16, FOOT SHAO YIN KIDNEY MERIDIAN

Location

In a supine position, the point is located 0.5 inch lateral to the umbilicus.

Needle and moxibustion method

Perpendicular insertion 0.5–1.0 inch.
— *Needle sensation:* local distension and heaviness.
— *Moxibustion dosage:* 3–5 cones; stick 10 minutes.

Cross-sectional anatomy of the needle passage

a. *Skin:* the branches containing fibers from the ninth intercostal nerve innervate the skin.

b. *Subcutaneous tissue:* includes the previously described skin nerve branches, and the inferior epigastric artery. The external iliac artery gives rise to the inferior epigastric artery.

c. *Rectus abdominis muscle and rectus sheath:* the branches containing fibers from the seventh to twelfth intercostal nerves innervate the muscle.

d. *Tendons of external and internal oblique muscles:* the branches containing fibers from the eighth to twelfth intercostal, the iliohypogastric, and the ilioinguinal nerves innervate the muscles.

e. *Tendon of transversus muscle:* the branches containing fibers from the seventh to twelfth intercostal, the iliohypogastric, and the ilioinguinal nerves innervate the muscle.

Warning

If the needle is inserted through the abdominal wall, it may puncture into the small intestine. Vigorous lifting, thrusting, and twirling of the needle may cause intestinal contents to drain into the peritoneal cavity, irritating the peritoneum and causing tension and rebound pain.

Functions

Tonifies the function of the Kidney, strengthens the function of the Spleen, and induces diuresis for treating strangury.

Clinical indications

Constipation, abdominal pain, abdominal distension, vomiting, dysentery, periumbilical colic due to invasion of Cold.

127.

(CHUNGCHU) ZHONGZHU, KI 15, FOOT SHAO YIN KIDNEY MERIDIAN

Location

In a supine position, the point is located 1 inch below the umbilicus, and 0.5 inch lateral to Yinjiao [CV 7].

Needle and moxibustion method

Perpendicular insertion 0.5–1.0 inch.
— *Needle sensation:* local distension and numbness.
— *Moxibustion dosage:* 3–5 cones; stick 15 minutes.

Cross-sectional anatomy of the needle passage

a. *Skin:* the branches containing fibers from the tenth intercostal nerve innervate the skin.
b. *Subcutaneous tissue:* includes the previously described skin nerve branches and inferior epigastric artery. The external iliac artery gives rise to the inferior epigastric artery.
c. *Rectus abdominis muscle and rectus sheath:* the branches containing fibers from the seventh to twelfth intercostal nerves innervate the muscle.
d. *Tendons of external and internal oblique muscles:* the branches containing fibers from the eighth to twelfth intercostal, the iliohypogastric, and the ilioinguinal nerves innervate the muscles.
e. *Tendon of transversus muscle:* the branches containing fibers from the seventh to twelfth intercostal, the iliohypogastric, and the ilioinguinal nerves innervate the muscle.

Warning

If the needle is inserted through the abdominal wall, it may puncture into the small intestine. Vigorous lifting, thrusting, and twirling of the needle may cause intestinal contents to drain into the peritoneal cavity, irritating the peritoneum and causing tension and rebound pain.

Functions

Tonifies the function of the Kidney and nourishes the Liver.

Clinical indications

Irregular menstruation, abdominal pain, constipation, cystitis, gonorrhea, orchitis, dysmenorrhea, enteritis.

128.

(SZUMAN) SIMAN, KI 14, FOOT SHAO YIN KIDNEY MERIDIAN

Location

In a supine position, the point is located 2 inches below the umbilicus and 0.5 inch lateral to Shimen [CV 5].

Needle and moxibustion method

Perpendicular insertion 0.5–1.0 inch.
— *Needle sensation:* local numbness and distension.
— *Moxibustion dosage:* 3–5 cones; stick 10 minutes.

Cross-sectional anatomy of the needle passage

a. *Skin:* the branches containing fibers from the eleventh intercostal nerve innervate the skin.
b. *Subcutaneous tissue:* includes the previously described skin nerve branches and the inferior epigastric artery. The external iliac artery gives rise to the inferior epigastric artery.
c. *Rectus abdominis muscle and rectus sheath:* the branches containing fibers from the seventh to twelfth intercostal nerves innervate the muscle.
d. *Tendons of external and internal oblique muscles:* the branches containing fibers from the eighth to twelfth intercostal, the iliohypogastric, and the ilioinguinal nerves innervate the muscles.
e. *Tendon of the transversus muscle:* the branches containing fibers from the seventh to twelfth intercostal, the iliohypogastric, and the ilioinguinal nerves innervate the muscle.

Warning

If the needle is inserted through the abdominal wall, it may puncture into the small intestine. Vigorous lifting, thrusting, and twirling of the needle may cause intestinal contents to drain into the peritoneal cavity, irritating the peritoneum and causing tension and rebound pain.

Functions

Tonifies the function of the Kidney, strengthens the function of the Spleen, reduces Heat and removes Dampness.

Clinical indications

Abdominal pain, abdominal distension, dysentery, seminal emission, irregular menstruation, dysmenorrhea, constipation, ascites due to liver cirrhosis, enteritis, cystitis, proctitis.

129.

(CHIHSHUEH) QIXUE, KI 13, FOOT SHAO YIN KIDNEY MERIDIAN

Location

In a supine position, the point is located 3 inches below the umbilicus and 0.5 inch lateral to Guanyuan [CV 4].

Needle and moxibustion method

Perpendicular insertion 0.5–1.0 inch.
— *Needle sensation:* local distension and numbness radiating inferiorly.
— *Moxibustion dosage:* 3–5 cones; stick 10 minutes.

Cross-sectional anatomy of the needle passage

a. *Skin:* the branches containing fibers from the twelfth intercostal nerve innervate the skin.
b. *Subcutaneous tissue:* includes the previously described skin nerve branches and the muscular branches of the inferior epigastric artery. The external iliac artery gives rise to the inferior epigastric artery.
c. *Rectus abdominis muscle and rectus sheath:* the branches containing fibers from the seventh to twelfth intercostal nerves innervate the muscle.
d. *Tendons of the external and internal oblique muscles:* the branches containing fibers from the eighth to twelfth intercostal, the iliohypogastric, and the ilioinguinal nerves innervate the muscles.
e. *Tendon of transversus muscle:* the branches containing fibers from the seventh to twelfth intercostal, the iliohypogastric, and the ilioinguinal nerves innervate the muscle.

Warning

If the needle is inserted through the abdominal wall, it may puncture into the small intestine. Vigorous lifting, thrusting, and twirling of the needle may cause intestinal contents to drain into the peritoneal cavity, irritating the peritoneum and causing tension and pain.

Functions

Regulates menstruation and the flow of Qi, arrests bleeding and restores the Original Qi.

Clinical indications

Irregular menstruation, dysmenorrhea, abdominal pain, dysentery, back pain, lumbago.

130.

(TAHO) DAHE, KI 12, FOOT SHAO YIN KIDNEY MERIDIAN

Location

In a supine position, the point is located 4 inches below the umbilicus and 0.5 inch lateral to Zhongji [CV 3].

Needle and moxibustion method

Perpendicular insertion 0.5–1.0 inch.
— *Needle sensation:* local distension and numbness radiating inferiorly.
— *Moxibustion dosage:* 3–5 cones; stick 10 minutes.

Cross-sectional anatomy of the needle passage

a. *Skin:* the iliohypogastric branches of the twelfth thoracic and first lumbar nerves (T12, L1) innervate the skin.
b. *Subcutaneous tissue:* includes the previously described skin nerve branches and muscular branches of the inferior epigastric artery. The external iliac artery gives rise to the inferior epigastric artery.
c. *Rectus abdominis muscle and rectus sheath:* the branches containing fibers from the seventh to twelfth intercostal nerves innervate the muscle.
d. *Tendons of external and internal oblique muscles:* the branches containing fibers from the eighth to twelfth intercostal, the iliohypogastric, and the ilioinguinal nerves innervate the muscles.
e. *Tendon of transversus muscle:* the branches containing fibers from the seventh to twelfth intercostal, the iliohypogastric, and the ilioinguinal nerves innervate the muscle.

Warning

If the needle is inserted through the abdominal wall, it may puncture into the small intestine or the fundus of the urinary bladder. Vigorous lifting, thrusting, or twirling of the needle may cause intestinal contents to drain into the peritoneal cavity, irritating the peritoneum and causing tension and pain.

Functions

Tonifies the function of the Kidney, regulates menstruation and reduces Heat to induce diuresis.

Clinical indications

Penile pain, leukorrhea, seminal emission, impotence, vaginitis, irregular menstruation.

131.

(HENGKU) HENGGU, KI 11, FOOT SHAO YIN KIDNEY MERIDIAN

Location
In a supine position, the point is located 5 inches below the umbilicus and 0.5 inch lateral to Qugu [CV 2] at the superior margin of the pubic symphysis.

Needle and moxibustion method
Perpendicular insertion 0.5–1.0 inch.
— *Needle sensation:* local numbness and distension.
— *Moxibustion dosage:* 3–5 cones; stick 10 minutes.

Cross-sectional anatomy of the needle passage
a. *Skin:* the iliohypogastric branches containing fibers from the twelfth thoracic and first lumbar nerves (T12, L1) innervate the skin.
b. *Subcutaneous tissue:* includes the previously described skin nerve branches, the inferior epigastric artery, and the external pudendal artery. The external iliac artery gives rise to the inferior epigastric artery. The femoral artery gives rise to the external pudendal artery.
c. *Pyramidalis muscle:* the needle is inserted on the lateral side of the pyramidalis muscle. The branches containing fibers from the twelfth thoracic nerve (T12) innervate the muscle.
d. *Rectus abdominis muscle and rectus sheath:* the branches containing fibers from the seventh to twelfth intercostal nerves innervate the muscle.
e. *Tendons of external and internal oblique muscles:* the branches containing fibers from the eighth to twelfth intercostal, the iliohypogastric, and the ilioinguinal nerves innervate the muscles.
f. *Tendon of transversus muscle:* the branches containing fibers from the seventh to twelfth intercostal, the iliohypogastric, and the ilioinguinal nerves innervate the muscle.

Warning
If the needle is inserted through the abdominal wall, it may puncture into the small intestine or the fundus of the urinary bladder. Vigorous lifting, thrusting, and twirling of the needle may cause intestinal contents to drain into the peritoneal cavity, irritating the peritoneum and causing tension and pain.

Functions
Tonifies the function of the Kidney, strengthens the function of the Spleen, and clears away Damp Heat.

Clinical indications
Genital pain, difficulty in urination, seminal emission, impotence.

132.

(YUANYEH) YUANYE, GB 22, FOOT SHAO YANG GALLBLADDER MERIDIAN

Location
In a seated position with the arm abducted, the point is located 3 inches inferior to the anterior axillary line and in the fifth intercostal space.

Needle and moxibustion method
Oblique insertion 0.3–0.5 inch.
— *Needle sensation:* local distension.
— *Moxibustion dosage:* 3–5 cones; stick 5 minutes.

Cross-sectional anatomy of the needle passage
a. *Skin:* the lateral cutaneous branches containing fibers from the fourth intercostal nerve innervate the skin.
b. *Subcutaneous tissue:* includes the previously described skin nerve branches.
c. *Anterior serratus muscle:* the long thoracic branches of the brachial plexus containing fibers from the fifth to seventh cervical nerves (C5, C6, C7) innervate the muscle.
d. *External and internal intercostal muscles:* the branches containing fibers from the fifth intercostal nerve innervate the muscles.

Warning
Directly beneath the point is the lung, so oblique insertion is safer than perpendicular insertion. The angle between the needle and skin should be no greater than 25° as a steeper angle may puncture through and damage the lung, causing pneumothorax. Mild symptoms, which may heal spontaneously, are cough and chest pain. Severe symptoms are progressive respiratory difficulty and cyanosis.

Functions
Reduces fever, removes masses, and regulates the flow of Qi to resolve Phlegm.

Clinical indications
Axillary pain, sensation of fullness in the chest, cough, chills and fever.

133.

(CHECHIN) ZHEJIN, GB 23, FOOT SHAO YANG GALLBLADDER MERIDIAN

Location
In a lateral recumbent position, the point is located 3 inches inferior to the anterior axillary line and 1 inch

anterior to Yuanyeh [GB 22] in the fifth intercostal space, approximately level with the nipple.

Needle and moxibustion method
Oblique insertion 0.3–0.5 inch.
— *Needle sensation:* local numbness and distension.
— *Moxibustion dosage:* 3–5 cones; stick 15 minutes.

Cross-sectional anatomy of the needle passage
a. *Skin:* the lateral cutaneous branches containing fibers from the fifth intercostal nerve innervate the skin.
b. *Subcutaneous tissue:* includes the previously described skin nerve branches.
c. *Pectoralis major muscle:* the needle is inserted at the inferior margin of the muscle. The medial and lateral pectoral branches of the brachial plexus containing fibers from the fifth cervical to first thoracic nerves (C5, C6, C7, C8, T1) innervate the muscle.
d. *Anterior serratus muscle:* the long thoracic branches of the brachial plexus containing fibers from the fifth to seventh cervical nerves (C5, C6, C7) innervate the muscle.
e. *External and internal intercostal muscles:* the branches containing fibers from the fifth intercostal nerve innervate the muscles.

Warning
Directly beneath the point is the lung, so oblique insertion is safer than perpendicular insertion. The angle between the needle and skin should be no greater than 25° as a steeper angle may puncture through and damage the lung, causing pneumothorax. Mild symptoms, which may heal spontaneously, are cough and chest pain. Severe symptoms are progressive respiratory difficulty and cyanosis.

Functions
Clears Heat from the Liver, regulates the function of the Stomach, and treats hiccup and arrests asthma.

Clinical indications
Sensation of fullness in the chest, asthma, vomiting, gastritis, gastric ulcer, enteritis.

134.

(CHINGMEN) JINGMEN, GB 25, FOOT SHAO YANG GALLBLADDER MERIDIAN

Location
In a lateral recumbent position, the point is located in the lateral lumbar region inferior to the anterior tip of the twelfth floating rib.

Needle and moxibustion method
Perpendicular insertion 0.3–0.5 inch.
— *Needle sensation:* local numbness and distension.
— *Moxibustion dosage:* 3–7 cones; stick 10 minutes.

Cross-sectional anatomy of the needle passage
a. *Skin:* the branches containing fibers from the eleventh intercostal nerve innervate the skin.
b. *Subcutaneous tissue:* includes the previously described skin nerve branches.
c. *External and internal oblique muscles:* the branches containing fibers from the eighth to twelfth intercostal, the iliohypogastric, and the ilioinguinal nerves innervate the muscles.
d. *Transversus muscle:* the branches containing fibers from the seventh to twelfth intercostal, the iliohypogastric and the ilioinguinal nerves innervate the muscle.

Warning
If the needle is inserted through the abdominal wall, it may puncture into the ascending and descending colon at the right and left sides, respectively. Vigorous lifting, thrusting, or twirling of the needle may cause intestinal contents to drain into the peritoneal cavity, irritating the peritoneum and causing pain and tension.

Functions
Clears away Heat from the Liver, regulates the flow of Qi, and reduces Heat to induce diuresis.

Clinical indications
Abdominal distension, diarrhea, lumbar pain, vomiting, facial edema.

135.

(TAIMAI) DAIMAI, GB 26, FOOT SHAO YANG GALLBLADDER MERIDIAN

Location
In a lateral recumbent position, the point is located in the lateral lumbar region at the intersection of a vertical line from Zhangmen [Liv 13] and a horizontal line from the umbilicus; or 1.8 inches inferior to the anterior tip of the eleventh rib.

Needle and moxibustion method
Perpendicular insertion 0.5–0.8 inch.
— *Needle sensation:* soreness and distension in the lateral lumbar region.
— *Moxibustion dosage:* 5–7 cones; stick 15 minutes.

Cross-sectional anatomy of the needle passage
a. *Skin:* the branches containing fibers from the twelfth intercostal nerve innervate the skin.

b. *Subcutaneous tissue:* includes the previously described skin nerve branches.

c. *External and internal oblique muscles:* the branches containing fibers from the eighth to twelfth intercostal, the iliohypogastric, and the ilioinguinal nerves innervate the muscles.

d. *Transversus muscle:* the branches containing fibers from the seventh to twelfth intercostal, the iliohypogastric, and the ilioinguinal nerves innervate the muscle.

Warning

If the needle is inserted through the abdominal wall, it may puncture into the ascending and descending colon at the right and left sides respectively. Vigorous lifting, thrusting, and twirling of the needle may cause intestinal contents to drain into the peritoneal cavity, irritating the peritoneum and causing pain and tension.

Functions

Regulates menstruation, arrests leukorrhea, and reduces Dampness and Heat.

Clinical indications

Intestinal hernia pain, diarrhea, irregular menstruation, leukorrhea, lumbar pain.

136.

(WUSHU) WUSHU, GB 27, FOOT SHAO YANG GALLBLADDER MERIDIAN

Location

In a lateral recumbent or supine position, the point is located 3 inches below Daimai [GB 26], lateral to Guanyuan [CV 4] and 0.5 inches anterior to the anterior superior iliac crest.

Needle and moxibustion method

Perpendicular insertion 0.5–1.0 inch.
— *Needle sensation:* local numbness and distension.
— *Moxibustion dosage:* 5–10 cones; stick 15 minutes.

Cross-sectional anatomy of the needle passage

a. *Skin:* the branches containing fibers from the iliohypogastric nerve innervate the skin.

b. *Subcutaneous tissue:* includes the previously described skin nerve branches.

c. *Superficial and deep circumflex iliac artery and vein:* the femoral artery gives rise to the superficial and deep circumflex iliac artery and vein.

d. *External and internal oblique muscles:* the branches containing fibers from the eighth to twelfth intercostal, the iliohypogastric, and the ilioinguinal nerves innervate the muscles.

e. *Transversus muscle:* the branches containing fibers from the seventh to twelfth intercostal, the iliohypogastric, and the ilioinguinal nerves innervate the muscle.

Functions

Clears away Heat from the Liver, tonifies the function of the Kidney, and regulates and promotes the Lower Jiao (Lower Warmer).

Clinical indications

Lumbar pain, abdominal pain, leukorrhea, constipation, periumbilical cold due to Cold invasion.

137.

(WEITAO) WEIDAO, GB 28, FOOT SHAO YANG GALLBLADDER MERIDIAN

Location

In a lateral recumbent or supine position, the point is located in the medial inferior margin of the anterior superior iliac crest, and 0.5 inch anterior and inferior to Wushu [GB 27].

Needle and moxibustion method

Perpendicular insertion 1.0–1.5 inches.
— *Needle sensation:* local numbness and distension.
— *Moxibustion dosage:* 3–5 cones; stick 10 minutes.

Cross-sectional anatomy of the needle passage

a. *Skin:* the branches containing fibers from the ilioinguinal nerve innervate the skin.

b. *Subcutaneous tissue:* includes the previously described skin nerve branches.

c. *Superficial and deep circumflex iliac artery and vein:* the femoral artery gives rise to the superficial and deep circumflex iliac artery and vein.

d. *External and internal oblique muscles:* the branches containing fibers from the eighth to twelfth intercostal, the iliohypogastric, and the ilioinguinal nerves innervate the muscles.

e. *Transversus muscle:* the branches containing fibers from the seventh to twelfth intercostal, the iliohypogastric, and the ilioinguinal nerves innervate the muscle.

Functions

Removes Heat from the Liver, regulates the function of the Stomach, and regulates the function of the Intestine to facilitate bowel movement.

Clinical indications

Leukorrhea, lower abdominal pain, hernia, prolapse of the uterus.

Cross-sectional anatomy of high risk acupoints

Many ancient classic acupuncture textbooks described anatomical contraindications when using certain acupoints. The *Huang Di Nei Jing* (The Yellow Emperor's Internal Classic) stated 'care should be taken with needle manipulation over the important fragile internal organs'; 'needle penetration to the thoracic region (pectoral muscle) might perforate the lung causing pneumothorax with cough and difficulty of breath'; 'needle penetration to the urinary bladder of the lower abdomen might perforate to the bladder, causing urine to drain into the lower abdomen'; 'needle penetration to the supraorbital foramen might perforate to the supraorbital vessels inducing massive bleeding and causing blindness'; and 'needle penetration to the skull might perforate to the brain, inducing brain damage or massive bleeding which may lead to immediate death'. The other classic acupuncture textbooks, such as *Zhen Jiu Jia Yi Jing* (A B C Classic of Acupuncture and Moxibustion), *Tong Ren Shu Xue Zhen Jiu Tu Jing* (Illustrated Manual of Acupoints of the Bronze Figure), *Zhen Jiu Da Cheng* (Great Compendium of Acupuncture and Moxibustion), and *Yi Zong Jin Jian* (The Golden Mirror of Medicine) have also described the contraindications and precautions required when using certain acupoints.

In this chapter, 15 commonly used acupoints are described, explaining how to control and manipulate the needle direction, depth, and manipulation in clinic. Included is:

a. Information from classic acupuncture textbooks which describe the acupoints where it is absolutely prohibited to manipulate the needle i.e. Quepen [ST 12, Chuehpen] and Yamen [GV 15, Yamen]. In ancient times, owing to inadequate knowledge of anatomy, these acupoints were absolutely prohibited to needle, or only shallow needle penetration was permitted in most ancient classic acupuncture textbooks.

b. Some acupoints which were not absolutely prohibited to needle in most ancient classic acupuncture textbooks, have been shown from the modern anatomical point of view, to have risks of puncturing or perforating vital organs such as the lung, liver,

spleen, kidney, urinary bladder, and large blood vessels. Dangers are increased if the depth of the needle insertion is too deep, or the direction of the needle is wrong, or the needle manipulation method is not correct. Also some diseases can induce an adverse acupuncture reaction which do not occur in a normal healthy person. Deep needle manipulation at some acupoints can damage the central nervous system such as the spinal cord, medulla oblongata and cerebellum. Not only may accidental damage be caused to the organs but also the patient's life may be threatened. For these reasons special care should be taken when using the following points.

1.

(CHINGMING) JINGMING, BL 1, FOOT TAI YANG BLADDER MERIDIAN

Location
With the eyes closed, the point is located in the fossa 0.1 inch superior to and lateral to the medial angle of the eye.

Needle and moxibustion method
Use the fingers to press the eyeball gently to the lateral side then the needle is slowly inserted posteriorly and laterally at an angle of 85° to the medial bony orbit of the eye to a depth of between 0.2–0.6 inch. No vigorous lifting, thrusting, or twirling the needle is permitted. Slight needle resistance is felt, after the needle has penetrated the eyelid.
— *Needle sensation:* Local distension and soreness, or sensation radiating to the posterior part of the eyeball and into the surrounding region.

Cross-sectional anatomy of the needle passage
(Fig. 6.1)
a. *Skin:* the skin of the eyelid is very thin, about 0.1 cm. The supratrochlear nerve containing fibers of the frontal nerve originating from the ophthalmic branch of the trigeminal nerve (CN V) innervates the skin.

b. *Subcutaneous tissue:* includes the previously described skin nerve branches. The subcutaneous tissue consists of a large amount of loose connective tissue and a small amount of adipose tissue. When the tissue is bleeding or inflamed, it will show obvious ecchymosis or edema. The supraorbital branch of the ophthalmic artery and the terminal branch of the facial artery supply the subcutaneous tissue. If the needle is inserted into the vessels, it will produce ecchymosis and a green-purple color.

c. *Orbicularis oculi muscle:* below the subcutaneous tissue of the upper and lower eyelids. The temporal and zygomatic branches containing fibers from the facial nerve (CN VII) innervate the muscle. If the needle is inserted superficially at Jingming [BL 1] it can treat spasm of the orbicularis oculi muscle.

d. *Adipose body of orbit:* between the eyeballs, the orbital muscles, and the periorbit are spaces filled with adipose tissue. The function of the adipose tissue is to provide an elastic cushion for the eyeballs. No needle resistance is felt when the needle is inserted through the structure.

e. The needle is inserted between the medial rectus muscle and the medial wall of the orbit. Sometimes the needle may puncture into the medial rectus muscle.

The structures surrounding the needle passage

a. *Medial rectus muscle:* on the lateral side of the needle. The inferior branches containing fibers from the oculomotor nerve (CN III) innervate the muscle.

The medial rectus muscle is surrounded by the orbital fascia. Needle resistance may be felt, if the needle penetrates the orbital fascia.

If the needle is inserted into the muscle, the needle sensation of the patient is soreness, distension, and heaviness.

If the needle is inserted into the muscle, it is able to improve external strabismus.

b. *Medial wall of orbit:* on the medial side of the needle. The wall is an arrowhead-shaped structure, with a wide anterior part and gradually narrowing posteriorly to the orbital apex. The middle and posterior walls contain the anterior and posterior ethmoidal

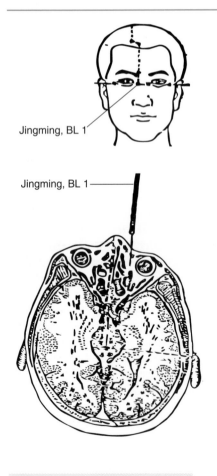

Jingming, BL 1

Jingming, BL 1

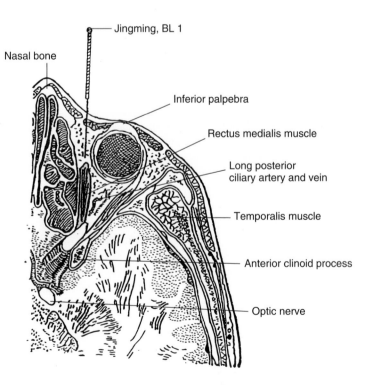

Jingming, BL 1

Nasal bone

Inferior palpebra

Rectus medialis muscle

Long posterior ciliary artery and vein

Temporalis muscle

Anterior clinoid process

Optic nerve

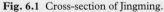

Fig. 6.1 Cross-section of Jingming.

foramina, containing the anterior ethmoidal artery and nerve and the posterior ethmoidal artery and nerve. The anterior and posterior ethmoidal arteries arise from the ophthalmic artery. The anterior and posterior ethmoidal nerves are branches from the ophthalmic divisions from the trigeminal nerve (CN V).

c. *Common tendinous ring, optic foramen and its contents:* the common tendinous ring is surrounded by and attached to the optic foramen and the tendons of the superior orbital fissure. It is the origin of the tendons of the rectus muscles of the eyes and is located posteriorly, slightly lateral to the needle passage.

The optic foramen, which is a short bony canal about 5 cm (2 inches) long, is in the orbital apex. The optic nerve, together with the ophthalmic artery, passes through the optic foramen.

The optic nerve is covered by the inner, middle and external fascia which are the continuation of the three meninges of the brain – the pia mater, the arachnoid, and the dura mater. The external fascia is the continuation of the dura mater, which is composed of dense, strong, fibrous tissue. The fascia covers the whole optic nerve and continues to the posterior eyeball. It then transits to become the sclera of the eyeball.

Complications, prevention and treatment

a. *Bleeding:* the subcutaneous tissue contains loose connective tissue and a small artery and vein. The space of the loose connective tissue is sufficiently large so that if the needle is not inserted too quickly, it will not cause severe damage. If the needle is inserted into these blood vessels use the finger to press the point and limit the bleeding. The most severe complication is local ecchymosis.

If the needle is inserted more than 2 cm (0.8 inch) to 3.2 cm (1.2 inches), it will be very close to the medial wall of the orbit and may puncture into the anterior and posterior ethmoidal arteries. If these two arteries are damaged, they will bleed very easily. The chief signs are swollen eyeballs and evagination. Heavy bleeding will drain into the loose connective tissue, causing purple ecchymosis of the superior and inferior eyelids. To prevent this, don't insert the needle too close to the medial wall of the orbit.

To manage the bleeding, use a cold ice pad compress first, then a hot pad compress, and a hemostat to decrease bleeding and increase absorption.

b. *Puncture into the eyeball:* this may happen while inserting the needle if the eyeball is not pressed laterally, or if the needle is too close to the eyeball. The external sclera of the eyeball is very strong so it is not easy to puncture through the structure especially if the needle is inserted slowly. It is very easy to puncture into the largest transverse diameter of the eyeball, which presents the thinnest part of the sclera. If the needle is inserted into the eyeball, the patient must be transferred to a physician immediately.

c. *Common tendinous ring and optic nerve:* if the needle is inserted more than 4.5 cm (1.8 inches), it could penetrate into the common tendinous ring and the optic nerve very easily. The optic nerve is covered by strong fibrous connective tissue, a continuation of the dura mater, and a sticky needle resistance will be felt if the needle punctures into the structure. If the needle is inserted into the optic nerve, the patient may complain of flashing before the eyes, headache, dizziness, vomiting, and nausea. Withdraw the needle immediately, and treat the symptoms.

d. *Ophthalmic artery and vein:* the ophthalmic artery is a terminal branch of the carotid artery which, together with the optic nerve, passes through the optic canal into the orbital cavity. It supplies nutrient to the eyeballs, is surrounded by the common tendinous ring, and is in the middle of the muscular funnel formed by the external eyeball muscle. The ophthalmic artery, together with the ophthalmic vein, is located lateral and inferior to the optic nerve. When inserting the needle, the needle direction must be on the medial side of the optic nerve in order to prevent puncturing into the ophthalmic artery. The muscular branches and long posterior ciliary arteries of the ophthalmic artery are very close to the needle pathway and very small in diameter. They are distributed in the loose adipose body of the orbit, which is mobile. To prevent inserting the needle into the long posterior ciliary arteries, don't insert the needle too quickly and do not use a thrusting movement.

e. *Superior orbital fissure and its deep contents:* if the needle is inserted posteriorly and laterally more than 5.0 cm (2 inches) in men and 4.8 cm in women, it may puncture through the superior orbital fissure. The oculomotor nerve (CN III), the trochlear nerve (CN IV), the abducens nerve (CN VI), and the ophthalmic branch of the trigeminal nerve (CN V) pass through the superior orbital fissure. If the needle is passed through the superior orbital fissure, it may puncture into the cavernous sinus of the middle cranial fossa and damage the frontal lobe of the cerebrum, causing intracranial bleeding leading to dizziness, headache, nausea, vomiting, shock, and even death. The deeper the needle is penetrated and the heavier the manipulation, the more dangerous it is.

Functions

Expels Wind and reduces Heat, and clears the collaterals to improve acuity of vision.

Clinical indications

Conjunctivitis, keratitis, myopia, optic neuritis, optic nerve atrophy, glaucoma, vitreous opacity.

2.

(CHENGCHI) CHENGQI, ST 1, FOOT YANG MING STOMACH MERIDIAN

Location

When the eye is looking straight ahead the point is located directly inferior to the pupil, between the inferior margin of the orbit and the eyeball.

Needle and moxibustion method

Ask the patient to look upward, the needle is then inserted in a perpendicular direction along the inferior orbital margin 1.0–1.5 inches.

Insert the needle in a medially posterior superior direction to the orbital apex 1.0–1.5 inches, but don't go too close to the inferior orbital wall.

Insert the needle into the subcutaneous tissue of the eyelids, then in a horizontal direction along the skin to the medial angle of the eye (treating spasm of the orbicularis oculi muscles).

— *Needle sensation:* Local distension and soreness, or sometimes salivation.

Cross-sectional anatomy of the needle passage

(Figs 6.2 & 6.3)

a. *Skin:* very thin. The maxillary branch of the trigeminal nerve (CN V) innervates the skin.

b. *Subcutaneous tissue:* includes the previously described skin nerve branch and the zygomatic branches containing fibers from the facial nerve (CN VII).

The smaller arteries branch off from the infraorbital artery, which in turn is a branch of the maxillary artery. The smaller veins drain into the infraorbital vein, and then into the inferior ophthalmic vein.

c. *Orbicularis oculi muscle:* below the subcutaneous tissue of the upper and lower eyelids. The temporal and zygomatic branches containing fibers from the facial nerve (CN VII) innervate the muscle.

d. *Adipose body of the orbit:* the spaces between the eyeballs, the orbital muscle, and the periorbit are filled with adipose tissue. The function of the adipose body of the orbit is to provide an elastic cushion for the eyelids. No needle resistance is felt when the needle is punctured through the structure.

e. *Inferior oblique muscle:* the inferior branches containing fibers from the oculomotor nerve (CN III) innervate the muscle.

f. *Inferior rectus muscle:* the inferior branches containing fibers from the oculomotor nerve (CN III) innervate the muscle.

The structures surrounding the needle passage

a. *Inferior oblique and inferior rectus muscles:* the needle is inserted through the adipose body of the orbit into the inferior oblique muscle. The inferior oblique muscle is one of the external muscles of the eyeball. The origin of the muscle is the medial part of the infraorbital wall, the insertion is the lateral sclera of the posterior eyeball, and the function is to turn the eye to the lateral superior direction.

If the needle is directed slightly towards the eyeball, it will puncture into the inferior rectus muscle. The inferior rectus muscle is one of the four rectus muscles of the eyeball, innervated by the inferior branches containing fibers from the oculomotor nerve (CN III). The origin of the muscle is

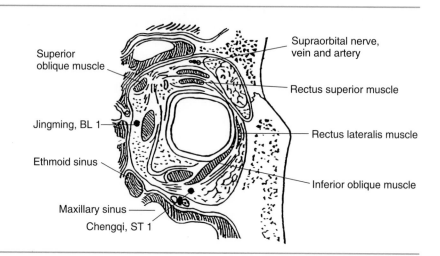

Fig. 6.2 Frontal section of Jingming and Chengqi.

Superior oblique muscle

Supraorbital nerve, vein and artery

Rectus superior muscle

Jingming, BL 1

Rectus lateralis muscle

Ethmoid sinus

Inferior oblique muscle

Maxillary sinus

Chengqi, ST 1

the common tendinous ring, the insertion is the anterior part of the inferior portion of the sclera of the eyeball, and the function is to turn the eyeball in an inferior direction.

Nerve branches containing fibers from the inferior divisions of the oculomotor nerve (CN III) innervate both muscles and the muscular branches of the ophthalmic artery supply the muscles. If the needle is inserted into the artery, it will bleed into the adipose body of the orbit and the inferior orbit wall.

If the needle is inserted into the muscles, a mild needle resistance may be felt. The patient may complain of soreness, distension, and heaviness.

b. *Infraorbital groove and canal, and contents:* in the middle of the infraorbital wall. From the posterior to anterior, there is a horizontal bony groove, the infraorbital groove, and an opening in the inferior margin of the infraorbital wall, called the infraorbital foramen. The infraorbital nerve, artery, and vein pass through the infraorbital groove and canal to the infraorbital foramen, and into the subcutaneous tissue.

The infraorbital nerve arises from the maxillary division of the trigeminal nerve (CN V). The infraorbital artery, together with the infraorbital vein, is a terminal branch of the maxillary artery. The previously described structures pass through the lateral part of the pterygoid fossa, continue through the infraorbital fissure into the orbital cavity, and then enter the bony structure of the infraorbital groove into the infraorbital canal. There is very little variation in the location of these structures. If the needle is punctured into these, it may cause severe complications.

Complications, prevention and treatment

a. *Bleeding of the inferior wall of the orbit:* if the needle is inserted into the infraorbital groove, it will damage the infraorbital artery and vein. The average distance from the midpoint of the inferior margin of the orbit to the infraorbital groove and canal is 1 cm (0.4 inch) and the average length of the infraorbital groove is 1.6 cm (0.63 inch). If the needle is inserted more than 1 cm (0.4 inch), it may pass very close to the infraorbital groove and penetrate into the infraorbital artery and vein, causing massive bleeding. To prevent this complication, while inserting the needle deeply, don't penetrate too close to the infraorbital wall, or in the orbital apex direction.

b. *Insertion into the eyeball:* this may happen while inserting the needle if the eyeball is not pressed upwards, or if the needle is too close to the eyeball.

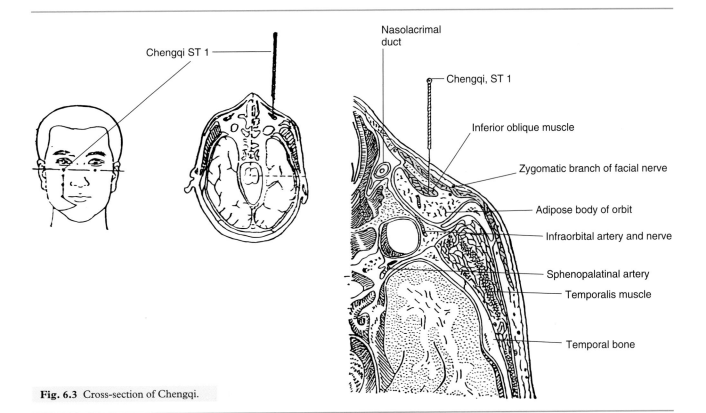

Fig. 6.3 Cross-section of Chengqi.

The external sclera of the eyeball is very strong and if the needle is inserted slowly, it is not easy to puncture through the sclera. However, it is very easy to puncture into the largest transverse diameter of the eyeball, the thinnest part of the sclera. If the needle is inserted into the eyeball, the patient must be transferred to a physician immediately.

c. *Puncture into common tendinous ring and optic nerve:* if the needle is inserted more than 4.5 cm (1.8 inches), it will puncture into the common tendinous ring and the optic nerve very easily. The optic nerve is covered by strong fibrous connective tissue, a continuation of the dura mater, and a sticky needle resistance will be felt if the needle punctures into the nerve. The patient may complain of flashes before the eyes, headache, dizziness, vomiting, and nausea. Withdraw the needle immediately, and treat the symptoms.

d. *Damaging ophthalmic artery:* the ophthalmic artery, together with the optic nerve, passes through the orbital cavity. The first part of the ophthalmic artery is at the inferior lateral side of the optic nerve, and then turns to the superior side of the nerve. Don't insert the needle more than 3.8 cm (1.5 inches), as it may puncture through the ophthalmic artery.

e. *Damaging superior orbital fissure and its contents:* if the needle is directed posteriorly and laterally more than 4.9 cm (1.93 inches) in men and 4.7 cm (1.85 inches) in women, it will puncture through the superior orbital fissure. The oculomotor nerve (CN III), the trochlear nerve (CN IV), the abducens nerve (CN VI), and the ophthalmic branch of the trigeminal nerve (CN V) pass through the superior orbital fissure. If the needle is inserted through the fissure, it may puncture into the cavernous sinus of the middle cranial fossa and damage the frontal lobe of the cerebrum, causing intracranial bleeding leading to dizziness, headache, nausea, vomiting, shock, or even death. The deeper the needle is penetrated and the heavier the manipulation, the more dangerous it is.

Functions
Expels Wind to activate the collaterals, improves acuity of vision.

Clinical indications
Myopia, optic nerve atrophy, spasm of orbicularis oculi muscle, keratitis.

3.

(SZUPAI) SIBAI, ST 2, FOOT YANG MING STOMACH MERIDIAN

Location
In a seated or supine position, the point is located with the eye looking straight ahead. It is directly inferior to the pupil at the midpoint between the lateral orbital angle and the tip of the nose, and in the fossa of the infraorbital foramen; or 0.3 inches below Chengqi (ST 1).

Needle and moxibustion method
Perpendicular insertion 0.2–0.3 inch.

Inferior oblique insertion along Yang Ming Stomach Meridian 1.0 inch (treating trigeminal neuralgia).
— *Needle sensation:* electrical sensation radiating to the upper lip.
WARNING: the point is in the infraorbital foramen, so don't insert too deeply.

Cross-sectional anatomy of the needle passage
(Fig. 6.4)
a. *Skin:* the infraorbital branches containing fibers from the maxillary branch of the trigeminal nerve (CN V) innervate the skin.
b. *Subcutaneous tissue:* includes the previously described skin nerve branches, and the zygomatic branches containing fibers from the facial nerve (CN VII). The infraorbital artery, a branch from the facial artery, supplies the subcutaneous tissue.
c. *Orbicularis oculi and levator labii superioris muscles:* the zygomatic and maxillary branches of the facial nerve (CN VII) innervate the orbicularis oculi muscle. The buccal branches of the facial nerve (CN VII) innervate the levator labii superioris muscle.
d. *Levator anguli oris muscle:* in the deep layer of the levator labii superioris muscle. Inferior oblique medial insertion of the needle can puncture into the muscle. The buccal branches containing fibers from the facial nerve (CN VII) innervate the muscle.
e. *Infraorbital foramen and maxilla:* inserting the needle into the three previously described muscles can treat facial palsy.

The structures surrounding the needle passage
The point is located at the infraorbital foramen, which contains the infraorbital artery and vein. If the needle is inserted directly into the foramen, it may damage the vessels, causing heavy bleeding.

Functions
Expels Wind to clear the collaterals, and improves acuity of vision.

Clinical indications

Facial palsy, facial muscle spasm, trigeminal neuralgia, conjunctivitis, myopia, acupunture anesthesia during eye operations.

4.

(JENYING) RENYING, ST 9, FOOT YANG MING STOMACH MERIDIAN

Location

In a seated or supine position, the point is located on the anterior margin of the sternocleidomastoid muscle, at the same height as the larynx. Press deep and feel the pulsation of the carotid artery. The needle is inserted medial to the carotid artery.

WARNING: Avoid puncturing the needle into the common carotid artery.

Needle and moxibustion method

Anterior or medial perpendicular insertion 0.2–0.4 inch.

— *Needle sensation:* local distension and soreness, or radiating to the shoulder.

— *Moxibustion dosage:* stick 10 minutes.

Cross-sectional anatomy of the needle passage

(Fig. 4.1)

a. *Skin:* the transverse nerve of the neck containing fibers from the cervical plexus of second and third cervical nerves (C2, C3) innervates the skin.

b. *Subcutaneous tissue:* includes the previously described skin nerve branches, and the platysma muscle. The cervical branches containing fibers from the facial nerve (CN VII) innervate the platysma muscle.

c. *Superficial layer of the deep cervical fascia:* the fascia covers the anterior margin of the sternocleidomastoid muscle. The deep layer of the fascia is very close to the carotid sheath.

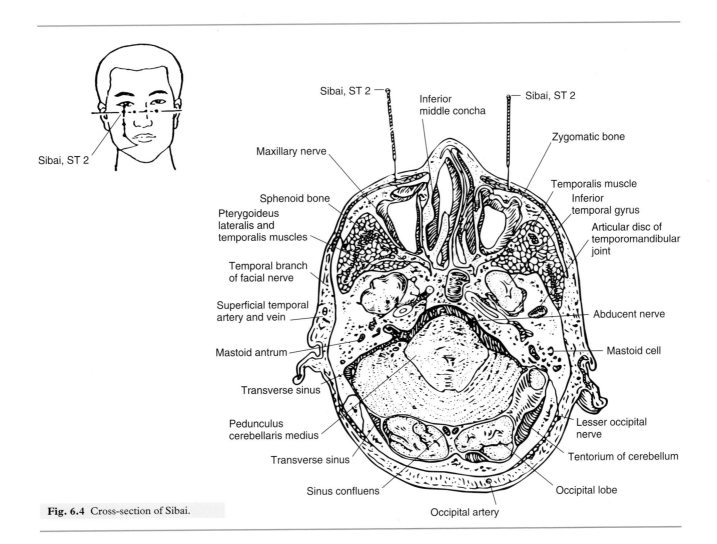

Fig. 6.4 Cross-section of Sibai.

d. *Constrictor pharynges muscle:* attached to the thyroid cartilage, a pharyngeal muscle. The pharyngeal branches containing fibers from the vagus nerve (CN X) innervate the muscle.

The structures surrounding the needle passage

a. *Sternocleidomastoid and infrahyoid muscles:* the needle is passed posteriorly and medially to the sternocleidomastoid muscle, and anteriorly and laterally to the infrahyoid muscle. The branches of the spinal accessory nerve (CN XI) innervate the sternocleidomastoid muscle. The branches of the hypoglossal nerve (CN XII) innervate the infrahyoid muscle.

b. *Carotid sheath:* the vessels and nerve are encircled by the carotid sheath which is formed by the deep cervical fascia, a connective tissue sheath. The needle is inserted anterior to the area covered by the sternocleidomastoid muscle. The carotid sheath contains the common carotid artery, the internal jugular vein, and the vagal nerve. The common carotid artery is located anteriorly and medially, the internal jugular vein posteriorly and laterally, and the vagal nerve posterior to the common carotid artery and the internal jugular vein.

   The correct direction of deep needle insertion for Renying [ST 9] is anterior and medial to the carotid sheath. If the needle is inserted in a lateral direction, it will puncture into the the common carotid artery, the largest artery of the neck. If the needle is inserted into the artery, an obvious pulsation will be felt. If the needle is inserted in a moderately lateral direction, it may pass posteriorly and laterally to the common carotid artery, through the internal jugular vein, and even into the vagal nerve, causing severe complications.

c. *Deep contents of the carotid artery sheath:* the deep carotid sheath consists of the sympathetic trunk, the deep cervical muscle, the vertebral artery, and the fourth cervical nerve. If the needle is not inserted more than 1 inch, it will not puncture these structures.

Complications, prevention and treatment

a. *Insertion into the common carotid artery:* this consists of dense connective tissue and thickened blood vessel wall. If the needle is inserted into the vessel, a resistance and an obvious pulsation are felt. Withdraw the needle immediately. The blood vessel wall is very strong so it is not easy to damage it. If bleeding is suspected, compress the vessel with the hand to prevent massive bleeding.

b. *Stimulating the vagal nerve:* if the needle is inserted in a moderately lateral direction, it will puncture through the internal jugular vein, and into the vagal nerve. The vein pressure is so low that there is seldom obvious bleeding. The vagal nerve contains the parasympathetic nerve fibers which regulate the heart beat. If the needle stimulates the nerve, it will suppress heart activity, causing a decrease in heart beat, coronary artery constriction, tachycardia, chest distress, facial pallor, or even death. To avoid this, don't insert the needle too laterally or too deeply, and don't manipulate too heavily.

Functions

Clears the channels to regulate the flow of Qi, reduces fever and relieves asthma.

Clinical indications

Hypertension, hypotension, asthma, hyperthyroidism, sore throat, hoarseness of the voice.

5.

(JINGBI) JINGBI, EX-HN 41, EXTRA POINT OF THE HEAD AND NECK

Location

One inch above the medial third of the clavicle, at the posterior margin of the clavicular head of the sternocleidomastoid muscle.

Needle and moxibustion method

Horizontal posterior perpendicular insertion 0.5–1.0 inch. Don't insert the needle in inferior oblique or inferior medial directions, as it may puncture into the pleura and the apex of the lung, causing pneumothorax.

Cross-sectional anatomy of the needle passage

(Fig. 6.5)

a. *Skin:* thin. The branches of the transverse nerve of the neck and the medial branches of the supraclavicular nerve from the brachial plexus of the third and fourth cervical nerves (C3, C4) innervate the skin.

b. *Subcutaneous tissue:* includes the previously described skin nerve branches, and the platysma muscle. The cervical branches containing fibers from the facial nerve (CN VII) innervate the platysma muscle. The external jugular vein passes proximal to the needle passage. Avoid puncturing the needle into the vein.

c. *Superior margin of clavicle and lateral side of clavicular head of sternocleidomastoid muscle:* the branches containing fibers from the spinal accessory nerve (CN XI) innervate the muscle.

d. *Brachial plexus and the margin of the anterior scalene muscle:* the needle is passed deep between the brachial plexus and the lateral margin of the anterior scalene muscle.

The fissure of the scalene muscle is surrounded by the anterior scalene, the middle scalene muscles, and the superior margin of the first rib. The brachial plexus and the subclavicular artery pass through the fissure of the scalene muscle to the axilla and are located superiorly and inferiorly, respectively.

The brachial plexus containing fibers from the anterior divisions of the fifth cervical to first thoracic nerves supplies the upper extremities and shoulders. After the brachial plexus passes through the fissure of the scalene muscle, it divides into the upper, middle, and lower trunks. The needle is passed towards the area of the upper trunk. If the needle is inserted into the brachial plexus, a very strong needle response radiates to the whole of the upper extremities.

e. *Middle and posterior scalene muscles:* these muscles are located posterior to the brachial plexus.

The structures surrounding the needle passage

a. *First rib:* the insertions of the anterior and middle scalene muscles are the scalene tuberosity and the middle part of the first rib. If the needle is inserted in an inferior oblique direction, it will puncture through the brachial plexus to the first rib. A strong needle response and needle resistance are felt.

b. *Cupola of the pleura and apex of the lung:* the cupola of the pleura is formed by the parietal pleura of the intrathoracic wall and the apex of the lung. The cupola of the pleura and the apex of the lung are located in the medial one third of the clavicle. They become dome-shaped at the superior aperture of the thorax, and are 2 or 3 centimeters (1 inch) above the clavicle, and are covered anteriorly and laterally by the anterior and middle scalene muscles. The needle passess very close to the cupola of the pleura and the apex of the lung. If the needle is inserted in a medial inferior direction, it may easily puncture through these structures.

Complications, prevention and treatment

As previously described, the direction of the needle must be controlled carefully. Don't insert the needle in inferior oblique or inferior medial directions, as it may puncture through the cupola of the pleura and the apex of the lung, causing pneumothorax. To avoid this complication, don't insert the needle deeply, especially in an emphysema patient. If the patient has difficulty in breathing after needle penetration, pneumothorax must be suspected.

Clinical indications

Arm numbness, paralysis of the upper extremities.

6.

(CHUEHPEN) QUEPEN, ST 12, FOOT YANG MING STOMACH MERIDIAN

Location

In a seated or supine position, the point is located in the middle of the supraclavicular fossa 4 inches lateral to the anterior midline directly above the nipples (male).

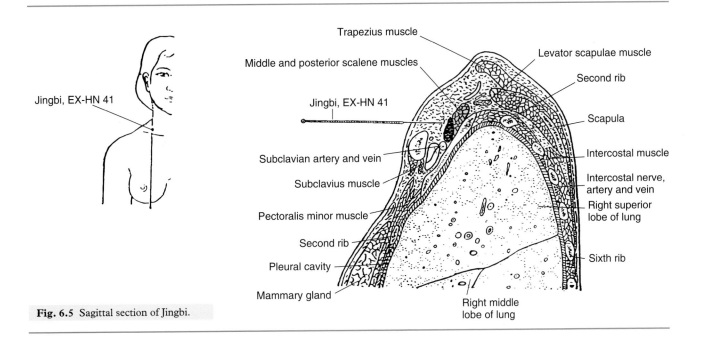

Fig. 6.5 Sagittal section of Jingbi.

Jingbi, EX-HN 41

Trapezius muscle

Middle and posterior scalene muscles

Levator scapulae muscle

Second rib

Jingbi, EX-HN 41

Scapula

Subclavian artery and vein

Intercostal muscle

Subclavius muscle

Intercostal nerve, artery and vein

Right superior lobe of lung

Pectoralis minor muscle

Second rib

Sixth rib

Pleural cavity

Mammary gland

Right middle lobe of lung

Needle and moxibustion method
Perpendicular insertion 0.3–0.4 inch.
WARNING: Don't insert the needle deeply.
— *Needle sensation:* local numbness and distension.
— *Moxibustion dosage:* 3–5 cones; stick 15 minutes.

Cross-sectional anatomy of the needle passage
(Fig. 6.6)
a. *Skin:* the supraclavicular branches containing fibers from the third and fourth cervical nerves (C3, C4) innervate the skin.
b. *Subcutaneous tissue:* includes the previously described skin nerve branches, and the platysma muscle. The platysma muscle is a cutaneous muscle, and is innervated by the cervical branches containing fibers from the facial nerve (CN VII).
c. *Trapezius muscle:* the needle is passed superior and anterior to the trapezius muscle which is located superior and posterior to the clavicle. The trapezius muscle is a superficial muscle of the back. The branches containing fibers from the spinal root of the spinal accessory nerve (CN XI) and the anterior branches containing fibers from the third and fourth cervical nerves (C3, C4) innervate the trapezius muscle.
d. *Subclavius muscle:* the needle is passed posterior to the subclavius muscle. The subclavicular branches of the brachial plexus containing fibers from the fifth

and sixth cervical nerves (C5, C6) innervate the muscle.
e. *Suprascapular artery, vein, and nerve:* the suprascapular artery is a branch of the thyrocervical trunk. The suprascapular vein, together with the suprascapular artery, joins the subclavian vein.

The structures surrounding the needle passage
The needle is inserted anterior to the trapezius muscle and between the clavicle and the subclavius and supraspinatus muscles. If the needle is inserted in a posterior inferior oblique direction, it will puncture through the supraspinatus muscle into the infraspinous fossa. If the needle is inserted in an inferior perpendicular direction, it will puncture into the suprascapular nerve and, if inserted deeply, anteriorly through the infraspinatus muscle to the anterior serratus muscle.

Complications, prevention and treatment
Don't insert the needle too deeply, as it may puncture through the anterior serratus muscle, the intercostal muscle, the parietal pleura, the pleural space and the visceral pleura into the lung, causing pneumothorax.

Functions
Soothes chest oppression, improves disorders of the diaphragm, and relieves cough and asthma.

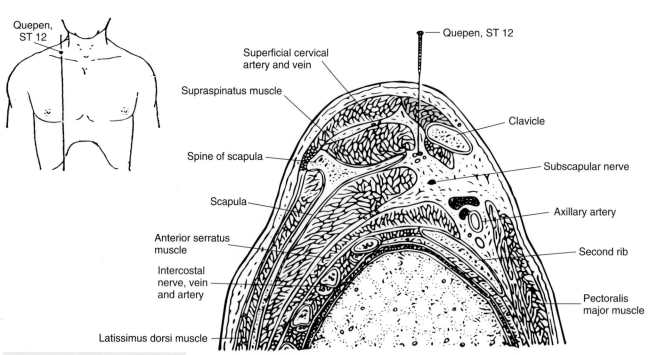

Fig. 6.6 Sagittal section of Quepen.

Clinical indications

Cough, asthma, shoulder pain, tuberculosis of the lymph nodes.

7.

(CHIENCHING) JIANJING, GB 21, FOOT SHAO YANG GALLBLADDER MERIDIAN

Location

In a seated position, the point is located on the shoulder at the midpoint between Dazhui [GV 14] and the acromion of the scapula.

Needle and moxibustion method

Perpendicular insertion 0.5–0.8 inch.
— *Needle sensation:* distension and soreness radiating to the dorsal shoulder.
— *Moxibustion dosage:* 3–7 cones; stick 15 minutes.

WARNING: Don't use deep perpendicular or deep anterior medial oblique insertion because of the risk of pneumothorax.

Cross-sectional anatomy of the needle passage

(Fig. 6.7)
a. *Skin:* the lateral branches containing fibers from the supraclavicular nerve innervate the skin.
b. *Subcutaneous tissue:* includes the previously described skin nerve branches. The transverse cervical artery supplies the tissue.
c. *Trapezius muscle:* the branches containing fibers from the spinal roots of the spinal accessory nerve (CN XI) innervate the muscle.

The structures surrounding the needle passage

a. *Anterior serratus muscle:* the anterior serratus muscle is located in the deep layer of the trapezius muscle. The point is located in the anterior serratus muscle

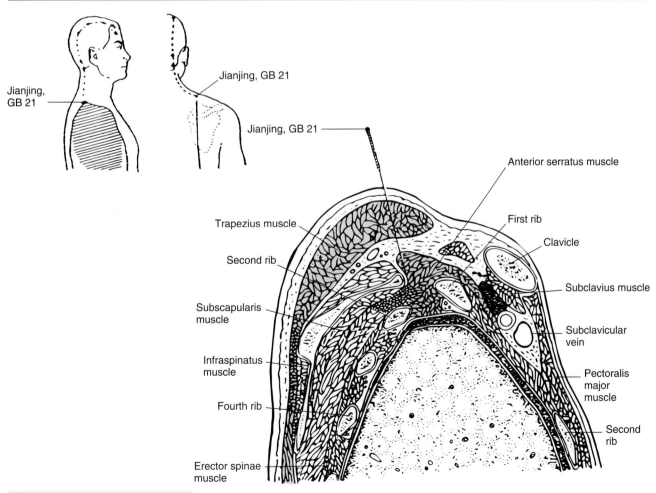

Fig. 6.7 Sagittal section of Jianjing.

between the first and second ribs.

b. *Ribs and intercostal space:* in the deep layer of the anterior serratus muscle. The positions from inferior to superior are the second rib, the first intercostal space, and the first rib. The intercostal space contains the external and internal intercostal muscles, and the intercostal artery and vein.

c. *Pleura and upper lobe of the lung:* the rib and the intercostal space are covered by the parietal pleura and the upper lobe of the lung.

d. *Cupola of pleura and apex of the lung:* if the needle is inserted in an anterior medial direction it may penetrate the cupola of the pleura and the apex of the lung.

Complications, prevention and treatment

If the needle is inserted deeply in the anterior inferior direction, it may elicit strong needle resistance when punctured towards the first and second ribs. If the needle is punctured through the first intercostal space, it may damage the parietal pleura and the upper lobe of the lung.

If the needle is inserted deeply in the anterior medial direction, it may pass superior to the first rib and may puncture through the cupola of the pleura and the apex of the lung, causing pneumothorax.

Functions

Clears the channels to regulate the flow of Qi, reduces Heat and removes masses.

Clinical indications

Hemiplegia, mastitis, functional uterine hemorrhage, tuberculosis of the lymph node, shoulder and back pain.

8.

(TIENTU) TIANTU, CV 22, CONCEPTION VESSEL

Location

In a seated or supine position, the point is located 0.5 inch above the middle of the fossa at the superior margin of the jugular notch of the sternum.

Needle and moxibustion method

Shallow insertion: perpendicular insertion 0.3–0.5 inches (child).
— *Needle sensation:* local soreness and distension.

Deep insertion: first perpendicular insertion 0.3 inch along the skin of the anterior neck to the posterior sternum, then inferior insertion 1.0–1.5 inches. Don't insert too deeply. The needle must be very close to the sternum, but should not penetrate from oblique to posterior direction and should not be too close to the trachea. In the inferior perpendicular direction, keep the needle central, and don't angle the needle to the right or left. If the needle is inserted deeply the patient may complain of throat tightness.
— *Needle sensation:* local distension and soreness, or a throat fullness that feels like suffocation.
— *Moxibustion method:* 3–5 cones; stick 15 minutes.

Cross-sectional anatomy of the needle passage
(Fig. 5.2)

a. *Skin:* the transverse nerve section of the anterior branches of the second and third cervical nerves (C2, C3) innervate the skin.

b. *Subcutaneous tissue:* includes loose connective tissue and adipose tissue and the previously described skin nerve branches. The inferior thyroid artery supplies the subcutaneous tissue. Some people have one superficial anterior cervical median vein in the anterior midline.

c. *Cervical line and sternothyroid muscle:* after the needle passes the subcutaneous tissue, it will reach the cervical line. The cervical line is composed of the deep fascia of the infrahyoid muscle. When the needle passes this layer, needle resistance is felt.

d. *Anterior space of trachea:* the space between the infrahyoid muscle and the cervical part of the trachea. It is filled with loose connective tissue. While deeply inserted, the needle changes its direction at this point to an inferior angle. The needle is inserted along the space at the superior aperture of the thorax, and penetrates inferiorly to the phlegmon and the thymus of the superior mediastinum. The needle sensation is a hollow feeling.

e. *Thymus:* a lymphatic organ with an endocrine function in the anterior and bilateral trachea. In the adult it is atrophied, becoming adipose tissue and lacking blood vessels. The branches containing fibers from the vagus nerve and sympathetic trunk supply the gland. The sensory branches containing fibers from the phrenic nerve supply the capsule.

The structures surrounding the needle passage

a. *Trachea:* if the needle is inserted perpendicularly more than 0.5 inch, it may puncture into the cartilage rings and the ligaments between the cartilage rings of the trachea. If the needle punctures the cartilage of the trachea, it will elicit a strong resistance. If the needle punctures through the ligament between the cartilage rings, the needle will feel sticky. If the needle punctures the mucosa of the trachea, it may cause severe cough.

b. *Aortic arch, brachiocephalic artery and left common carotid artery:* the aortic arch and its branches are located anterior and lateral to the trachea. If the needle is inserted in a slightly oblique posterior direction, it may puncture into the aortic arch. If the needle is inserted in an obliquely lateral direction, it may puncture into the brachiocephalic and common carotid arteries at the right and left, respectively. Because these three arteries are very large, obvious pulsation is felt when puncturing the vessels.

c. *Prezone of pleura and anterior margin of lung:* if the needle is inserted too deeply at the same height as the sternal angle, it may puncture into the anterior margin of the lung. If the needle is inserted in the bilateral direction or during treatment of an emphysema patient, don't insert deeply as it is much easier to puncture into the anterior margin of the lung.

Complications, prevention and treatment

a. If perpendicular insertion of the needle is too deep and punctures the cartilage of the trachea, slightly withdraw the needle, and it will not affect the treatment. If the needle is inserted into the ligament between the cartilage rings of the trachea, it may puncture through the tracheal wall and damage the mucosa of the trachea. A severe cough may result. Withdraw the needle immediately. Usually there is no severe complication.

b. On posterior deep insertion, the needle may puncture into the aortic arch and its branches. The pulsation is very obvious and the needle must be withdrawn immediately. Usually there is no severe complication such as bleeding.

If the patient complains of chest tightness and pain he or she must be observed very carefully. If there is any suspicion of massive bleeding, transfer the patient to a hospital. To prevent this complication, don't puncture the needle too deeply in a posterior direction.

c. *Puncture of the prezone of the lung causing pneumothorax:* this usually happens if the needle is inserted too deeply and in too posterior a direction to the sternum or in a bilateral direction. If the patient has suspected emphysema, don't insert deeply. If the patient complains of gradual difficulty in breathing, after the needle is inserted, pneumothorax must be suspected and the patient should be referred to hospital.

Functions

Regulates the function of the Lung to relieve asthma, reduces Heat and removes Dampness.

Clinical indications

Bronchial asthma, acute and chronic bronchitis, pharyngitis, hiccough.

9.

(FENGCHIH) FENGCHI, GB 20, FOOT SHAO YANG GALLBLADDER MERIDIAN

Location

In a seated position and with the head bent forward, the point is located at the posterior, lateral aspect of the neck at the same height as Fengfu [GV 16], in the fossa between the superior margins of the trapezius and sternocleidomastoid muscles.

Needle and moxibustion method

The needle is directed towards the medial canthus of the eye on the opposite side: perpendicular insertion 0.8–1.0 inch.
— *Needle sensation:* local distension and soreness radiating to the top of the head, lateral head, front of the head, or the orbital region.
— *Moxibustion dosage:* 3–7 cones; stick 10–15 minutes.

Cross-sectional anatomy of the needle passage
(Fig. 6.8)

a. *Skin:* the lesser occipital branches of the third cervical nerve (C3) innervate the skin.

b. *Subcutaneous tissue:* consists of adipose tissue and fibrous connective tissue and includes the previously described skin nerve branches, and the subcutaneous vein.

c. *Lateral side of trapezius muscle:* the branches containing fibers from the spinal roots of the spinal accessory nerve (CN XI) innervate the muscle which consists of connective tissue. The needle response and resistance are less strong than the skin.

d. *Splenius muscle:* the superficial layer of the splenius muscle is very close to the sternocleidomastoid and trapezius muscles. The posterior branches containing fibers from the lateral divisions of the second to fifth cervical nerves innervate the muscle. The needle is inserted lateral and superior to the muscle.

e. *Semispinalis capitis muscle:* the muscle is located at the deep layer of the splenius muscle. The branches containing fibers from the dorsal divisions of the thoracic nerve innervate the muscle.

f. *Occipital triangle:* at the deep layer of the semispinalis capitis muscle. It is filled with adipose connective tissue. The occipital nerve innervates the occipital triangle and the needle is passed through the midpoint of the lateral margin of the triangle. It is much safer not to insert the needle through the triangle.

The structures surrounding the needle passage
(The surrounding structures at the deep midpoint of the lateral margin of the suboccipital triangle.)

a. *Deep layer:* the atlanto-occipital articulation is

composed of the occipital condyle and the superior articular fovea of the atlas. The posterior atlanto-occipital membrane is located medially posterior to the joint capsule. At the medial side of the joint capsule and behind the posterior atlanto-occipital membrane is the base of the medulla. The vertebral artery passes lateral to the joint capsule.

b. *Superior side:* occipital condyle. It is oval-shaped and located lateral to the occipital magnum.

c. *Inferior side:* lateral mass of the atlas. It is located in the anterior and posterior arches of the atlas forming a kidney-shaped joint fossa, and articulates with the occipital condyle.

Complications, prevention and treatment

The deep layer contains important structures such as the medulla and the vertebral artery located at the medial and lateral parts of the atlanto-occipital joint, respectively. The depth from the skin to these structures is about 1.5 inches on average so it is much safer not to puncture the needle more than 1.2 inches. The correct direction is to insert the needle towards the ipsilateral atlanto-occipital articulation. If the needle is inserted contralaterally towards the lateral angle of the opposite eye, the needle may puncture into the medulla. Because the superficial to deep layers of the needle passage are the occipital triangle, the posterior

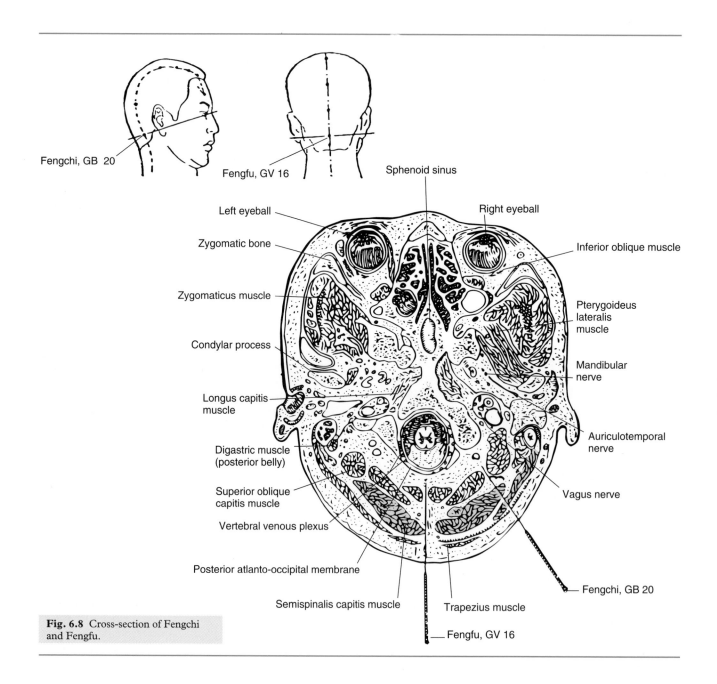

Fig. 6.8 Cross-section of Fengchi and Fengfu.

Fengchi, GB 20

Fengfu, GV 16

Sphenoid sinus

Left eyeball

Right eyeball

Zygomatic bone

Inferior oblique muscle

Zygomaticus muscle

Pterygoideus lateralis muscle

Condylar process

Mandibular nerve

Longus capitis muscle

Auriculotemporal nerve

Digastric muscle (posterior belly)

Vagus nerve

Superior oblique capitis muscle

Fengchi, GB 20

Vertebral venous plexus

Posterior atlanto-occipital membrane

Semispinalis capitis muscle

Trapezius muscle

Fengfu, GV 16

atlanto-occipital membrane, the dura mater and the medulla, the needle responses are soft resistance, strong resistance, breakthrough sensation and soft resistance, respectively.

If the needle is inserted into the medulla, the patient may complain of body-wide electrical sensation and may exhibit panic, crying and mental disturbance. Mild symptoms are neck stiffness, dizziness, panic, sweating, and vomiting. If the patient is not treated immediately, difficulty of breathing and coma may ensue. Cardio-pulmonary resuscitation must be applied to the patient immediately or death may become inevitable.

If the needle is inserted ipsilaterally to the medial angle of the eye, the direction of the needle is towards the ipsilateral vertebral artery. To avoid damaging the artery, don't insert the needle too deeply, or lift, thrust, or twirl the needle too vigorously. If the needle punctures into the vertebral artery, a pulsation will be felt. Withdraw the needle immediately for a few minutes. The patient may complain of headache, dizzi-ness, and decreasing blood pressure, in which case vertebral artery bleeding must be suspected. Use a local cold pad to prevent further bleeding.

Functions
Dispels Wind to remove Exterior Syndromes, and refreshes the Mind.

Clinical indications
Sequelae of cerebrovascular accident, neuropsychosis, epilepsy, neurological headache, common cold, rhinitis, hypertension.

10.

(FENGFU) FENGFU, GV 16, GOVERNING VESSEL

Location
In a seated position with the head bent forward, the point is located on the posterior midline in the inferior fossa of the external occipital protuberance of the occipital bone.

Needle and moxibustion method
Perpendicular insertion in the direction of the mental protuberance of the mandible 0.5–1.0 inch.
— *Needle sensation:* local distension and numbness radiating to the head.
— *Moxibustion dosage:* 3–5 cones.
Slow insertion. No thrusting or twirling permitted.

Cross-sectional anatomy of the needle passage
(Figs 6.8 & 6.9)
a. *Skin:* thickened, causing moderate needle resistance. The greater occipital branch of the second cervical nerve (C2) and the third occipital branch of the third cervical nerve (C3) innervate the skin.
b. *Subcutaneous tissue:* thickened, with a large amount of loose connective tissue and adipose tissue. The cutaneous branches of the second and third cervical nerves, and the subcutaneous vein pass through the tissue. The resistance of the needle passage through this layer is less than that of the skin.
c. *Nuchal ligament:* a triangular elastic fibrous membrane of dense connective tissue. A strong resis-

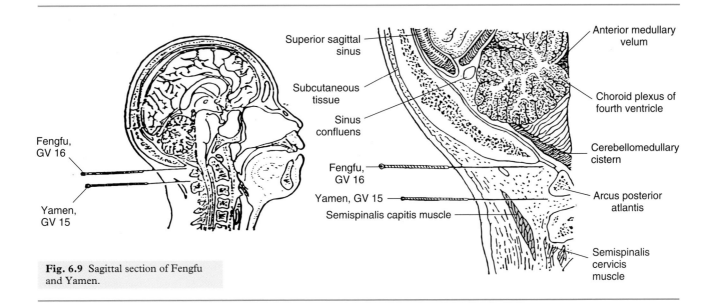

Fig. 6.9 Sagittal section of Fengfu and Yamen.

tance to the needle passage are felt. The needle should not puncture through this ligament.

The structures surrounding the needle passage

a. *Deep layer:* the deep layers of the nuchal ligament from superficial to deep are the posterior atlanto-occipital membrane, the dura mater, the arachnoid, the pia mater, and the medulla.

   i. *Posterior atlanto-occipital membrane:* a dense connective tissue membrane situated between the posterior margin of the foramen magnum and the superior margin of the posterior atlantis arch. Anteriorly attached to the dura mater.

   ii. *Dura mater:* external membrane of the brain and the spinal cord, thickened and strong. It consists of collagenous and elastic fibers.

   iii. *Arachnoid:* a thin transparent connective tissue membrane, the middle membrane of the brain and the spinal cord.

   iv. *Pia mater:* attached to the surface of the brain and the spinal cord. Between the arachnoid and pia mater is the subarachnoid space, which is filled with the cerebrospinal fluid. The subarachnoid space of the dorsal medulla is expanded to become a cerebellomedullary cistern.

   v. *Medulla:* inferior part of the brain stem, in the foramen magnum continuing to the spinal cord. The major functions of the medulla are regulation of the respiratory, vomiting and cardiovascular centers.

b. *Superior part:* the posterior margin of the foramen magnum.

c. *Inferior part:* the posterior atlantis tubercle. The anterior and posterior arches of the atlas are fused to become the posterior atlantis tubercle.

d. *Lateral part:* the vertebral artery and the suboccipital nerve. The vertebral artery passes and ascends up the posterior atlanto-occipital arch and the attached lateral mass of the posterior part of the vertebral groove and then, via the foramen magnum, it enters the cranial cavity.

Complications, prevention and treatment

The point is located in the back of the neck where there are very important structures. It is much safer not to puncture the needle more than 1.5 inches, in order to avoid the posterior atlanto-occipital membrane, the dura mater, the arachnoid and the pia mater and the medulla. If the needle is inserted through the posterior atlanto-occipital membrane, the subarachnoid space and into the medulla, strong needle resistance, a breakthrough sensation and a soft sensation respectively are felt. At the same time, the patient will complain of an electrical sensation and may exhibit panic, crying, and mental disturbance. The mild symptoms are neck stiff-ness, dizziness, panic, sweating, and vomiting. If the patient is not treated immediately, difficulty of breathing and coma may ensue. If these symptoms are shown, withdraw the needle immediately or death may become inevitable.

It is much safer to puncture the needle in the direction of the mental protuberance of the mandible. Don't insert the needle in the direction of the nose, as it may puncture into the medulla. If the needle is inserted too laterally, it is very easy to puncture into the vertebral artery. A pulsation of the needle will be felt. Withdraw the needle immediately, and press the point for a few minutes. If the vertebral artery is still bleeding, use an ice bag compress to decrease bleeding. The patient may complain of headache, dizziness, and decreasing blood pressure.

Functions

Reduces fever and dispels Wind, and refreshes the brain to induce resuscitation.

Clinical indications

Sequelae of cerebrovascular disease, epilepsy, hysteria, neurologic headache, spondylitis, neck strain.

11.

(YAMEN) YAMEN, GV 15, GOVERNING VESSEL

Location

In a seated position and with the head bent forward, the point is located on the posterior midline in the superior margin of the spinous process of the axis.

Needle and moxibustion method

Perpendicular insertion along the superior margin of the spinous process of the second cervical vertebra 0.5–1.2 inches.

Inferior oblique insertion 0.5–1.0 inch.

— *Needle sensation:* If an electrical shock is felt, the needle must be withdrawn immediately.

— *Moxibustion dosage:* 3–5 cones.

Cross-sectional anatomy of the needle passage

(Fig. 6.9)

a. *Skin:* thickened, with hair. The greater occipital branches of the second cervical nerve (C2), and the third occipital branch of the third cervical nerve (C3) innervate the skin.

b. *Subcutaneous tissue:* thickened. It includes the previously described skin nerve branches, and the subcutaneous vein. It consists of loose connective tissue and adipose tissue. When the needle is inserted, a weak resistance is felt.

c. *Trapezius muscle:* the needle is passed between the right and left trapezius muscles. The branches containing fibers from the spinal accessory nerve (CN XI), and the anterior divisions of the third and fourth cervical nerves (C3, C4) innervate the muscle.

d. *Nuchal ligament:* a triangular elastic fibrous membrane of dense connective tissue. A strong resistance to the needle passage is felt.

e. *Splenius muscle:* the needle is passed between the right and left splenius muscles.The dorsal branches containing fibers from the cervical nerve innervate the muscle.

f. *Semispinalis capitis muscle:* the needle is passed between right and left semispinalis capitis muscles. The dorsal branches containing fibers from the cervical nerve innervate the muscle.

The structures surrounding the needle passage

a. *Deep layer:* the structures from superficial to deep layers are the posterior atlanto-occipital membrane, the dura mater, the arachnoid, the pia mater, and the medulla.

    i. *Posterior atlanto-occipital membrane:* thin and broad. At the deep layer of the nuchal ligament, and between the atlas and the axis. A weak resistance to the needle passage is felt.

    ii. *Dura mater:* the external membrane of the spinal cords, thickened and strong. Between the dura mater and the periosteum of the innervate side of the vertebral canal is the epidural space which is filled with connective tissue and veins.

    iii. *Arachnoid mater:* thin and reticular connective tissue. Between the arachnoid and the pia mater is subarachnoid space which is filled with cerebrospinal fluid. A sudden decrease in resistance is felt if the needle is punctured through this structure.

    iv. *Pia mater:* a thin membrane rich with blood vessels, and closely attached to the spinal cord.

    v. *Spinal cord:* in the vertebral canal. It is a continuation of the medulla. A soft resistance is felt if the needle is punctured into the spinal cord.

b. *Superior part:* the posterior tubercle of the atlas.

c. *Inferior part:* the spinous process of the axis.

d. *Bilateral part:* first intervertebral joint which is composed of the inferior articular facet of the atlas and the superior articular facet of the axis.

Complications, prevention and treatment

Because the deep layer of the point consists of important vital organs such as the spinal cord, don't insert the needle more than 1.5 inches. Insert the needle slowly, or it may penetrate through the dorsal atlanto-epistrophic membrane into the spinal cord in the neck. The patient may complain of an electrical shock from the neck to the coccyx or even to all the extremities. Some patients don't have any symptoms, and some have mild symptoms such as headache, dizziness, and vomiting. Withdraw the needle immediately. Other complications include subarachnoid hemorrhage and damage to the spinal cord. The patient may complain of severe headache, vomiting, or even functional disturbance of the extremities. Observe the patient carefully, and treat appropriately according to symptoms.

If the needle is inserted in the direction of the nose, it may puncture through the posterior atlanto-occipital membrane into the medulla. The patient may complain of an electrical sensation and exhibit panic, crying, and mental disturbance. A mild symptom is neck stiffness. If the patient is not treated immediately, difficulty of breathing and coma may ensue. Withdraw the needle immediately. Cardiovascular resuscitation must be applied without delay if necessary or death may become inevitable.

If the needle is inserted in a lateral direction, it may puncture into the first intervertebral joint. No symptoms will be shown.

If the needle is inserted in an inferior oblique direction it may reach the vertebral arch and the spinous process of the axis. No symptoms will be observed.

Functions

Tranquilizes the Mind to stop convulsions, and invigorates the power of speech.

Clinical indications

Cerebrovascular disease, hysteria, epilepsy, schizophrenia, cerebral dysgenesis, deafness, neurogenic headache, hoarseness of the voice, epistaxis, soft tissue damage of the neck.

12.

(JUKEN) RUGEN, ST 18, FOOT YANG MING STOMACH MERIDIAN

Location

In a supine position, the point is located in the fifth intercostal space directly below the nipple, 4 inches beside the mid-abdominal line.

Needle and moxibustion method

Oblique insertion 0.5–1.0 inch.

— *Needle sensation:* local distension and pain.

— *Moxibustion dosage:* 3–5 cones; stick 15 minutes.

Cross-sectional anatomy of the needle passage
(Figs 6.10 & 6.11)

a. *Skin:* the cutaneous branches containing fibers from the fourth to sixth intercostal nerves innervate the skin.

b. *Subcutaneous tissue:* thickened cellular tissue. It includes the cutaneous branches of the intercostal nerve, and the cutaneous veins. The point in the female is within breast tissue which consists of cellular adipose tissue and the saccular lobule. Slight resistance to the needle passage is felt.

c. *Pectoralis major muscle and lateral margin of pectoralis major muscle:* the branches of the medial and lateral anterior thoracic nerves containing fibers from the fifth cervical to first thoracic nerves (C5–T1) innervate the muscle. The needle resistance at this level is stronger than that of the skin.

d. *Internal and external intercostal muscles:* at the intercostal space between two ribs. The branches containing fibers from the intercostal nerve innervate the muscle. The deep layer of the internal and external intercostal muscles is fascia and the lung so do not puncture through these muscles.

The structures surrounding the needle passage

a. *Deep layer:* the deep layer structures from superficial to deep are the endothoracic fascia, the costal pleura, and the lung.

   i. *Endothoracic fascia:* a thin connective tissue attached to the inner side of the chest wall.

   ii. *Costal pleura:* closely attached to the deep layer of the endothoracic fascia. The branches containing fibers from the intercostal nerve innervate the fascia. Because this layer is rich in nerve tissues, it is very sensitive. The pleural cavity is composed of an outer parietal and inner visceral pleural. During inspiration the pleural space diminishes and the two layers of the pleura are almost closed together, so it is very easy on the inbreath to puncture the needle into and damage the pleura and the lung.

   iii. *Lung:* in the thoracic cavity. The lung is supplied by the vagal nerve and the phrenic nerve. If the needle penetrates into the lung, no obvious pain will be felt. Because the lung is mostly composed of alveoli, no resistance or a hollow needle sensation is felt if the needle is passed into the lung.

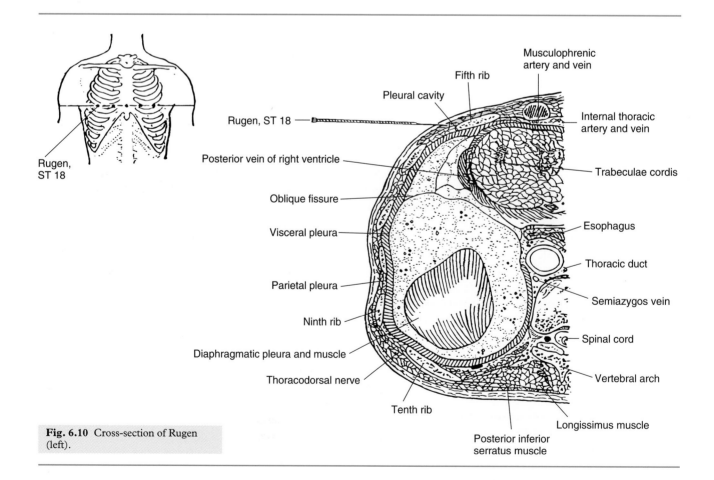

Fig. 6.10 Cross-section of Rugen (left).

b. The superior and inferior parts of the internal intercostal muscle, and the superior and inferior ribs. If the needle is inserted to the ribs, a strong resistance is felt.

Complications, prevention and treatment

Directly beneath the point is the lung so oblique insertion is better than perpendicular insertion. The angle between the needle and skin should not be greater than 25° as a steeper angle may puncture through the lung, causing pneumothorax. Mild symptoms are cough, chest tightness, and chest pain and a small pneumothorax may heal spontaneously. Severe symptoms are progressive respiratory difficulty and cyanosis and tension pneumothorax may cause tachycardia, hypotension, and shock. The standard pneumothorax treatment must be applied to prevent shock or respiratory failure may ensue, endangering the patient's life.

Functions

Promotes lactation, and increases Blood circulation to remove Blood Stasis.

Clinical indications

Bronchitis, intercostal neuralgia, mastitis.

13.

(JIHYUEH) RIYUE, GB 24, FOOT SHAO YIN GALLBLADDER MERIDIAN, FRONT-MU POINT OF THE GALLBLADDER

Location

In a supine position, the point is located in the seventh intercostal space directly below the nipple, and in the midclavicular line.

Needle and moxibustion method

Oblique insertion 0.5–0.8 inch.
— *Needle sensation:* local numbness and distension.
— *Moxibustion dosage:* 3–5 cones; stick 10 minutes.

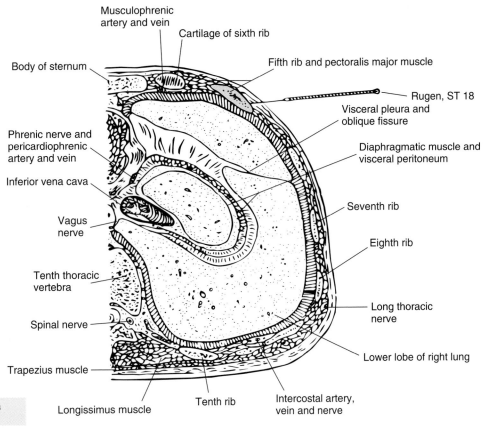

Fig. 6.11 Cross-section of Rugen (right).

Labels: Musculophrenic artery and vein · Cartilage of sixth rib · Body of sternum · Fifth rib and pectoralis major muscle · Rugen, ST 18 · Visceral pleura and oblique fissure · Phrenic nerve and pericardiophrenic artery and vein · Diaphragmatic muscle and visceral peritoneum · Inferior vena cava · Seventh rib · Vagus nerve · Eighth rib · Tenth thoracic vertebra · Spinal nerve · Long thoracic nerve · Trapezius muscle · Lower lobe of right lung · Longissimus muscle · Tenth rib · Intercostal artery, vein and nerve

Cross-sectional anatomy of the needle passage
(Fig. 5.5)

a. *Skin:* thin and well supplied with nerves. The cutaneous intercostal branches of the thoracic nerve innervate the skin.

b. *Subcutaneous tissue:* includes the cutaneous branches of the intercostal nerve and cutaneous veins. Mild needle resistance is felt at this level.

c. *External oblique muscle:* the superficial layer of the anterior external abdominal wall. The needle is passed through the origins of the external oblique muscle at the seventh and eighth ribs.

d. *External intercostal muscle:* the superficial layer of the intercostal space. The branches of the intercostal nerve innervate the muscle.

e. *Internal intercostal muscle:* the deep layer of the external intercostal muscle. The branches of the intercostal nerve innervate the muscle.

f. *Transversus muscle:* in the deepest layer of the anterior external abdominal wall. To avoid damage to the internal organs, don't puncture the needle through this muscle.

The structures surrounding the needle passage
The structures from superficial to deep are endo-thoracic fascia, costal pleura, costophrenic sinus, diaphragm, and the liver or stomach.

a. *Endothoracic fascia:* covering the inner part of the thoracic wall and continuing to the diaphragmatic fascia of the diaphragm.

b. *Costal pleura:* inner part of endothoracic fascia and rich with nerve tissue.

c. *Costophrenic sinus:* a space at the corner between the costal and parietal pleura.

d. *Diaphragm:* between the thoracic and abdominal cavity. A dome-shaped flat muscle with the concave side facing down, attached to the costal and parietal pleura superficially. The phrenic branches from the third to fifth cervical nerves innervate the muscle.

e. *Liver:* just below the diaphragm. The largest organ in the body. The right Riyue [GB 24] is at the anterior margin of the liver. The liver is innervated by the splanchnic nerve and is not very sensitive to pain.

f. *Stomach:* the stomach, a hollow organ, is in the deep layer of the left Riyue [GB 24]. The point is located in the greater curvature near the fundus of the stomach. The splanchnic nerve innervates the stomach.

Complications, prevention and treatment
The thoracic wall at the point is very thin, and the deep layer has many important vital organs so don't use perpendicular insertion. The angle between the needle and the skin should not be greater than 25° as a steeper angle may puncture into the thoracic cavity. If needle resistance suddenly disappears and a hollow needle sensation is felt, withdraw the needle immediately. If the needle is inserted further, it will puncture through the diaphragm into the liver and the stomach at the right and left, respectively. Usually the patient will feel nothing or only slight pain.

Hard thrusting or twirling of the needle may damage the liver and the stomach. The complications of liver damage are pain in the liver region, or a small mass of blood or bile. If the liver capsule is damaged, a small amount of blood or bile may drain into the peritoneal cavity, irritating the peritoneum and causing tension and pain at the right upper hypochondriac region. The severe complication of stomach damage is a small amount of stomach contents draining into the peritoneal cavity, irritating the peritoneum and causing tension and pain in the left upper hypochondriac region. As the liver and stomach are large organs, medial, lateral, or inferior oblique deep insertion may puncture them. Superior oblique insertion may pass under the seventh rib, and oblique insertion can pass through the costophrenic sinuses both causing pneumothorax.

Functions
Clears Heat from the Liver and the Gallbladder, treats hiccup and stops vomiting.

Clinical indications
Hepatitis, gastritis, cholecystitis, intercostal neuralgia, periarthritis of shoulder.

14.

(HSINSHU) XINSHU, BL 15, FOOT TAI YANG BLADDER MERIDIAN, BACK-SHU POINT OF THE HEART

Location
In a prone position, the point is located in the inferior part of the spinous process of the fifth thoracic bone, and 1.5 inches lateral to Shendao [GV 11].

Needle and moxibustion method
Medial perpendicular insertion 0.5–1.0 inch.
— *Needle sensation:* local distension and soreness, sometimes radiating to the intercostal rib.
— *Moxibustion dosage:* 3–5 cones; stick 10 minutes.

Cross-sectional anatomy of the needle passage
(Fig. 5.6)

a. *Skin:* the cutaneous branches containing fibers from the dorsal division of the fifth thoracic nerve innervate the skin.

b. *Subcutaneous tissue:* includes the previously described skin nerve branches, and the subcutaneous vein.

c. *Trapezius muscle:* superficial muscle of the back. The needle is inserted at the transition part of the muscular and tendon parts of the trapezius muscle. The needle resistance is stronger than the skin. The branches containing fibers from the spinal accessory nerve (CN XI) innervate the muscle.

d. *Rhomboid muscle:* at a deeper layer than the trapezius muscle. The dorsal scapular branches of the fourth to sixth cervical nerves (C4, C5, C6) innervate the muscle. The needle is inserted at the inferior margin of the muscle.

e. *Sacrospinalis (erector spinae) muscle:* in the bilateral parts of the spinal vertebra and the deeper muscle of the back. The dorsal primary branches of the spinal nerves innervate the muscle. The muscular groups consist of the iliocostocervicalis muscle anteriorly, the spinalis muscle posteriorly, and the longissimus muscle in the middle. The needle is inserted into the longissimus muscle. It is much safer not to puncture the needle through the muscle.

The structures surrounding the needle passage

The deepest surrounding structures of the point with perpendicular insertion.

a. *Deep part:* the deep layers of the sacrospinalis muscle from superficial to deep are the levator muscle of the ribs, the internal intercostal ligaments, the endothoracic fascia, the costal pleura, and the lung.

   i. *Levator muscle of ribs:* on both sides of the spine. The point is located at the lateral margin of the muscle.

   ii. *Internal intercostal ligaments:* underneath the levator muscle of the ribs. The internal intercostal muscle transits posteriorly in the costal angle to become the aponeurosis. It is a thin connective tissue membrane.

   iii. *Endothoracic fascia:* on the medial side of the thoracic wall. The superficial and deep layers are the internal intercostal ligament and costal pleura, which are closely attached to the endothoracic fascia. Only a slight needle resistance is felt. As the deeper structure is the pleural space, a sudden hollow sensation is felt when the needle punctures into the space.

   iv. *Lung:* branches containing fibers from the splanchnic nerve supply the lung nerve. This nerve is not very sensitive to pain. The lung is mainly composed of alveoli, so only slight resistance and a sudden hollow sensation are felt on needle puncture.

b. *Upper part:* the transverse process articulation of the fifth rib, which is also reinforced by the ligaments, is composed of the articulate part of the tubercle of the fifth rib and the transverse costal fovea of the fifth thoracic vertebra. If the needle is inserted in the superior oblique direction, it may penetrate to the joint. A strong needle resistance is felt.

c. *Inferior part:* the transverse process articulation of the sixth rib.

d. *Lateral part:* the lateral intercostal muscle and the internal intercostal ligament.

e. *Medial part:* the thoracic vertebral arch.

Complications, prevention and treatment

Because the lung underlies the point, the needle should not puncture perpendicularly deeper than 1.0 inch. It is much safer to insert the needle in the medial oblique direction (towards the spine).

If the needle punctures the lung, pneumothorax may result. Mild symptoms are cough, chest tightness, and chest pain and a small pneumothorax may heal spontaneously. Severe symptoms are progressive respiratory difficulty and cyanosis. Tension pneumothorax may cause tachycardia, hypotension, and shock.

Functions

Regulates the function of the Heart meridian, and relieves mental stress.

Clinical indications

Heart problems such as atrial fibrillation and tachycardia, intercostal neuralgia, soft tissue injury of the back.

15.

(HUANGMEN) HUANGMEN, BL 51, FOOT TAI YANG BLADDER MERIDIAN

Location

In a prone position, the point is located level with the inferior border of the spinous process of the first lumbar vertebra, and 3 inches lateral to the midline of the back.

Needle and moxibustion method

Perpendicular insertion 0.6–1.0 inch.
— *Needle sensation:* local numbness and distension.
— *Moxibustion dosage:* 3–5 cones; stick 10 minutes.

Cross-sectional anatomy of the needle passage

(Fig. 6.12)

a. *Skin:* the lateral branches of the dorsal division of the first lumbar nerve (L1) innervate the skin.

b. *Subcutaneous tissue:* thickened. If includes cutaneous branches containing fibers from the twelfth thoracic nerve, and the subcutaneous vein.

c. *Latissimus dorsi muscle:* a superficial muscle. The thoracodorsal branches of the fifth to seventh cervical nerves (C5, C6, C7) innervate the muscle. The needle is inserted at the external inferior margin of the muscle. The point is located at the transition point between the muscular and tendinous parts of the latissimus muscle.

d. *Inferior posterior serratus muscle:* in the deeper layer of the latissimus dorsi muscle. The needle is inserted at the inferior margin of the muscle.

e. *Superficial layer of thoracolumbar fascia:* a dense connective tissue. The point includes the deep layer of the fascia of the inferior posterior serratus muscle.

f. *Sacrospinalis (erector spinae) muscle:* a deep muscle of the back. The dorsal primary branches of the spinal nerve innervate the muscle. The needle is inserted at the lateral part of the muscle. A moderate needle resistance is felt on needle insertion.

g. *Deep layer of thoracolumbar fascia:* in the deep layer of the sacrospinalis muscle, a thin connective tissue membrane.

h. *Quadratus lumborum muscle:* rectangular muscle at the posterior abdominal wall. Separated by the deep layer of the thoracolumbar fascia and the sacrospinalis muscle. The branches containing fibers from the twelfth thoracic and first lumbar nerves (T12, L1) innervate the muscle. The needle is inserted at the lateral margin of the muscle. In order to avoid puncturing into the kidney and the surrounding structures, don't penetrate the muscle deeply.

The structures surrounding the needle passage

a. *Deep part:* the structures from the superficial to deep layers are the lumbar fascia, the kidney fascia, the adipose capsule of the kidney, the renal fibrous membrane, and the kidney.

  i. *Lumbar fascia:* intra-abdominal fascia attached to the lumbar area. The upper part of the lumbar fascia becomes the diaphragmatic fascia whilst the lower parts become the pelvic fascia.

  ii. *Kidney fascia:* the external connective fascia membrane of the kidney. Kidney fascia is fixed to and protects the kidney.

  iii. *Adipose capsule of the kidney:* adipose tissue between the kidney fascia and the renal fibrous membrane. A hollow needle resistance is felt if inserted to this level.

  iv. *Renal fibrous membrane:* fixed fibrous membrane of the kidney, closely attached to the external kidney.

  v. *Kidney:* covered by the fascia, the adipose capsule, and the fibrous membrane. The point is located at the inferior border of the left kidney, and the middle part of the right kidney.

b. *Superior part:* at the twelfth rib attached to the diaphragm. The anterior costodiaphragmatic recess, elongated from the pleural cavity, is attached to the diaphragm and the superior part of the kidney. The needle can be punctured superiorly through the costodiaphragmatic recess, the diaphragm, and into the kidney.

c. *Inferior part:* the right Huangmen [BL 51] is level with the inferior border of the kidney, and the left

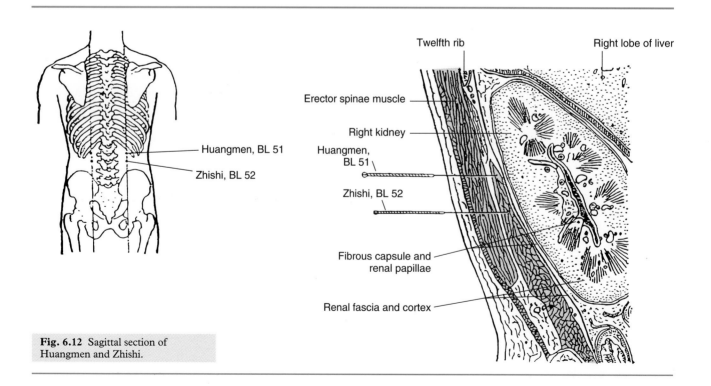

Fig. 6.12 Sagittal section of Huangmen and Zhishi.

Huangmen [BL 51] is over the colon. If the needle is punctured too deeply, it will penetrate into the kidney and the colon on the right and left sides, respectively.

d. *Medial part:* the middle part (longissimus muscle) and posterior part (spinalis muscle) of the sacrospinalis muscle. The anterior medial part of the needle passage is the psoas major and quadratus lumborum muscles. It is much safer to insert the needle towards the medial direction.

e. *External part:* three layers of the platysma muscles and the iliocostal muscle are in the external wall of the abdomen.

Complications, prevention and treatment

Directly beneath the point is the kidney so it is better not to use perpendicular insertion for more than 1.2 inches or the needle may penetrate through the posterior wall of the peritoneum into the kidney. The structures from superficial to deep layers are the thick muscular tissue, the dense connective tissue, and the loose adipose capsule of the kidney. The needle resistance is from strong to slight, to a hollow sensation respectively. If a hollow sensation is felt, stop inserting and withdraw the needle immediately. If the needle is inserted further, it will puncture into the kidney, and a strong needle resistance will be felt. Most patients do not feel uncomfortable but some may complain of lumbar or abdominal pain.

Hard thrusting and twirling of the needle may tear the capsule or the parenchyma of the kidney. The blood and urine of the ruptured parenchyma may drain into the pelvis or from the capsule of the kidney into the perirenal area. In mild cases bleeding may be stopped by compressing the outer organs, and blood may be re-absorbed slowly by itself. Severe cases may result in hematoma and the formation of a mass and referral to a specialist is necessary.

Functions

Regulates the function of the Stomach and Intestine, and removes Blood Stasis and local masses.

Clinical indications

Gastritis, gastric ulcer, habitual constipation, mastitis.

Point index

Page numbers in bold print refer to illustrations.

Meridian index

Page numbers in bold print refer to illustrations.

Subject index